INFERIORITY FEELINGS

Founded by C. K. Ogden

The International Library of Psychology

ABNORMAL AND CLINICAL PSYCHOLOGY
In 19 Volumes

INFERIORITY FEELINGS

In the Individual and the Group

OLIVER BRACHFELD

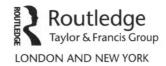

LONDON AND NEW YORK

First published in 1951 by
Routledge and Kegan Paul Ltd
2 Park Square, Milton Park, Abingdon, Oxfordshire OX14 4RN
711 Third Avenue, New York, NY 10017

First issued in paperback 2014

Routledge is an imprint of the Taylor and Francis Group, an informa business

© 1951 Oliver Brachfeld
Translated from the French by Marjorie Gabain

British Library Cataloguing in Publication Data
A CIP catalogue record for this book
is available from the British Library

Inferiority Feelings

ISBN 978-1-138-88237-9 (pbk)
ISBN 978-0415-20921-2 (hbk)

Abnormal and Clinical Psychology: 19 Volumes
ISBN 0415-21123-9
The International Library of Psychology: 204 Volumes
ISBN 0415-19132-7

CONTENTS

5

CONTENTS

PREFACE

THIS book will be more in the nature of an inventory than of a synthesis. My aim has been to unite in a single volume the most essential information on the subject generally denoted as the *Feelings of Inferiority* or *Inferiority Complex*. Everyone will agree that the subject is beset with difficulty. We are dealing here with a notion which, before it has gained official status in professional psychiatry, is used by the man in the street, haunts the columns of the popular press, and appears in the conversation of the educated public. *Habent sua fata* . . . for words, too, have a fate of their own. There are terms which, having been created by and for scientists, escape from the laboratories and studies of the specialists like the evil genius that issued from the bottle that held it imprisoned. We need only recall the fate of such words as 'neurasthenia', 'psychosis', 'complex'. In the old days the vulgar tongue used to borrow its terms from the language of the Church; nowadays it takes them from the psychiatric clinics. Is this a sign of the times? Let the cynic decide.

Only a tiny minority in England, France and the U.S.A. is beginning to rebel against 'the power of words'; Stuart Chase looks to Semantics as the most important of the recent acquisitions of civilisation and if we begin with the expression 'feeling of inferiority', we shall soon see how vague, elusive and unprecise it is. Born, one could almost say, of the marriage of chance and confusion, it might well, on closer analysis, prove to be completely devoid of meaning.

And yet at the back of it all there lies one of the most important ideas of our epoch. Not for centuries has humanity been so deeply plunged in uncertainty and insecurity. Even the faithful creatures of our own making—the machines—have turned against us and submitted us to the most painful of all feelings, that of our own impotence. We have been very poor sorcerer apprentices.

There are some terms that are put into circulation under a signature which guarantees their possessing high value, rather like the name of the issuing bank on a banknote. You speak of Relativity in physics, and you know that the truth of the idea is guaranteed by Einstein. 'Oedipus complex' makes you think of Freud; you read of the *élan vital*, and immediately remember Bergson. These notions or expressions will have for you exactly the value which you attach to the body of theories propounded by their respective authors; their credit rises or falls with that of the thinkers who first coined the words in question. But if you say the words 'inferiority complex' it will be like trying to cash a cheque at a bank with no cash cover. Only the initiated, apart from the specialists, will know the name of him who rightly or wrongly has been called the true father of the inferiority complex—I am speaking of Alfred Adler. When a new idea circulates among people without the name of him who first conceived it, there is a certain grandeur about this anonymity. But Adler's finest and most fertile idea was not the 'complex' which, owing to the insecurity of the times, has achieved such sad popularity; it was the idea of *compensation*. 'Inferiority complex' is, after all, only an ugly phrase, whether it be used by a specialist or a layman. I shall endeavour in the sequel to delimit its exact value whether literary, scientific, or utilitarian.

The first part of this study will therefore be purely historical. I shall investigate the history of this term, so often used and so rarely understood; I shall then trace its literary career, its press, or more exactly, its publicity. In the second place I shall give a short account of the ideas that preceded and led up to the notion embodied in the term. In the third place I shall use it as a kind of network of research, applying it to the surface of the human soul, both individual and collective. In some places the notion will be of the greatest use, in others it will not apply at all. True, there is in man's psyche much more than feelings of inferiority, their derivatives and their compensations. Nevertheless, as a working hypothesis, as a fictitious form of measurement like the latitude and longitude of the geographer, it can undoubtedly serve as a unique and fundamental principle of research.

The more vague and general a subject is, the greater the number of domains to which it appertains, the harder will be the labour of circumscribing and defining it. In the hands of a single author it will prove a thankless task, but it is one that must nevertheless be undertaken. Feelings of inferiority, we are told, belong to psychology, and more particularly to pathological psychology. And yet they are closely connected with such notions as shame, nervousness, timidity, as well as those of honour and vanity. An experimental psychologist—and there are no others nowadays—would scorn to interest himself in such disreputable subjects, which he would contemptuously relegate to the sphere of Ethics. We are prepared, however, to stand our ground and defy those meticulous specialists who, like Georges Dumas and his collaborators, can compile a learned 'Treatise of Psychology' without once mentioning a term which appears over and over again in the biographies of our famous men.

Our subject is certainly ethical, and philosophical as well, though we have not thought fit to take the reader further than the threshold of these avenues of thought. I have given more attention to the pedagogic aspect of the subject and, since nowadays no one can escape the political and sociological approach, we have been careful to include it in our study.

In a number of Paris newspapers we once saw a curious advertisement accompanied by a series of photographs. The first of these represented the tiny figure of a man standing before three enormous male figures talking to each other; the picture gave an almost surrealist impression of the distress one feels at being small and insignificant. The second photograph represented the same little man kneeling before a gigantic female figure of irreproachable elegance, like Gulliver before the giant daughter of Brobdingnag. In the third photograph the same homunculus, standing on a gigantic basin, stretches his arms towards a bottle of the Lotion X, the sale of which these faked photographs are designed to promote. The last picture shows us our diminutive hero after he has used the lotion in question. This time it is he who is the giant. He stands there with his hands in his pockets, looking down with smiling satisfaction at the former giants and giantesses, who are now reduced to the size of dwarfs.[1]

This is perhaps the most typical of the many examples showing the use that is made by clever publicity experts of the *feeling of inferiority*. They skilfully compel the public to undergo the following psychological process: Whoever does not use a certain face cream, or wear a certain make of ties, drive in cars of a specific brand, or take his holiday in a particular bathing resort, must feel ill at ease, uncertain of his place in the social hierarchy, *he must feel inferior*. This is the essence of the greater part of commercial and political propaganda.

Totalitarian regimes owe their success to the use of violence as their

[1] Marcel Vértes, the great Hungarian caricaturist living in America, recently published in a book a caricature which has been widely reproduced in the American press. It represents a small bearded psycho-analyst of bohemian appearance coming to his front-door, which has the brass-plate 'Dr. Schmalz, M.D., Psychicoco'. He is being accosted by a gigantic hotel porter in uniform who asks him, 'Doctor, may I talk to you some day about my inferiority complex?' Thus even caricaturists busy themselves with our subject.

chief weapon of publicity. Acts of violence—often unpunished—impress upon the minds, or rather the unconscious minds, of the public the superiority of the aggressors. Especially if these aggressors dress themselves up in uniforms, hoist military insignia of all sorts, and use every device to convince themselves and the public that they are strong, terrible and immune from punishment. A characteristic example of this was the fashion indulged in by the early Fascists of wearing long hair and long beards. We have it from Aldous Huxley that when questioned as to the reason for this growth on their faces they replied 'per essere piu terribili!' In this way do men overcome their own feeling of inferiority, and then produce in the amorphous neutral mass that constitutes the raw material of all political movements, the feeling that *only by belonging to the faction of violence can they overcome their own feeling of littleness*; only so can one acquire a 'superiority complex'.

For those who like to 'give to the anecdote the value of a category' (D'Ors), for those who can espy significant symbols in the trivial phenomena of daily life, the photographic advertisement described above is charged with meaning. Only one detail was lacking in the text (which incidentally made use of the term 'feeling of inferiority'). The manikin should have been christened Gulliver. For the psychological complex at the back of the phenomena of modern life to which we have briefly alluded ought really to be called the 'Gulliver Complex'. For we are all Gullivers. At one moment we are oppressed with the sense of our weakness and impotence in the face of problems which only giants could solve. At the next moment—especially if we have just had a drink, or seen a Tyrone Power film, or read the account of a victory brought off by our armies or even our favourite football team— we feel like Swift's hero in the country of Lilliput. We live under the sign of Gulliver, and if Unamuno were alive to-day, he would certainly address his prayers to 'Our blessed Saint Gulliver'. This Gulliverian feeling about life has nothing to do with the Promethean or even the Faustian feeling of earlier epochs. It could more easily be compared to that curious *antithetic feeling of life* which, according to the most distinguished specialists in Romantic literature,[1] inspired the Spanish *edad de oro*, or on a wider scale, all the Baroque that is worthy of the name. In the words of one of the greatest masters in the knowledge of the human heart, 'To be a man is to be tormented with feelings of in-

---

[1] Cf. the long and thoroughgoing answer which Mr. Léo Spitzer was kind enough to make to my note on '*Belengabor; une curieuse erreur de Gracián*' in the *Revista de Filologia Española*, 1930.

feriority and to tend towards situations of superiority.' This sentence of Adler's stands at the head of the Spanish edition of this work, and if there is one thing with which we can reproach our revered master it is that instead of calling his system by the ambiguous title of 'Comparative Individual Psychology' he did not call it 'Psycho-synthesis' and substitute 'Gulliver Complex' for 'Inferiority and Superiority Complex'. So named, his theories would have penetrated the public mind more easily and people would have been more readily able to understand the mechanisms (hateful word to a psychologist!) of their psychic life.

Gulliver—symbol of human relativity—would certainly never have come to life if Dean Swift had not been the intimate friend of Bishop Berkeley and had not read the latter's *Essay towards a New Theory of Vision* (1709). This seems to have been very clearly grasped by the Abbé Desfontaines, who writes in his preface to the first French edition of *Gulliver's Travels*: 'The first two Travels are based on the idea of an undisputed principle of physics, namely, that there is no absolute magnitude and that all measurement is relative. . . . In these two Travels he seems in a manner to be considering men with the aid of a telescope. First he looks through the big lens and consequently sees them very small; this is the Journey to Lilliput. Turning his telescope round the other way he sees men very big; this is the Journey to Brobdingnag.' In our days, when the heated debates on physical relativity were soon to be followed by the slogan of the relativity of all things, the *Gulliverian sense of life* is a fact that can no longer be denied. When one analyses neurotic patients who are always minimising or magnifying themselves, the conception can easily serve as the scaffolding of a whole theory. And it was after reading *Gulliver* that Doctor Johnson remarked, 'When once you have thought of big men and little men, it is very easy to do all the rest.'

But there is another reason in favour of using the name of Gulliver in connection with the complex that concerns us here. It has become a habit with many to speak of the inferiority and the superiority complex as though they were opposed, when in fact one is the result of the other. The superiority complex is very often a cloak for a very deep inferiority complex and is therefore only one of its symptoms. The two closely connected phenomena could thus be expressed in a single symbol, and nothing would seem so appropriate for the purpose as the name of Gulliver. Moreover, it has become a custom to designate various complexes by names taken from legend or literature, witness the

Oedipus, the Electra, the Diana and even the Brunhilde complex. Gulliver is a more universally familiar figure than any of these, and the Gulliverian feeling of being either too little or too big is one which everyone must have experienced in the course of his life. It is essentially one which consists in a change of focus, and this change of focus is inherent in all human life. It is, moreover, the aim of all psychological analysis, for what we try to do there is to change the patient's point of view, to make him 'turn round the telescope', as the good Abbé Desfontaines would have put it. Generally speaking, it is a question of making light of a difficulty which the patient is over-estimating, or of magnifying the sense of his own value where this has fallen below a certain level. Novels written by neurotic authors generally represent a series of Gulliverian situations. As, for example, André Gide's *École des Femmes*, where the hero, Robert, first strikes his wife as being inordinately big and is eventually reduced in size to the point of caricature (Brunhilde Complex).

It is interesting to note how little study has been made in the past of this complex, which is so fundamental an element in our psychological make-up. Even among those who were privileged to know Alfred Adler personally, I was the first who attempted a monograph, incomplete though it was, on this fundamental subject. In general bibliography it only comes up occasionally, and is treated in an unmethodical spirit. It almost seems as though the feeling of inferiority were something so painful to own to and submit to a diagnosis, that writers would rather avoid it than examine it *sine ira et cum studio* from the point of view of scientific investigation. The term "inferiority complex" appears frequently in the columns of the press and in the speeches of political men. Paul Reynaud has given it official consideration, so to speak, from the political viewpoint by mentioning it in one of his speeches at the American Club in Paris (1939); a well-known actor has avowedly based his interpretation of Othello on the complex of racial inferiority; there is a novelist who builds up his plots on the cases described by Adler; and André Maurois himself would like to see the work of the 'père du complexe d'infériorité' translated into every language. (We shall examine later Adler's claim to this title.) Great strides have been made in the teaching of modern languages owing to the principle that the first thing to do is to eliminate the pupil's feeling of linguistic inferiority. Thus in every branch of mental activity this notion, so long neglected by science, has acquired increasing importance.

At times, indeed, the idea is carried too far, especially in America. But what matter? When a great river overflows, the flooding waters bring fertile seeds to the land around. In the same way, ideas can be brought to the mind of the masses. All that matters is that the seed should grow. And this brings us to a very important point, one which the psychologists themselves have ignored. Adler and his disciples looked upon the inferiority feelings or complexes as a great evil weighing upon humanity. It never occurred to them to try to tame or control these undesirable feelings. Instead, they had a mystical faith in the possibility of doing away with these feelings by education, of rooting them out and eliminating them from human existence—a thankless and impossible task. Adler himself, towards the end of his life, realised that he and his followers had erred through idealism—a cardinal sin in these days of realism, and it was undoubtedly what made him say, 'To be man means to feel oneself inferior.' If, then, the feeling of inferiority is inherent in our human condition—as religious people will be the first to admit, for is not man imperfect and inferior before God?—if this be so, is it not futile to try to remove these feelings of distress from the depths of our soul? This, of course, is the starting-point of the Existentialist philosophy, so much in fashion, which has been expounded by Kierkegaard, Heidegger and Jaspers. . . . No, we must not seek to do away with these feelings. Rather must it be our task to control them and direct them, so as to use them to the best possible advantage that we can in a new and better world founded on the Science of Man.

You sometimes feel worried; things are not going as you would wish, you are not 'feeling yourself', you are irritable, can't settle down. . . . 'I feel very nervy to-day,' you remark. But the nerviness is not dispelled by being admitted. At the best it will serve as an excuse to yourself and to others. ('Don't bother him; don't you see how nervy he is?') And on those terms you are content to be labelled 'nervous', for you have read your Proust and remember the old doctor's eloquent defence of nervous people as the salt of the earth.

You meet some friends in a restaurant. They are waiting for you, and you sit down opposite them with your back to the rest of the room. Very soon you are overcome by a disagreeable feeling, a growing *malaise*. At last you realise what it is. 'Do you mind if I change places? It makes me nervous to sit with my back to a crowd.' So you get up and sit with your back to the wall like the others. Your nerves calm down.

Suddenly you are 'off your food'. Something may have annoyed you, at home, at your office or factory. And now your stomach betrays you and refuses to accept what you eat. You take a cachet or a sedative, but the trouble persists and you finally run to a doctor. 'Nothing much the matter,' he says with professional heartiness; 'don't worry about it, it's only your nerves.' True, the phrase does not act like magic, although, in spite of your education, you had hoped that it would. All the doctor can suggest is a little rest, a change, a holiday abroad, which of course you cannot afford. Then suddenly, as you are listlessly glancing through a magazine, your eye is caught by the words —'Inferiority Complex. That is what you are suffering from. Have the courage to admit it. *We can help you.* . . . Write for our pamphlet, etc. . . .'

A whole trade has been skilfully built up on the term. As though we were not threatened enough by a life shaken with far-reaching social and political changes, as though we had not sufficient reason already to feel inferior, weak, depressed, without being expressly invited to do so by the daily or weekly press. If by any chance you were not 'nervy', if you were happily free from any 'inferiority complex', these artfully repeated advertisements would certainly end by shaking your confidence. For in the monopolistic phase of capitalism in which we live the war of nerves is carried on from within as well as from without.

Jean Richard Bloch was probably one of the first, some fifteen years ago, to denounce the *psychological offensive* to which modern men are subjected by their governments. World War II certainly showed that an enemy could be reduced not only by bombs and other projectiles, but also by psychological weapons. Stuart Chase has never ceased to maintain that Japan was defeated not only by the atomic bomb but also by psychological warfare.

It is time that professional psychologists should accept the challenge and stem this rising tide of danger. For there are other factors in this 'war of nerves'. On the side of the enemy are two powerful allies— the passion for speed and the machines. Some psychologists, indeed, have shouldered the task, thankless enough, as their efforts were seconded by no one. Charles Baudouin, of the Geneva *Institut Psychagogique*, Paul Plottke in Paris, and Dr. Fritz Künkel and his pupils in Berlin have given us models of psychological treatment by correspondence. But the illicit competition of the pseudo-institutes makes the efforts of these men of good will seem too reticent, and naturally they did not wish to resort to advertisement. The psycho-analytical school, which had free ambulatory clinics in Berlin, Vienna and Budapest, did not supply the same unpaid services in Paris, where, in any case, the personnel was too cosmopolitan. Secularisation has destroyed the faith of millions and has given them nothing in return; they have no moral equivalent, unless it be a handful of hollow phrases. Happy are those who can find a political creed that will act as a psychological protective armour for them.

Other psychologists have shouldered the task of overcoming the phenomenon of 'nerves' which, though it has always existed, has in the last hundred years become a collective illness. The disease, it is not without interest to note, has come to us from America, and its victims are chiefly to be found among the leisured classes. Dr. Oczeret in Switzerland, the sociologist Folkert Wilken[1] in Baden, and the Adlerian school in Austria have given us, in their time, very interesting studies on the subject. But it was a young Hungarian psychologist, Paul Schiller de Harka, who attempted to master the phenomena of 'nerves' by experimental methods, or rather by a method of 'questionnaires'.[2]

His research led to the most instructive results. In the first place he found that each subject, when questioned, gave different causes for his 'nerves'. This seemed to imply that 'nerviness' as a category did not exist, since there were as many ways of being 'nervy' as there were

[1] Folkert Wilken, *Die nervöse Erkränkung als sinnvolle Erscheinung unseres gegenwärtigen Kulturzeitraumes.* Munich, 1927.

[2] Cf. Paul Schiller de Harka and I. Molnár, *Everyday Nervousness as a Drive to Act.* Lélektani Tanulmányok, I, Budapest, 1937. We reproduce the text of the principal questionnaire. 1. Could you point out what habitually makes you nervy? 2. Have you noticed that you are more apt to get nervy at some times than at others—e.g. in the evening; when out of sorts; in the Spring, etc.? 3. Since when have you noticed that you get into nervous states—e.g. Since you were a child? Since you were married? Since you have been working in an office? Since fate has dealt you a serious blow, etc? 4. Are there certain impressions that regularly make you nervy—e.g. colours, smells, the touch of certain surfaces, rhythms, ugliness or untidiness, etc.? 5. Do other people's manners and behaviour make you nervy, and when—e.g. bad manners, self-important or pretentious behaviour, injustice, nervousness, etc.? 6. When does your *personal* situation or behaviour make you nervy—e.g. uncertainty, inability to act, waiting, constraint, disagreement, joy, boredom, etc.? 8. Which among the things that generally make people nervy are those that do not affect you in this way? 9. Sum up what 'gets on your nerves'. 10. In general, how do you show your nerviness? 11. After all this, what would you say was the *essential* thing that made you 'nervy' and the essential nature of nerviness?

The study from which I have quoted contains statistical tables obtained from the examination of one thousand nervous situations.

types of human beings. (Cf. *Zeitschrift für angewandte Psychologie*, 49, 1935.) After carrying out the same experiments on a number of subjects in Barcelona, I personally came to the same conclusion as my friend and colleague. The first results gave three groups of causes productive of 'nerviness'. Here are some typical examples. (*a*) The professor draws a line across the blackboard with the chalk making a noise that sets our teeth on edge. (*b*) A man sitting beside us at table eats 'like a pig', chewing loudly and putting his knife into his mouth. (*c*) We have an urgent appointment to keep and it so happens that no bus turns up or that there is a hold-up on the Underground.

Further studies, however, produced more interesting results. Observation was made of typically 'nervy' behaviour, such as walking up and down the room, fiddling with one's wedding ring, drumming with one's fingers, etc. And it was found that most 'nervy' actions expressed tendencies to flight. The subject appears to be seeking for a way out of a nerve-racking situation (38 per cent of nervous actions). We must add that he seeks to escape from them by inadequate means, by actions that have no definite aim. Another group of such actions clearly expresses the desire 'to do something or other', but here again the nerve-racking situation remains unchanged. The subject does not get beyond the desire or tendency. Women succumb less easily than men to nerve-racking situations, probably for social and self-interested motives. On the other hand, they are more generally impressionable, with consequent nervous reactions. In Jewish subjects the 'tendency' category is the weakest and the 'activity' category the strongest. Our authors seek to explain this by the psychology of race instead of referring it to the sociological situation that has been created for Jews. The factors present in nerviness are: will, evaluation, and need, i.e. the three factors that urge man to activity in general. In a nerve-racking experience there is something that opposes my will, my way of attributing value, and my needs. Such conflicts provoke the tendency to 'do something or other', but unfortunately the cause which arouses this tendency or desire is the very thing that prevents me from doing what I would like to do. It is this conflict which leads to the formation of nervous attitudes. For instance, I am in a situation which obliges me to act, but at the same time it prevents me from doing the one thing that would enable me to escape from it. So I fall back upon *Ersatz* actions, more or less acute affective explosions, definite cenaesthesias, etc. 'Nerviness' is therefore in the last analysis an imperious need to act in face of the impossibility to do so; and it can thus be regarded as an 'inadequate psychic factor'. We are in the presence here of a disturbance in the 'domestic economy of the soul'. Any tendency to act which becomes inhibited calls forth nerviness. Whether this symptom appears or not, in what situations it does appear, at what moments and with what intensity, will depend on the previous data in the subject's general make-up, i.e. his constitution, his temperament, his volitional, estimative and necessitative orientation in general. Such are in brief the conclusions reached by Schiller de Harka and Molnár.

Once again the experimental and statistical method proves what Adler and his school have always claimed, viz. that all nervous complaints, whether they take the form of neurasthenia or some psychic or moral crisis, are due in the last resort to a painful *sense of impotence*, more generally known as feeling of inferiority, arising directly from our inability to produce an adequate reaction to an external or internal challenge. Thus, apart from complaints like neuralgia, etc. (though they too can be influenced by moral factors), all genuine nervous illnesses have their roots in the domain of the feelings of inferiority, with all their infinite variants, for this is the fertile soil where the neuroses take root and grow to full stature.

This statement shows us the enormous scope of the problem before us. It explains the special interest taken in it by the quacks, whether they be graphologists, characterologists, or dispensers of 'practical' psycho-therapy; and it accounts for the success of the weekly or daily column of advice printed by newspapers in answer to letters asking for help in their personal difficulties. It is therefore high time that we should attack the problem from a less interested and more serious point of view, and that we should determine more precisely the place occupied by the feelings of inferiority in our individual and social life.

OLIVER BRACHFELD

Barcelona, 1950.

CHAPTER I

THE PRINCIPLE OF SECURITY
AND THE FEELING OF IMPOTENCE[1]

'But why do all the people here shrink into themselves, why do they want
to turn themselves into small change, take up as little room as possible, make
themselves scarce: I don't exist, I don't exist at all. I am hiding, please pass on
and take no notice of me. Pretend you have not seen me. Pass on, pass on.
—But of whom are you speaking? Who is shrinking into himself?
—Why, the Bourgeois.
—He? Good Heavens, he is king, he is the Third Estate, he is everything,
and you talk of shrinking!'
                    Dostoyevsky, *Le Bourgeois de Paris*, in his Essays on
                    the bourgeois, after the French translation by Guter-
                    man, Paris (Kra) 1925.

THROUGHOUT the centuries the bourgeois class, in its gradual
ascent to pre-eminence, has been haunted by an uneasy conscience, a curious feeling of insecurity. Dostoievsky had the
penetration to discern this in his time, and it is often noted by the sociologists of to-day. And yet this class has always neglected the examination of its problem so long as it felt no external threat to its security.
To-day, however, this security has become problematic, even where it
survives, while in many countries it has completely disappeared.
Never have internal social upheavals and external political complications challenged the accepted order on so vast a scale nor for such a
rapidly increasing population. Never have so many human beings been
subjected to violence, driven from their homes, exposed to all sorts of
physical and psychological shocks, and submitted to the painful but inevitable vexations of an increasing bureaucracy. Whole nations are
struggling in an agony of insecurity, society is involved in the desperate
attempt to rectify the dislocation that has taken place between the

[1] This chapter was written in its first Spanish version early in 1935, when the
claims for security were not so generally recognised as they are now. In Spain, then
a pacific country, the first spontaneously to disarm after 1931, confident as it was
in the League of Nations, my ideas were received with scepticism, but since then
they have been the subject of frequent comment by Spanish writers.

machine and what is contemptuously called 'the human factor', and to some regimes war appears to be the only way out of their economic difficulties. To some sociologists the gigantic upheavals we are witnessing in the world to-day mark *the phase of transition from the era of unorganised insecurity to that of organised insecurity*.[1] It is not for us to pronounce upon the correctness of such a diagnosis; what interests us about the social and economic world crisis of to-day is its repercussions in human psychology. In the present state of our knowledge it does not seem possible to relate a state of crisis in human psychology to collective, economic or social causes. We see the results but can only guess at what brought them about. The psycho-analysis of collectivities, the *Social Psycho-analysis*, which in one form or another is beginning to haunt so many minds, and minds of no mean order, is a science that is not yet born.[2] And yet no large-scale psychological phenomenon can be understood unless we can point not only to its individual causes but also—in broad outline, and as a cautious approximation—to the great sociological processes which have gone before it.

In order really to understand the question of the inferiority feelings we shall have to cast a rapid glance at the origin and growth of the interest which the idea has evoked. Before theoreticians turn their attention to a given idea, certain values must have become problematic, they must have been doubted, even threatened. The value that is challenged to-day is security, the fundamental principle of all bourgeois society, its supreme and hitherto most envied asset.

[1] Cf. Karl Mannheim's study in *Peaceful Change*, a work edited by C. A. W. Manning.

[2] The periodical *L'Hygiène mentale* mentioned before the last war a group formed in Paris for the study of Collective Psychology under the leadership of the well-known psycho-analyst Dr. René Allendy. In London the Hungarian sociologist Karl Mannheim has for several years been urging the necessity for a Collective Psychology which he proposes to call *Social Technique*. The *Institut de Psychagogie* in Geneva, so ably directed by M. Charles Baudouin, received an official subsidy in order to pursue its researches in the same field (see *Action et Pensée*, the official bulletin of the Institute). The American technique practised by M. Gallup's Institute of Public Enquiry and the Mass Observation carried out in England are working roughly on the same line. The first number of *Zeitschrift für freie Deutsche Forschung*, a review published by German émigrés in France, mentions a lecture given by M. J. L. Schmidt on 'Buts, moyens et méthodes pour influencer les masses,' which led to the formation of study groups. Finally, mention should be made of the Swiss movement for Psycho-hygiene with its excellent book series edited by the well-known psycho-analyst Dr. H. Meng.

THE PRINCIPLE OF SECURITY

THE ORIGINS OF BOURGEOIS SOCIETY

The world to-day is far more deeply plunged in insecurity than in past centuries. The end of the nineteenth century and (since the flow of humanity's life pays scant respect to the divisions of the calendar) the opening of the twentieth still appear to us *The Happy Generation*,[1] simply because the majority of people then lived according to a pre-established pattern in a state of security only slightly overshadowed by the incalculable and the uncertain. Since then, humanity has witnessed a ghastly procession of catastrophes, in which millions have been annihilated, whole sets of values overthrown with incredible swiftness, vast regions devastated, and in which, finally, this *feeling of security* previously enjoyed by individuals, social classes, nations and even continents has been finally destroyed. 'Chaos is come again.'[2]

The beginnings of the fourteenth century saw the emergence of a new social class in Europe—the bourgeoisie. A principle was in-augurated, which, though not entirely new, had never dominated men's minds to the same extent before, nor marked so strongly every phase of social life. New forms of life superseded the old, and the search for security now took shape in the bourgeois way of life. Formerly, in a predominantly feudal Europe, human existence centred round the stronghold or castle and the small number of powerful persons residing in it—the noblemen. The feudal lord was absolute master of his serfs and of all those who lived in or passed through the territory adjoining his castle or lands. In return, the vassals, though subject to the caprice of their master, could count on his protection in case of danger, for he was obliged—in his own interest—to guarantee them a certain security against major disasters, epidemics, and attacks by other feudal lords. The common man, serf or peasant, was, as it were, handed over to the justice and mercy and very often too to the whims of his over-lord. All the same, a strong community feeling or at any rate a sense of mutual dependence had reigned over the human group that centred round the castle.

As the bourgeoisie advances, however, and feudalism falls into decay,

[1] This is the title of a novel by F. Körmendi which has been translated into several languages. The appearance of such books dealing with the pre-1914–1918 period, such as *1900*, by Paul Morand, is certainly not fortuitous.

[2] Title of a novel by the excellent writer Claude Houghton, in which English society is depicted as the victim, since 1918, of a wide inferiority complex. Note, too, his novel *I am Jonathan Scrivener*, and others. It was my privilege to introduce this excellent author to the Spanish public.

a new mode of living suddenly emerges involving far larger numbers than before. Kings and princes support the development and consolidation of the town-dwelling population, hoping to find in it a defence against the kinglets and other petty tyrants, all too prone to assert their own sovereignty. Henceforth, groups of men and women, free and autonomous, though bound by a whole system of tenure and services, lead a new kind of existence within powerful walls which protect them against perils and surprises that are growing fewer every day.

Forms of life that have lain dormant since ancient Rome come to light again. Once more the *pater familias* reigns supreme in the home, and though he no longer has the right of life and death over the members of his family, he is in every other respect their lord and master. The family emerges as the community life of feudal times on a smaller scale. The father commands but he also protects. And his protection extends to those who live under his roof, work at his trade, and are regarded as members of his household. The house fences the family in; and the city is fenced in by walls, of which the guard is entrusted to all the valid males of the community, the different bastions being in the hands of the various corporations or guilds. *Thus the bourgeois appears as a man who lives behind protective fences, in security.* The very etymology of his name gives its stamp to his whole style of life, of which the essence will be to live in security, to enjoy it, and when it is lost or in jeopardy to seek to re-establish it in its pristine integrity. No need now to run to the cellars and vaults of the seigneurial castle in the hour of danger. The life of the burgh—the castle held by all—develops along fixed norms. Every night heavy gates are closed so that the burgher may sleep in peace while armed watches guard his security. Certain towns even obtain rights and privileges over the king himself; thus there is a tradition which survives, at least in form, to this day that the King of England cannot leave his residence to walk through the streets of London without the permission of the Lord Mayor. Those enjoying this new kind of life no longer require the protection of the castle. 'My house is my castle' is the proud saying of the enfranchised burgher.

And yet in the early days of the bourgeoisie people find themselves obliged to forgo certain forms of security which had been enjoyed by their fathers. Urged by a feeling of social inferiority, the artisan longs to turn bourgeois, and the bourgeois aspires to the dignity of the knight, gentleman, or *caballero*. To Molière's bourgeois his own condition is painful and contemptible. Yet even at the beginning of the fourteenth century the bourgeois was clearly on a higher rung of the social hierarchy than the artisan. To rise in this hierarchy, to leave a sphere of life which one knows and can control for one less sure, because less familiar and less easy to control, is to expose oneself to all kinds of surprises and uncertainties. These are accepted, however, for the sake of the higher rank, the desired superiority. But the man who wants to appear superior to what he is in reality no longer treads on familiar ground, his steps will falter, and he may easily stumble. From the point of security at any rate he stands to lose. Ramon Llull, who lived during the period when the craftsman was being transformed into the bourgeois, raised his voice in protest against the folly of those who turned their backs on the solid security of the *mester* or craft, blinded as they were by the lure of an apparently superior form of life.[1]

SECURITY IN PERIL

As the centuries passed, the securities which the bourgeoisie had brought to man become more and more extended, reaching their zenith in the conquest of the Rights of Man in the French Revolution. Never before had man felt so sure of the future, never had the paths of life seemed to him so free, never had he trusted so proudly in the power of divine Reason. Modern science, which emerged and developed with astonishing rapidity, sought to give a lasting and even philosophic

[1] Ramon Llull, or Raymundus Lullus (in Spanish Raimundo Lulio) the Majorcan *doctor illuminatus*, perhaps the greatest Catalan genius of all times and one of the few Spanish philosophers with an acute social conscience. In the first issue of my Spanish periodical *Europa*, 1933, I published the text of his *De las Artes Mecanicas*, which I had rediscovered and translated into Spanish from the Old Catalan. What he calls " Mechanical Art" is identical with the Old French *mester* (métier) or craft. He was a vehement critic of the *burgés* class, the new social group then in formation, and he anticipated in the fourteenth century the famous theory of the 'three bourgeois generations'. Here are some characteristic utterances:
'The bourgeois derives from the trades because originally his ancestors were in a trade, and some forebear made money and became a bourgeois, and then his line began to decline because the bourgeois wastes and does not make, and he has sons and they are idle and all want to be bourgeois and their money is not enough for them all.'
'Much more safely rich is he who enriches his sons with some craft than he who leaves them money and possessions, because all other riches abandon a man except only a craft; therefore, my son, I advise you to learn some craft by which you can live in case of need.'

formulation to this quest for security and to the illusion of having already attained it. The sociology of Comte defined science simply as a means of ensuring man's security : 'To know in order to foresee; to foresee in order to forestall.' Technique, physical comforts, sensational discoveries—all contributed to confirm man in his sense of security until we reach the beginning of the present century. So far, humanity could echo Sophocles in saying:

Πολλὰ τὰ δεινὰ κ' οὐδὲν ἀνθρώπου δεινότερον πέλει

'There are many powerful things, but none more powerful than man.'

But free and independent minds were already conscious of the decay to which this excessive security was leading. Artists, writers and thinkers raised their voices in execration of this Philistine existence from which all risk and all danger were excluded, and Nietzsche uttered the famous words, 'Live dangerously'. Astute political leaders were later to exploit this phrase for their own ends, but on their lips it was no new programme, it was an *a posteriori* justification of an accomplished fact, a theoretical superstructure built over the dangerous life to which we had been condemned since the First World War. 'At this time no one lived in security': these words stand at the opening of a lovely little Russian novel written at the time of the Revolution, and they might well appear in some history manuals of the future to describe the present phase in human life. In the time of Ramon Llull it was the *craft* which gave security to life, that semi-mystical craft which even the sons of monarchs were obliged to learn so that they might be equipped with a means of livelihood in case of a reversal of fortune. But in the capitalistic and bourgeois phase of humanity before the First World War there was only one form of security—*money*. Since then whole countries have been through the bitter experience of finding that neither banknotes nor even gold itself represented sure and solid values. No attempt has been made to estimate even approximately the incalculable damage done by monetary devaluation to the millions of human souls for whom it represented the overthrow of the last positive and tangible value. 'Make the world safe for democracy', President Wilson had cried on the morrow of the First World War. Since then, unfortunately, the world has only become less and less safe, and the enormous material advances of our civilisation which ought to assure our existence are actually fresh means for rendering it more and more precarious. *Security as a problem and as a psychological postulate* has never been really evaluated. And yet it is one of the most urgent needs of the

23

bourgeois form of life, which to-day is the form adopted by all civilised humanity, not excluding Soviet Russia.

'Security', to quote the Vienna psycho-analyst Wittels,[1] 'means liberty. . . . Everything in our modern epoch tends towards security. Our journeys are carried out not only with increased speed but with an incomparably greater degree of technical security. We know to the last kilogramme the carrying capacity of our bridges, we know that our boilers will not explode, that our trains will not collide, that neither storm nor flood will destroy our roads. And in so far as such dangers still exist a whole army of specialists is at hand to overcome them. Our hygiene has made such progress that certain illnesses which were the scourge of former epochs have been almost completely wiped out in civilised parts. *Everywhere security is asked for, everywhere it is obtained.* Only the simplest form of security does not exist, although everyone is straining after it: for the individual only rarely has the luck to realise his economic aim, the security of his own existence. Society does not help him in the matter.'

And yet the writer does not seem to have noticed a rather obvious consequence of this feverish search. The greater our security, the more painful will the least encroachment upon it be, even if the resulting lack of security is negligible when compared to that existing at earlier epochs of history. Since the modern inhabitant of towns and even villages has included electricity among the list of his securities, he suffers more from the black-out than did his ancestors from their primitive means of lighting, and he will be inordinately upset if his car breaks down for a few minutes on the road. So that even the extraordinary growth of our securities has contributed only to undermine their mental counterpart, the feeling of security, thus occasioning in us an increased dose of insecurity or inferiority complexes.

FAMILY AND SECURITY

In the bourgeois world one of the safest things that existed was undoubtedly the *family*. Ever since the home has ceased to be the place where grandparents, parents, sons, daughters, and even sons-in-law met to work in common, ever since the family has ceased to be self-supporting and each of its members has had to seek sources of revenue outside the home, this social institution has inevitably suffered the fate to which all others sooner or later succumb, viz. 'functional loss'.

[1] 'Edelnarzissismus' in *Almanach der Psychoanalyse* 1932.

The fathers of to-day are very far from being home-birds, and very often they are unable to ensure their children's livelihood. The son who earns his living and thus helps to support the family gains a certain autonomy and enjoys an enhanced prestige. Parents feel less sure of themselves than in the old days, but this, alas, does not help to promote a sense of security in the children. What has been called the 'problem of the clash of generations' has become more acute, and it is easy to show that in such periods of crisis feelings of inferiority are on the increase, and with them nervous tension and irritability both in fathers and sons.

And how could this 'functional loss' in the oldest and apparently the most solid institution (since it is based on purely natural feelings) fail to entail that in another closely linked to it—*marriage*? Formerly 'marriages were made in heaven', or at any rate before the earthly representative of divine power, thus acquiring a character of absolute security. If we isolate the institution of marriage from all its other psychological contents and study it from our own consciously one-sided approach, we must come to the conclusion that it represents in modern bourgeois society a means of *security*. This security the bourgeois will defend at all costs and with every means at his disposal; his social institutions serve no other end. Love might tend to make him take risks and lose his safety, and so he will dread nothing so much as love, while in theatre plays and cinemas no figure will exercise such terrifying fascination on him as the *femme fatale*, or vamp. These safety-partitions set up in the sphere of love are falling away one by one. We are not thinking of the peculiar increase in the number of divorces nor of the growing facility of obtaining divorce; we are simply noting the 'functional loss' suffered by the institution of matrimony. It is one more security gone by the board. Once again the legal prerogatives of the *pater familias* have been gravely impaired, and continue to dwindle, while new privileges accrue daily to his partner, the wife. Marriage is no longer an eternal bond, but tends more and more to be a purely business contract. Has not Mrs. Roosevelt urged married women to demand payment for their housework? Adultery and divorce no longer incur the opprobrium that formerly attended them. The *security* of marriage is in decline.

But it is not only in the life of the individual that security is diminishing; collective life shows a marked trend in the same direction. During the First World War, the hazards and suffering of those who stayed at home were as much in the picture as those of the men who were fighting at the front. After the war, unemployment, revolution and its aftermath of counter-revolution, strikes and social conflict produced waves of insecurity, first in Central and Eastern Europe and later in the West and in other continents.

It was then that the idea which is the object of our present study emerged and quickly spread. A new word came into being and became fashionable, first in German-speaking countries—*Minderwertigkeits-gefühl*, generally translated as 'Feeling of Inferiority'. The term had appeared before, but for the first time it fitted the situation. It fell on prepared soil, and a whole new theory arose around it. It cannot be re-garded as a mere chance that the theory of the feeling, or 'complex', of inferiority should have arisen at this period of history. It would not be hard to show that the 'Comparative Psychology of the Individual' (the name first given by Alfred Adler to the body of his theories) owes its appearance to that very Adlerian mechanism by which an Ego con-demned to inferiority develops tendencies towards over-compensa-tion and security. As Arthur Kronfeld wisely noted in 1926, it was chiefly the intellectuals of the last generation who groaned under the excessive pressure of economic and social conditions. But we would go further, and point to the extreme significance of the fact that Adler's theories, which took their start in medical science and were originally directed to purely therapeutic ends, should have grown and developed to the point of becoming a psychological interpretation of the whole of our present existence.

THE FEELING OF IMPOTENCE

If a man shuts himself up in an armour-plated room surrounded with barbed wire and watch-dogs, if he engages the best squad of detectives in the world to guard him, if he has two loaded revolvers lying on his table, and if he then declares that *he is not afraid*, do we believe him? Obviously not. We cannot know whether a man is brave or not until, voluntarily or involuntarily, he is deprived of all his securities. In the same way, the bourgeoisie of modern Europe has skilfully surrounded itself with a rampart of such securities, and then asserts that it 'is not afraid'. And yet under its parchments and privileges, behind its city gates, and in spite of its army and police force, insecurity lurks un-abated. It is not difficult to unearth the symptoms.

The man of our epoch, who has reached the final and most developed stage of the bourgeois form of life, falls a prey to all the insecurities which his race—or his class—have been dreading for centuries. What characterises him, therefore, is a profound feeling of impotence, of which, as yet, he is almost entirely unaware. Let us examine the testimony of modern sociologists such as Erich Fromm (*Zeitschrift für Sozialforschung*, No. 1, Paris, Alcan, 1937). The author, after considering a certain type of *religious man*, contrasts with him the *bourgeois man*, who is characterised by the feeling of impotence of which we spoke above, 'a feeling which could hardly be brought to light with the methods of descriptive psychology'. According to Fromm, a profound feeling of impotence marks the whole of bourgeois life,[1] and he regards the feeling as *unconscious*. I must point out here that the last term is ambiguous. It generally applies to experiences which were once conscious and have been since repressed. But it is clear that the author is referring to something deeper than the psychic layer which Freud has called the *unconscious*. Dr. Fromm has psycho-analysed a large number of people, in all of whom he discovered a curious feeling of impotence. In extreme cases the analysis resulted in the following admissions: 'I can have no influence on anyone, I can start nothing, I am incapable, of my own will, of changing anything either in the external world or in myself, I have no strength, I do not exist for others, they notice me as little as the air they breathe.' This sense of impotence, says Fromm, is not confined to our relations with other people. It can arise from our

---

[1] In the review in which Dr. Fromm's study appears the term *Ohnmachtsgefühl* is translated in the accompanying French résumé by *sentiments d'impuissance* (feelings of impotence). As often happens, there is a serious divergence between the original German term and its translations into languages of Latin origin. The *Ohnmacht* of the Germans is a phenomenon regarded by some as the 'very prototype of all neuroses'. Such is the opinion of M. Nils Antoni ('Vaso-vagale Synkope und Orthostatische Epilepsie' in *Acta Psychiatrica et Neurologica*, XII, 4, 1937 (Copenhagen)). The term *Ohnmacht* as used by German psychiatrists seems to describe a basic condition of the subject's constitution; a revolution of the vegetative system brought about by somatic rather than sensorial and emotional factors and producing finally a retroactive effect on the contents of consciousness. It would seem that here if anywhere there is a real 'flight into illness', a flight from reality, and of so intense a nature, the author maintains, that the subject finally disappears completely. For those interested in matters of terminology here are some of M. Nils Antoni's observations. The syndrome in question is called *svimming* in Swedish, *svime* or *besvimelse* in Norwegian and Danish, *Ohnmacht* in German, and in French it is rendered by *évanouissement* or *pâmoison*. Actually the last two words have not quite the same meaning. The first stresses the cause which brings about the phenomenon, viz. a physical collapse, whereas *pâmoison* is of purely psychological origin. In English the terms *Fainting* or *Fainting Fit* are used, and the international term is *syncope*. As the reader will see, the German *Ohnmacht* means much more than simply 'impotence'.

relation to ourselves or to inanimate objects. It produces primarily anguish, anger and feelings of inferiority. (The latter term is clearly used by the author to denote a concrete feeling of inferiority, resulting from a comparison.) But man cannot remain for long the prey to such disagreeable feelings of impotence. In order to mitigate them he has recourse to 'rationalisations'. This term, borrowed from Freud, is the equivalent of what the luckless Theodor Lessing described as *die Sinngebung des Sinnlosen*, i.e. the act of conferring *a posteriori* a meaning on something which either has none or has quite a different one. According to our author, these consoling rationalisations ('fictitious explanations' would be a better phrase, for nothing could be more contrary to reason than these phantasmagoria) bring about a belief in sudden miracles, or in changes wrought progressively throughout a long lapse of time; in short, they are a form of reaction which is so active, becomes so much a habit, that in the end it completely buries the sense of impotence, which therefore remains unconscious.

Highly complex social conditions, in Fromm's view, are very favourable to the growth of this sense of impotence. In the first place there is the fact that in bourgeois education the child, however affectionately he may be treated, is not taken seriously. And let us hasten to add that it is a feeling of inferiority in the parents which produces this form of education. For, and this is the second main cause of the trouble, the role of the adult in bourgeois society, his own impotence in the face of forces which he is unable to control or even recognise, deprives him of any real autonomy and efficacy.

The author carries his analysis of the various forms of the feeling of impotence very far, almost to the point of over-subtlety. He even regards *vertigo* as resulting from the feeling of helplessness (*Hilflosigkeit*), i.e. the sensation of not being able to control the impulses and feelings of anguish that arise in us.

The least pretext will serve to motivate feelings of such complete insufficiency. Adler, in such cases, used the French word *arrangement*, and I myself have used in Spanish the more engaging term *arreglito*. Freudian psycho-analysis, with its theory of the infantile trauma, has done much to unveil such 'pretexts'. There are people who try to explain their bad luck or their lack of success in life by the fact that they were smacked at the age of three or that when they were five an elder brother made fun of them.

There are many of us who deem ourselves incapable of giving or receiving love or affection. Others regard themselves as incapable of work of any kind, they cease to study or produce. Others again take refuge in a kind of pseudo-activity: they mistake restlessness for action, they are always busy, they never have time; at bottom they achieve nothing.

Many of these 'impotents' hope that time will bring a solution. A tragic event in their life or in that of the community does sometimes deliver them from the state of inertia in which they live. Such men greet war as 'the great adventure', as a welcome break in the monotony of daily routine. They are marked down as the supporters of totalitarian regimes.

This disease does not spare even those who are called to combat it— those modern directors of conscience which the psycho-analysts claim to be. Most of them seem deeply convinced—consciously or unconsciously (one can see it in their treatments)—of their own inability to help their fellow-beings, to cure their patients. So they take refuge in the 'magic gesture'. They impose upon their patients tasks that are to be literally carried out in every detail, and if the cure does not work they always have the easy excuse that their orders were not obeyed.

This feeling of impotence leads to masochism and its counterpart sadism. As its most direct derivative it releases rage, which, if repressed, changes into fear. Fear in its turn will only reinforce the initial feeling of impotence; and the process, which one could describe as an ever-rising vicious spiral, begins all over again.

All this, which we have exposed along the lines suggested by Fromm, tends to produce in humanity the Gulliverian feeling towards life: man is inadequately equipped to stand up, not to nature but to the social structure which binds him down. This Gulliverian feeling will differ in individuals according to age and social condition, but no one seems able to escape it. Society measures the personal worth of the individual in terms of his economic output; therefore children and old people have no claim to *Lebensraum* in the whole of the social area.

Much concern has been felt about the fate of the proletarian child (Otto Rühle and also Kanitz, who summed up the latter's works for the French reader in the short-lived *Revue de psychologie concrète*), but perhaps no one will ever know the psychological misery of the bourgeois child. It would seem that in spite of very real physical misery the working-class child and adolescent very often enjoy more freedom and find psychological compensation more easily, especially in the country surroundings.

The feeling of impotence experienced by the average adult of our present society is not gratuitous; for impotent he truly is in face of the opaque and highly complicated forces of our social structure. Present-day society is rather like a tragi-comical performance by millions of dwarfs of a play written for giants. Tell them that their troubles are their own fault, and you will only increase their sufferings. Montaigne used to say that he would suffer cruelly if he were forbidden access to a certain forgotten strip of territory in India. He had incidentally no occasion to go there, but the prohibition would have seemed like an obstacle to his liberty. What would he say to the present regime of passports and visas!

Actually there is nothing new in what Fromm describes in his study. Most of the facts he reports can be found described in even greater detail in the works of Alfred Adler or of his disciples. In Fromm's view, as in that of his great forerunner, the neurotic only presents in an extreme form the sense of impotence which weighs on us all, for the germ of the disease is present in normal man.

'The feeling of impotence', says Fromm, 'is very generally present in the neurotic, and constitutes so central a part in his individuality that it could be taken as the starting point in defining his neurosis.' And again, 'In every neurosis—whether symptomatic or a neurosis of character—we have a man who is incapable of performing certain definite functions, of doing what he ought to be able to do, and in whom this incapacity is linked with a deep conviction of his own weakness and powerlessness; the latter may be conscious or it may be an "unconscious conviction".'

This rediscovery of the results achieved by the Adlerian school is significant even from the methodological point of view. Fromm, indeed, stresses the point that 'the only road which will lead us to understand this socio-psychological phenomenon is that which starts from individual psycho-analysis'. This is open to question. In the meantime the claim remains unchallenged until someone has found a different and a better road.

Fromm has perceived very clearly a problem which is of decisive importance for our epoch. But it is doubtful whether the series of individual psycho-analyses which he has carried out can lead to any definite conclusions. Perhaps he has been in too great a hurry to reach results.

Before the 1914 war, obviously, one could deem oneself to be living in the best of worlds where all was going well. Everything could be understood, so, one felt, everything could be forgiven. The papers one read seemed to explain everything, whether economic processes or political events. Everywhere a splendid Chief of State watched over the interests of the country, assisted by excellent ministers and brave generals, not forgetting the police. Money was solid and stable, economic changes took place slowly, not at a breakneck speed. So the good bourgeois of Europe could enjoy his securities in peace. And these penetrated every sphere of his life. There were 'safety' matches and 'safety' pins; beards and moustaches gave an air of wisdom and dignity, even to fools; while the large hats and long skirts mercifully concealed many a defect in the weaker sex. Top-hats, walking-sticks, heavy rings all helped to produce a feeling of solidity. The thick glasses we drank out of (compare them to the carton container thrown away immediately after use!) felt as if they would last for ever. The very material of which clothes and footwear were made, the leather used for trunks, all produced the same feeling of solidity. Alas, vulcan fibre has taken the place of tan-coloured leather; instead of wearing a suit from five to ten years we get a new one every six months (when we can!); our shoes become unwearable after four months, and we can no longer pass our hats on to our sons. Who would have the folly to deny that our minds are not influenced by all these changes? As production has developed, new and inferior materials have been made utilisable by machines, so that the world in which we live, the world of objects that surround us, with its thin partitions separating us from our neighbours instead of the thick walls of the old days, cannot produce in us the feeling of permanence, of solidity, and of security that we formerly enjoyed. And yet another point. This same mechanised form of production requires us *not to use* such durable materials as in the past, for this might interfere with the constant demand, causing a drop in production, an increase in unemployment, and the vicious spiral (for it is no longer a circle, but an infinite spiral) of the economic and social crisis would begin to ascend. Mass production, the extreme form of mechanisation which appeared in the thirties of our era, tells the consumer very clearly, 'Wear your straw hat from morning to night, throw it away and buy another one to-morrow, throw away the carton container from which you have drunk a single time, sell your new car as scrap iron a few weeks after buying it', and so on. And it is perhaps no mere chance that this form of production, based on rapid destruction of its products, should have taken birth in Japan, the country where they have been building the lightest wooden and paper houses for centuries, where earthquakes do little to promote a feeling of security, and where the American bombardment of 1864 caused a collective 'inferiority complex' of such magnitude that history has not seen its like.

Thus economic production tends to spread feelings of instability among us. Instability is insecurity, and insecurity becomes *inferiority*. To-day the man in the street no longer understands 'world politics'. Formerly secret diplomacy was the only thing he thought himself incapable of understanding. And yet, to-day, when it is supposed to have been banished from international life, when those who rule our fate seem to be closely under the control of publicity, whether of the printed word, of the radio, or of the film, this 'secret diplomacy' has actually invaded every field of public life. Nothing could be more opaque. Economic processes are so complicated that we feel we cannot possibly understand, still less foresee them. The internal and, to an even greater extent, the external policy of a country, instead of flowing peacefully as between the banks of a river, takes place in fits and starts, by means of *coups de théâtre*, as a result of factors that are contradictory and incomprehensible to the vast majority of people. Listen, if it amuses you, to the conversation of experts in international politics or economics, compare their conclusions, and then compare these to current events. These men may be partly right, but no one of them can foresee *everything*. All will have made serious mistakes in estimating the situation. One need only recall the forecasts that were made on the subject of 'total war'. All this leads to a peculiar increase in psychological insecurity, and more than ever the souls of men are disposed to suffer from 'complexes' or, as they are very improperly called, 'psychoses'.

Economic forces, instead of being at the service of man, to be used by him with skill and cunning, have become indomitable genii, over which man, like the sorcerer-apprentice, has lost all control. We have come to regard ourselves as subject to them as to fate, the voice of Destiny seems to breathe through them. And yet if we are to think and act with autonomy, we must be free of fate; moreover, we must be able to *understand*. Otherwise we should only be increasing the number of *Putsches* and *coups de théâtre*.

Before concluding we would draw attention to two large-scale phenomena of inferiorisation in present-day humanity. One arises from the modern superstition that *only what is social is truly human*, and this entails the destruction of many no less human values which are not necessarily of a social order. It is time, therefore, to challenge this modern dogma, with all due respect to vast social reforms which we owe to it, and to remember the deep and genuine values that lie dormant in man as an individual.

The other phenomenon is the increasing *infantilisation* of the human being—a subject to which I hope to devote another work. This process has been going on on a vast scale in the twentieth century despite the fallacious theories of the so-called 'revolt of the masses'. So long as the masses believed in the omnipotence of God, the feeling of individual responsibility continued to subsist, as did also the sense of not being defenceless against superior hostile forces. Man could count on the protection of a personal God of infinite goodness. But since for vast sections of the population, grouped under different political flags, the idea of God has been replaced by that of an omnipotent, impersonal and bureaucratic state, the feeling of personal impotence has grown apace. Individuals are thus relieved of all personal responsibility and become transformed into marionettes to be manipulated by political demagogues, provided these are clever enough to pull the strings.

And the specialists in human behaviour, the psychologists, the psychiatrists, the theoreticians—how are they reacting to this vast and increasing complex of insecurity which we find in the world to-day? It is extremely instructive to examine what they have to say, but alas, they will not supply us with very edifying answers.

CHAPTER II

HISTORY OF A TERM AND OF AN IDEA

BIRTH OF A MODERN TERM

THE term which forms the subject of our enquiry has not yet attained civic status, and there is little chance of finding it in a dictionary. True, it is mentioned in the *Encyclopaedia Britannica*, but this is only the exception that proves the rule. And yet for the last twenty-odd years at least the 'Inferiority Complex' has been current coin in daily talk. It is all the more singular, therefore, that hardly anyone should have bothered to define it, let alone to trace its history.

The truth is that the idea is relatively new and that only the events taking place between the two wars have forced us to make current use of it. Used originally only as part of the psycho-analytic jargon, it is now on Mr. Everyman's lips, and it shares, indeed, the fate of many other terms which, by dint of constant use by the layman, have finally lost their precise and technical meaning. Psycho-pathology has supplied ordinary language with a number of such terms, especially since the turn of the century. Instead of admitting that we are irritable or even irritated we say that we are 'nervy'; aversions have given way to 'phobias'; instead of 'vapours' (originally a medical term born at the time when people still believed in 'humours') we have 'neuralgia', 'neurasthenia', even 'complexes'. As for the 'psychoses' so dear to the journalists, the term had for a time to be banned by specialists, so confused had the notion become. The same may be said of 'schizophrenia'; and if 'hysteria' dropped out for a time from the vocabulary of all self-respecting French psychiatrists only to be recently reintroduced, was this not because of the way the general public misused the word as a result of the studies made by Charcot?

The attempt has been made to estimate the time needed for a new scientific notion to penetrate the mind of the public. Some say that it needs fifty years, others say thirty. But to-day these figures have lost their significance. The radio, the aeroplane, the motor-car have become such integral parts of our lives that it needs some effort of the imagination to carry our minds back to the not so very distant time when they did not exist.

Now in the case of the 'Inferiority Feelings'—to say nothing of 'complexes'—this percolation into the public mind has been more than usually rapid. These terms are used in everyday talk before having been consecrated for the use of the manuals of psychology by a historical study or a clinical monograph. The devaluation has been too swift. A currency which ought to have been fixed runs the risk of losing all value for science for want of having ever been stabilised. A whole system of psychology, of psychiatry, of pedagogy, even of practical 'meliorism' has been based on this term, which seems to us so alarmingly complex and ambiguous: we are speaking of the 'Individual Psychology' of Alfred Adler. It all happened before the term had been submitted to minute analysis, and though later on people began to regard words with a certain suspicion, far too little care has been exercised in this direction.[1]

The bulk of Adler's work, both theoretical and practical, could equally well be named *Gemeinschafts-psychologie* (Community Psychology). The proof of this is that after Hitler's seizure of power the Adlerians still in Germany continued their work under this title under the direction of the veteran Leonhard Seif of Munich. Thanks to this change of name, which involved no change of theory or practice, they were left in peace.[2]

No term can become fashionable unless the phenomenon it denotes has become part of the public's daily life. Before the terms 'feeling of inferiority' or 'inferiority complex' could pass into ordinary language, the thing itself had to invade our daily life. It behoves us, therefore, to cast a rapid glance at the history of what only later became a subject of scientific reflection.

So long as man had a definitely theocentric conception of the world he could relate his feelings of insufficiency and inferiority to God. The fact that his feelings of inferiority were of a religious character put the problem on a purely ethical and not on a psychological plane. The Renaissance, which saw the appearance of the first of the famous

[1] Stuart Chase, *The Tyranny of Words*, Methuen, 1938.
[2] The *Individual Psychology Bulletin*, Chicago, 1944, quotes from Seelman's *Kin. Sexualität und Erziehung*, 'publishers unknown'. A curious thing is that every chapter is headed with a motto taken from Adler's writings, but all signed Leonhard Seif. This was done to outwit the Nazi censorship.

neurotics of history, brought a heightened sense of psychological penetration in its wake. Some give priority in this matter to Petrarch, others to Montaigne, while as regards deep understanding of human conduct what name springs more readily to the mind than that of Machiavelli?

MONTAIGNE

The first author in whom we find a fairly precise description of the phenomena which we now denote as feelings of inferiority is undoubtedly Montaigne. His psychological 'acquisitions' have been analysed with great subtlety, if with a certain lack of technical background, by my Danish friend, Professor Billeskov-Jansen. According to him, the psychological disorder we are examining appears quite clearly in Montaigne as a disturbance in the function of self-esteem. He writes: 'The moment that Montaigne is no longer content simply to note the difference which separates him from the observed object but begins to measure himself against it, he immediately experiences a *malaise*, a feeling of weakness which finds expression in an underestimation of himself and an over-estimation of what does not belong to him'.[1]

Montaigne carried the analysis of his ego to a degree of subtlety worthy of St. Augustine; it has been surpassed only in our own times in such writers as Marcel Proust and James Joyce. Sometimes his self-abasement seems merely a literary conceit: 'Rampant au limon de la terre je ne laisse pas de remarquer, presque dans les nues, la hauteur d'aucunes âmes héroiques.' At others, the strongly subjective note completely removes any conventional character from his 'confrontations'. He admits the existence of *bransles* (movements) of the body and of *bransles* of the soul.

'I cannot answer for the motions of my body, but concerning those of the soule, I will here ingenuously confess what I thinke of them. There are two parts in this glory; Which is to say for a man to esteeme himselfe overmuch, the other, not sufficiently to esteeme others. . . . I feel myself surcharged with one errour of mind, which both as bad, and much more as importunate, I utterly dislike. I endeavour to correct it; but I cannot displace it. It is because I abate the just value of those things

[1] Cf. F. J. Billeskov-Jansen, *Sources vives de la pensée de Montaigne*, Levine et Munksgaard, Copenhagen, 1935. This book contains everything which an intelligent historian of literature who is not himself a psychologist or a sociologist can extract from the *Essays* from the socio-psychological point of view.

which I possesse; and enhance the worth of things by how much they are more strange, absent and not mine owne. This humour extends itselfe very farre, and between two like workes, would I ever weigh against mine. Not so much that the jealousie of my preferment and amendment troubleth my judgment and hindereth me from pleasing myself, as that mastery her selfe begets a contempt of that which a man possesseth and oweth. . . . My neighbour's oeconomie, his house and his horse, though but of equal value, is more worth than mine by how much more it is not mine owne. Besides, because I am most ignorant in my own matters I admire the assurance and wonder at the promise that every man hath of himselfe, whereas there is almost nothing that I wot I know nor that I dare warrant my selfe to be able to doe. I have not my faculties in proposition, or by estate, and am not instructed in them but after the effect. As doubtfull of mine owne strength, as uncertaine of another's force. Whence it followeth if commendably I chance upon a piece of worke, I rather impute it to my fortune, than ascribe it to mine industry; forasmuch as I designe them all to hazard, and in feare.' (From the essay on 'Presumption', Vol. II, 17, in Florio's translation of the *Essays*, published in 1603.)

These, as can be seen, are genuine 'confrontations'. What Montaigne describes as an 'error of the mind' is really nothing more than a very subtle analysis of *envy* rather than of the feelings of inferiority proper. But in other places the sage of Périgord diagnoses very clearly the oscillations that take place in his feelings of self-esteem. His only consolation in this life, which is 'un mouvement inégal, irrégulier et confus', is the *confrontations*.

'What I find excusable in mine is not of it selfe and according to truth; but in comparison of other compositions worse than mine, to which I see some credit given.'
'I have ever an idea in mind which presents me with a better forme than that I have already framed, but I can neither lay hold on it nor effect it' (*loc. cit.*).

Montaigne also feels the universal uncertainty of things in this world which is nothing but a *branloire perenne*. But he is not ignorant of the *sense of being*. He speaks of the almost divine perfection of a frank enjoyment of one's being. But this must not be confused with what we refer to to-day as the Complex of Superiority, for in the essay from which we have already quoted he says,

37

'I remember then that even from my tenderest infancy some noted in me a kind of I know not what fashion of carrying my body and gestures witnessing a certain vain and foolish fierceness (French: *fierté*)' (*loc. cit.*).

'Montaigne', says Billeskov-Jansen (*loc. cit.*, p. 13), 'does not seem able to understand this inconsistency within his own mind, which is more inclined to undervalue itself than to rate itself too highly.' But I would say that the contradiction is only apparent, and disappears completely in the light of the modern psychology of the feelings of inferiority. 'It seems probable', continues the Danish author, 'that the child, without quite knowing why, put on a mask of pride with the object of defending himself against the emotions that assailed him on every side. Throughout his life we shall see him thus on guard against what seem the most trivial wounds which daily life might inflict upon him.'

Moreover, Montaigne himself will give us the explanation. After complaining of his low stature, his ignorance of music, swimming, fencing, vaulting and leaping, he continues the list of his failings:

'I perceive how the auditorie censureth me. . . . I cannot very wel close up a letter nor could I ever make a pen. I was never a good carver at table. I could never make ready nor arm a horse. Nor handsomely carry a Hawke upon my fist nor cast her off, or let her fly, nor could I ever speak to Dogges, to Birds, or to Horses. The conditions of my body are, in fine, very well agreeing with those of my minde' (*loc. cit.*).

And in an earlier essay he says of himself, 'I cannot well contain myself in mine owne possession and disposition.'

SHAKESPEARE

After Montaigne it is Shakespeare (how many of his heroes are the victims of complexes—Hamlet, Shylock, Othello!) who gives us the most masterly analysis of the same soul-sickness, but in a far graver and more pernicious form. I am thinking of his portrait of Richard III as it is presented in the powerful monologue at the opening of the play. The diagnosis has all the force of a mathematical axiom. The whole argument of the plot unfolds from it as an inevitable consequence. Adler looked upon this monologue as the quintessential schema of criminality. In writing it Shakespeare may have had in mind the ancient physiognomic rule: *distortum vultum sequitur distortio morum*.

But I, that am not shaped for sportive tricks,
Nor made to court an amorous looking-glass;
I that am rudely stamp'd, and want love's majesty,
To strut before a wanton ambling nymph;
I, that am curtailed of this fair proportion,
Cheated of feature, by dissembling nature,
Deform'd, unfinish'd, sent before my time
Into this breathing world, scarce half made up,
And that so lamely and unfashionable
That dogs bark at me as I halt by them;—
Why I, in this weak piping time of peace,
Have no delight to pass away the time,
Unless to spy my shadow in the sun,
And descant on mine own deformity;
And therefore—since I cannot prove a lover,
To entertain these fair well-spoken days—
I am determined to prove a villain,
And hate the idle pleasures of these days.
Plots have I laid, inductions dangerous,
By drunken prophecies, libels and dreams,
To set my brother Clarence and the king
In deadly hate the one against the other.

Richard III, Act I, Sc. i.

HOBBES

After Shakespeare we have to wait for Stendhal to show us with equal penetration a soul tortured with feelings of inferiority. In the intervening period these problems of the ego were chiefly the concern of moralists and 'philosophers'. The earliest of these is the political philosopher Thomas Hobbes (1588–1679), one of Adler's most important forerunners, though on a completely different plane. The Baron Seillière in a rather unsatisfactory book[1] has described Adler as the

---

[1] Seillière, *Psychanalyse ou Psychologie impérialiste Allemande*, Paris, 1928. I have written a detailed criticism of this book in the *Internat. Zeitsch. f. Ind. Psych.*, 1929. The author regarded Freudian psycho-analysis as a product of the Jewish Talmudic mind and Adler's ideas as characteristic of the Teutonic mind.(!) This reminds me of a certain little M.A. thesis by an American, Sumner, who compared Freud to Christ on account of his soft and feminine mentality, and Adler, 'hard even in his style', to Antichrist. After this last word he added in parenthesis '(Nietzsche)'.

prophet of the *libido dominandi*, as opposed to the Freudian *libido*. In a recent book,[1] Lewis Way recalls this resemblance. He writes:

'The theories of Hobbes, for instance, are based on his belief that men strive for power, and those of Bentham on the belief that they strive for pleasure. Among the moderns, Adler and Freud are the scientific representatives of these two traditions of thought. . . . Adler's psychology was designed with special reference to the neurotic patient and it ought not to be applied wholesale. The Will to Power, especially, is true only of the neurotic, and it has always seemed to me that Hobbes, Nietzsche, Machiavelli, and its other distinguished exponents overstate the matter when they try to make it fit a larger context.'

Adler, who so often saw his ideas identified with Nietzsche's Will to Power, used to say that people confused his psychology with that of his patients. He was anything but the psychologist of German Imperialism, as a brief comparison across the centuries of his ideas with those of Hobbes will show. And yet Hobbes in the seventeenth century and Adler in the first part of the twentieth set out from the same observations; only their interpretations were different.

Michael Oakeshott, in the introduction to his excellent edition of *Leviathan*,[2] writes as follows:

'Hobbes' philosophy is in all its parts pre-eminently a philosophy of *power*. . . . The end of philosophy itself is power—*scientia propter potentiam*. Man is a complex of powers; desire is a desire for power, pride is illusion about power, honour, opinion about power, life is unremitting exercise of power, and death the absolute loss of power.'

If for the word 'power' we substitute the term 'significance', suggested by Way, we shall come very close to the Adlerian *Geltungsstreben*, a 'tendency to make one's worth felt'; the Americans speak in the same sense of 'seeking personal importance'. And if for 'power' we put the word 'superiority', the term used by Adler, we shall find that Hobbes' ideas are almost identical with those of the great Viennese psychologist. In Hobbes' own words, '. . . In the first place, I put for a general inclination of all mankind, a perpetual and restless desire of power that ceaseth only in death' (*Leviathan*, p. 63). Adler, taking the psychology

[1] Allen and Unwin, 1948.
[2] *Leviathan, or the Matter, Form and Power of the Commonwealth*, by Thomas Hobbes (1651). Basil Blackwell, Oxford. All quotations will be from this edition.

of the neurotic as his starting-point only, regarded human life as an un-ceasing struggle for superiority by a being who feels himself in-feriorised. 'To be man is to feel oneself inferior and to strive for the goal of superiority.' That sums up his whole philosophy. Is it so very different from that of Hobbes?

On re-reading Hobbes we find, under the lumber of preoccupations peculiar to his epoch, a number of very modern ideas. Take, for instance, the passage on *laughter* which contains *in nuce* the somewhat over-simple but nevertheless very Adlerian theory recently expounded by Marcel Pagnol.[1] According to Hobbes (*loc. cit.*, p. 36), we laugh 'by observing the imperfections of other men. And therefore much laughter at the defects of others is a sign of pusillanimity.' Pagnol's theory that we laugh (*a*) when we feel superior to someone else, or (*b*) when we notice someone else's inferiority, or (*c*) at a combination of these two cases, is clearly anticipated by Hobbes, who ends on a moral or, one might even say, a philosophical note which is totally absent from Pagnol's amusing but superficial work.

Hobbes regarded life, as Adler did later, as *movement*, and he thought that this movement was set afoot by desire, desire being a will for power. As Oakeshott sums it up:

'Will is the last desire in deliberating. There can, then, be no final end, no *summum bonum* for a man's active powers; the appropriate achievement will be continual success in obtaining the things which a man from time to time desires, and this lies not in procuring what is desired, but also in the assurance that what will in the future be desired will also be procured. This success is called felicity, which is a condition of movement, not of rest or tranquillity. The means by which a man may obtain this success are called, comprehensively, his Power; and therefore there is in man *a perpetual and restless desire for power*, because power is the *sine qua non* of felicity' (*loc. cit.*, p. 31).

Like his contemporary, Spinoza, in whom some have seen a pre-cursor of Freud (B. Alexander), Hobbes looked upon desire as life's ruling principle.

'Nor can a man any more live, whose desires are at an end, than he whose senses and imagination are at a stand. Felicity is a continual pro-gress of the desire from one object to another; the attaining of the former being still but a way to the latter' (*loc. cit.*, p. 65).

Hobbes was clever enough not to confuse real power with the mere

[1] Marcel Pagnol, *Notes sur le Rire*, Nagel, Paris.

41

appearance of superiority. That is why he establishes a difference between 'pride' (which Mandeville called 'vanity' or 'vain-glory') and glory. Oakeshott sums up the question as follows:

'Glory, which is exaltation of the mind based upon a true estimate of a man's power to procure felicity, is a useful emotion; it is both the cause and the effect of well-grounded confidence. But pride is a man's false estimate of his own powers and the fore-runner of certain failure. Indeed, so fundamental a defect is pride, that it may be taken as the type of all hindrances to the achievement of felicity. The existence of other beings than myself and the impossibility of escaping their company is the first impediment in the pursuit of felicity, for another man is necessarily a competitor. ... There is ... a permanent potential enmity between men, a "perpetual contention for Honour, Riches and Authority". Superiority of strength . . . is nothing better than an illusion. The natural condition of man is one of the competition of equals for the things (necessarily scarce because of the desire for *superiority*) that belong to felicity' (*loc. cit.*, p. 34–5).

Hence the famous 'war of all against all'.

Pride, which since Adler we call the Superiority Complex, is a very serious encumbrance in life. For, to quote Oakeshott again, 'if pride, the excessive estimate of his own powers, hinders a man in choosing the best course of action when he is alone, it will be the most crippling of all handicaps when played upon by a competitor in the race.'

This brings us to the point of bifurcation between the ideas of Adler and those of Hobbes. The latter regarded man as essentially solitary. 'Man is solitary', he says; 'would that he were alone'; thus placing himself at the opposite pole from the early theories concerning the social nature of man, such as the 'social instinct' of Richard Cumberland or the 'social passions' of Adam Smith.

Adler held, on the contrary, that the child is born with a *community feeling* which can only be hampered by the various inferiority feelings. He maintains that the child is not a selfish little animal, for all the insistence placed upon childish egocentricity by the Bühlers and Piaget, and he thus revives the 'social instinct' theory of the early liberals.

This is not the place to draw a full-scale parallel between Hobbes and Adler, though it is surprising that the task has never been undertaken by the Adlerian school. We have simply pointed to Hobbes as a precursor, and have noted that he has much to say that is of interest to psychologists, as when he speaks of what he calls 'aversion', one of the extreme forms of which is *fear*. In any case, it is curious to note how these two thinkers, starting from the same point, with a wide divergency of background and epoch, were led to no less divergent conclusions. It has been said that the Jews (and Adler was one) are lacking in the sense of power, the sense that was so strong in Hobbes. But it cannot be denied that they possess a very fine flair for the power of others and for every degree of inferiority and superiority. Thus it would seem natural that Hobbes should be the prophet of the war of all against all, while Adler was the first to detect the varying shades of superiority in all the fictitious forms of it that exist in the neurotic.[1]

ROUSSEAU

The expression *esprit d'escalier* comes from Jean-Jacques Rousseau, one of the most typical examples of that micromania which is common to all *déclassés*. What are the *Confessions* but the reflection of a soul that is constantly being inferiorised, living parasitically on an aristocratic class touched with only a veneer of superficial culture? Nor has modern psychology failed to analyse Rousseau's character in the light of present knowledge (cf. Wexberg in *Heilen und Bilden*).

MANDEVILLE

Rousseau may have believed that man, a child of nature if left to himself, was fundamentally good; the moralists of the eighteenth century held, on the contrary, that he was evil, for they regarded him as essentially selfish. This theme recurs with almost wearisome iteration in the writings of the period. If for example we open F. L. von Hopfgarten's *Versuch über den Charakter des Menschen und eines Volkes überhaupt*, published by J. F. Junius in Leipzig in 1773, we find it stated that man's fundamental instinct is love of self (*Eigenliebe*), made up of greed and a desire for honour and pleasure. The moralists see the manifestation of this egoism in the thirst for power. It was named the 'instinct of sovereignty and self-liking' by the Dutch philosopher and physician Mandeville,

---

[1] In speaking of the Jews' 'lack of the sense of power' I am thinking of the ideas of the Jewish sociologist, G. Salomon-Delatour, and not of the *Leviathan*, written by the Nazi *Kronjurist*, Carl Schmitt, which is interesting to read but exaggerated in its conclusions.

whom we may regard as another forerunner of Adler.[1] According to him men are sociable, not from a *plus*, but from a *minus*. While Adler regards man as sociable because of the weakness of the species, in Mandeville's opinion he is sociable from wickedness. Sociability arises from man's vilest qualities. Our species distinguishes itself from others by the 'strange desire which all men have that others should think well of them', and in the Remarks to his famous *Fable of the Bees* (published in 1723) the author has subjected this idea to the most searching analysis. We want to impress others, so we seek honour. Translated into Adler's terminology this becomes the *Geltungsstreben*, the desire to make one's worth felt, to feel important, and not, as superficial commentators have so often tried to make us believe, the Nietzschean Will to Power. *Geltungsstreben* is quite content with the *appearance* of worth, and for the most part requires no effective power. 'Honour', says Mandeville, 'in its true and proper signification is nothing but the good opinion which other men have of our merit.'

The opposite of honour is dishonour, also called *ignominy* or *shame.*

'Shame', says Mandeville, 'signifies a passion that has its proper symptoms, over-rules our reason, and requires as much labour and self-denial to be subdued, as any of the rest; and since the most important actions of life often are regulated according to the influence this passion has upon us, a thorough understanding of it must help to illustrate the notions the world has of honour and ignominy; I shall therefore describe it at large. First to define the passion of shame I think it may be called a *sorrowful reflection on our own unworthiness, proceeding from an apprehension that others either do or might, if they knew all, deservedly despise us*' (From *The Fable of the Bees*, Remark C).

This feeling of shame, though it is not as clearly established as was later Janet's 'feeling of shame of self', is, however, something more than pure imagination, for 'Though the good and evil of honour and dishonour are imaginary, yet there is reality in shame'. The picture which Mandeville paints of this shame enables us to identify it fully with the feeling of inferiority so frequently mentioned to-day:

'The shame that raw, ignorant and ill-bred people, though seemingly without cause, discover before their betters, is always accom-

---

[1] The first to point this out was the late Robert Michels in his study on 'L'Economie eudémoniciste' in *Wirtschaft und Gesellschaft*, Frankfort, 1924, *Oppenheimer—Festschrift*.

panied with and proceeds from a consciousness of their weakness and inabilities' (*loc. cit.*).

Thus the feeling of shame seems in the last resort to be a negative principle which constantly disturbs our outward behaviour. Its source is purely internal and subjective, as Mandeville has cleverly discovered; our behaviour is therefore under the influence of a purely psychological factor. This older author therefore confronts us with that principle of psychic determinism which, to the educated public of the beginning of our century, seemed such a sensational novelty.

But Mandeville also discerns the opposite and more active principle in us, that of pride, which he seems to identify with honour.

'That these two passions (shame and pride), in which the seeds of most virtues are contained, are realities in our frame, and not imaginary qualities, is demonstrable from the plain and different effects, that in spite of our reason, are produced in us as soon as we are affected with either.

'When a man is overwhelmed with shame, he observes a sinking of the spirits, the heart feels cold and condensed, and the blood flies from it to the circumference of the body; the face glows, the neck and part of the breast partake of the fire; he is heavy as lead; the head is hung down; and the eyes through a mist of confusion are fixed on the ground: no injuries can move him; he is weary of his being, and heartily wishes he could make himself invisible' (*loc. cit.*).

And yet this feeling, so eloquently described, is not entirely to the prejudice, we will not say of man, but at any rate of humanity as a whole. To Mandeville shame appears to be the first step towards sociability, just as the feeling of inferiority did to Alfred Adler.

'It is incredible how necessary an ingredient shame is to make us sociable. It is a frailty in our nature; all the world, whenever it affects them, submit to it at regret, and would willingly prevent it if he could; yet the happiness of conversation depends upon it, and no society could be polished if the generality of mankind was not subject to it' (*loc. cit.*).

Moreover, society makes a point of stimulating this feeling of shame, so useful to her purposes. She uses the educators. Incidentally one cannot help being reminded of the reproaches levelled by the Adlerian School at traditional education, which unfortunately does so much to create and maintain feelings of inferiority in the young entrusted to its care. Mandeville speaks of man's propensity to throw off this feeling of shame:

'And therefore from infancy, throughout his education, we endeavour to increase instead of lessening or destroying this sense of shame; and the only remedy prescribed is a strict observance of certain rules to avoid those things that might bring this troublesome sense of shame upon him. But as to rid or cure him of it, the politician would sooner take away his life' (*loc. cit.*).

The abuse by politicians of those feelings which are their easiest prey appeared in full force in the horrifying results of German National Socialism. We shall deal with the subject later. In the meantime let us conclude this part of our sketch of pre-Adlerian theories concerning feelings of inferiority, with a final quotation from Mandeville. Here is the description he gives of the symptoms accompanying Pride, i.e. the manifestations of the *sentiment de l'être* in the terminology of Vauvenargues, or of the Superiority Complex in the language of Adler.

'But when, gratifying his vanity, he exults in his pride he discovers quite contrary symptoms: his spirits swell and fan the arterial blood, a more than ordinary warmth strengthens and dilates the heart; the extremities are cool; he feels light to himself and imagines he could tread on air; his head is held up, his eyes rolled about with sprightliness; he rejoices at his being, is prone to anger, and would be glad that all the world could take notice of him' (*loc. cit.*).

VAUVENARGUES

I do not know if anyone has ever compared this singular English medico-philosopher, who knew so much about self-esteem and vanity, with Luc de Clapiers, Marquis de Vauvenargues, who is considered one of the most searching of the French moralists, and who seems to be coming into fashion again in literary circles. It is very probable that he knew the *Fable of the Bees,* for we read in him sentences like these: 'One wonders whether the majority of vices do not contribute to the public good as well as the purest virtues. How would commerce flourish without vanity, avarice, etc.' Be that as it may, Vauvenargues had a very profound knowledge of the strength and the weakness of the human mind. In his view feeling is a deeper mode of knowledge than reason. He was born and brought up 'in a family that smiled but little and where everything was painted in the darkest colours'. His father was harsh, surly, and parsimonious. His own 'deplorable health' made him lonely and misanthropic; he disliked the company of women, and having come into the world 'too late', he was 'disgusted and discouraged' at feeling himself 'awkward and ridiculous' in it. (We are quoting from Gustave Michaut's *Vauvenargues, Réflexions et Maximes*, Cours de la Sorbonne, 1937–38, p. 12.) His fellow officers in the army nicknamed him 'le père', and indeed he was a spiritual director who had missed his vocation. He suffered inevitably from the futility of his profession, which he despised, and finally gave up a few years before dying in 1747 at the age of thirty-two. Writing in the *Revue des Deux Mondes*, 1919, Le Breton said of him, 'His life was a perpetual defeat'. Such was the man who first gave a name to the feelings which form the subject of our enquiry. He had a weak chest and defective eyesight, his life was poisoned by continual financial worries, he was terribly disfigured by smallpox, he suffered from lung trouble, and was afflicted with frozen feet during a campaign. Inferiorised himself to this degree, he outlined a theory of the strength and the weakness of the soul, which he thinks of as extended. One of his maxims, which he subsequently altered, reads 'Courage enlarges the soul'. In another (Maxim 43) he speaks of 'smallness of spirit'. 'There are passions', he says elsewhere, 'which shut in the soul and prevent it from moving; and there are those which enlarge it and let it spread abroad.' Voltaire labelled as obscure Maxim 196: 'We scorn many things in order not to scorn ourselves.' Vauvenargues' commentators, Gilbert and Michaut, have also interpreted it amiss. In our opinion, the words indicate the discovery of a very simple compensation formed by souls tortured with feelings of inferiority, those feelings which Janet and Adler were later to describe respectively as *péjoration* or 'tendency to devaluation'. Vauvenargues knew very well the oscillations of self-esteem. 'There are men', he writes in Maxim 236, 'who unconsciously form an idea of their appearance which they borrow from their prevailing sentiments'; and a little further on we read: 'However much we may be accused of vanity, we sometimes need to be assured of our worth and to have our most manifest advantages proven to us.' And the same idea recurs in the letter he wrote to his friend Mirabeau (the father of the tribune), 'for there is nothing so natural as to shape one's own image on the curious feeling with which one is filled'. Around him he sees the same ill by which he is tormented. 'The world is full of anxious spirits who

47

will be inexorably tormented till their death by the harshness of their condition and the desire to change their fortunes. . . .'

He was not content, however, to point to the evil in question: he supplied for the first time a theory that attempted to explain it. He distinguished in man two opposing feelings which generally appear in a singular combination: the 'sense of imperfection' (*sentiment de l'imperfection*) and the 'sense of being' (*sentiment de l'être*). M. Bernard Grasset has succeeded very well in tracing a parallel between the first and our 'feeling of inferiority'; the sense of being, on the other hand, could be compared to positive self-esteem based on an abundant if not on an exuberant vitality.

'We draw from the experience of our being', says Vauvenargues, 'an idea of greatness, of pleasure, of power which we would like to increase indefinitely; in the imperfection of our being we find an idea of smallness, subjection and misery which we seek to stifle; that is the sum total of our passions. There are men in whom the sense of being is stronger than that of their imperfection. Hence their cheerfulness and the moderation of their desires. There are others, in whom the sense of their imperfection is more lively than that of their being, hence anxiety, melancholy, etc. From the union of those two sentiments, i.e. that of our strength and that of our misery, all the greatest passions arise, because the feeling of misery urges us to go out of ourselves and the feeling of our resources encourages us and inclines us to hope. But those who feel only their misery without their strength will never excite themselves so much, for they dare not hope; nor will those who feel only their strength but not their helplessness, for they have too little to wish for. Thus what is needed is a mixture of courage and weakness, of sadness and presumption.'

Vauvenargues was truly French in postulating the right balance of the two elements—weakness and imperfection on the one hand, strength and a sense of being on the other. We therefore find in him the idea of an equilibrium, a notion which does not exist in Adler, who, though a practitioner of genius, was a poor theoretician. Vauvenargues knew well enough that, as Nicole had said, 'Il y a des esprits qui sont douloureux partout', just as on the other hand there are people who feel only their strength. But in his opinion (and in ours too in spite of the views of certain Adlerians) the ideal state is the coexistence in right proportion of the two feelings in question.

Vauvenargues can be regarded as a very modern as well as a very astute psychologist. At the age of twenty-five he foretold in almost prophetic terms that his contemporaries would tire of the natural and mathematical sciences and would turn their attention to the things of the soul. To-day something very similar is taking place, and the appearance of the Adlerian psychology is a first effect of this new trend, viz. to leave to biology and physiology their share of knowledge, but to return to that in man which eludes the analysis undertaken from the viewpoint of these two sciences.

The ideal which the Adlerian psychology aims at is *Understanding Human Nature* (that is the name of the most widely read and translated of Adler's books). The idea of a 'psychagogy' only occupies a secondary place, and has been more the concern of the disciples than of the master. We have repeatedly claimed that it is on human conduct that the psychology of character must fasten its attention, a view which has been openly acknowledged in Germany for the last twenty years. It was a view held too by Vauvenargues, the friend of Voltaire and of Mirabeau's father. He was a born spiritual director and his desire was to dominate men's minds so as to gain mastery of their wills. As Merlant has said in his *De Montaigne à Vauvenargues*, he made friends with men of outstanding merit because he would have liked to possess their souls.

STENDHAL

It is not by chance that Vauvenargues has often been compared to Stendhal. The *Réflexions et Maximes* was Henri Beyle's bedside book. He was the first to use the term 'feeling of inferiority'. Like Montaigne and Vauvenargues, he regarded it as an 'error of the mind', but he added that it was an error worthy of a superior man.[1] But if Stendhal had been asked to give a name to this malady of the soul he would have called it 'inverted imagination' (*imagination renversée*)[2]. To this day

[1] 'He himself had been loved by her but she had never seen how slight were his merits. "And indeed they are slight", Julien told himself with entire conviction. "I am, when all is said, a very dull creature, very common, very tedious to others, quite insupportable to myself." He was sick to death of all his own good qualities, of all the things he had loved with enthusiasm; and in this state of *inverted imagination* he set to work to criticise his work with his imagination. This is an error that stamps a superior person'. (From the translation of *Le Rouge et le Noir*, made by Scott Moncrieff. Vol. I, p. 168, Chatto and Windus.) This recalls Vauvenargues' 'On est très souvent injuste pour soi-même et on se condamne à tort', and Montaigne's 'Et de nos maladies la plus sauvage c'est de mespriser nostre être'.

[2] It is interesting to note that Adler, though he never paid any particular attention to *inverted imagination*, liked to quote a passage from *Macbeth* which expresses a similar idea. In his communication to the International Congress of Psychology at Oxford, *Advances in Individual Psychology*, we read, 'Nothing that man

Julien Sorel is the most perfect representative in literature of the inferiority complex. *Le Rouge et le Noir* is an anticipation of the Adlerian theories, just as Dostoievsky's novels anticipated the theories of Freud. Stendhal shows us very clearly how Julien, who was inferiorised in his home by the mere fact of being different from his brothers ('to be different breeds hatred', he writes somewhere), is later on concerned only to assert and more than assert his own worth. *Le Rouge et le Noir* is the story of a modern neurotic told with incomparable art. Thus love is used by the hero to convince himself of his own worth, to serve as an outlet for the resentment felt by the commoner for his social superiors. Or again, take the description of Julien Sorel's behaviour in the bourgeois home of M. Renal and in the aristocratic palace of the Marquis de la Mole; he is constantly on the alert, as though he were in an enemy country, feeling himself inferior both to masters and servants. These points, more than anything else in the book, and more even than much in the incomparable *De l'Amour*, bear witness to the vigour and penetration of Stendhal's psychology.

Two German precursors of the psychology of inferiority deserve mention, Th. G. von Hippel,[1] who drew attention to feelings of inferiority in women, and C. Ph. Moritz, director of the State School in Berlin, who discovered egotism before Stendhal, and with great intuition anticipated the Freudian complexes and the Adlerian 'plan of life'. After that, we reach the scientific phase in the study of these feelings. This phase begins with the work of the late Pierre Janet, honorary professor of the Collège de France.

He was the first, towards the end of the last century, to treat systematically certain nervous symptoms which are very much part and parcel of the subject we are studying,[2] and his contribution to it will therefore be dealt with in the next chapter.

experiences, nothing that he enjoys can be completely indifferent to him. "Fair is foul and foul is fair" sing the witches in *Macbeth*. . . .' And yet in the same address Adler regards the phenomenon of inverted imagination as inevitable, and an inherent part of human nature. 'Error', he says, 'can never be avoided, either in estimating our situation or in making a choice. . . .'

[1] Cf. the section on 'L'Amélioration bourgeoise des femmes' in his *Sämtliche Werke*, 1828. In the course of this work he develops a whole theory about the 'disagreeable sensation' which arises from the fact of being at a disadvantage, and the psychological 'pressure' which still weighs on the weaker sex. The feelings of inferiority in women are also attributed to their 'lack of physical strength and the limitation of their intelligence'.

[2] An excellent study of this subject will also be found in Viola Klein's book *The Feminine Character* (Kegan Paul).

CHAPTER III

PIERRE JANET, FORERUNNER OF THE THEORY OF THE FEELINGS OF INFERIORITY

PIERRE JANET[1] is in a sense a tragic figure in the history of modern psychology. Before Freud (whom incidentally he met at the Salpêtrière under Charcot), he clearly anticipated both the theory of *psychological determinism*, which asserts that one psychic event can be caused by another psychic event without the intervention of a physical factor, and also the psychiatric idea of the *unconscious*. Nevertheless, a certain diffidence, an excessive bourgeois intellectualism inclining to nominalism, prevented him from erecting a real system based on the innumerable observations he had made. He had not the courage to think out his discoveries, sensational though they were, to their logical conclusion, and so allowed Freud to steal his thunder from him by christening *psycho-analysis* what he had always called psychological analysis and by incorporating many of his results into the Freudian system, which, for all its mistakes, is none the less a brilliant achievement. There can be no doubt, and all the specialists are agreed upon this point, that without the previous work done by Janet the Freudian Unconscious would not have been possible.

Janet was never able to discard an old-fashioned psychiatric notion which his own theory of *psychasthenia* should have helped him to throw on the scrapheap. He still spoke the language of the nineteenth century and could see only 'ideas' where clearly the phenomena in question were of an affective order.

His approach is purely intellectual and moral, and he cannot bring himself to believe in 'what is worst in man'. He must therefore have lacked the sympathetic intuition required to enter into his patients' condition. He always remained an outside spectator. His habit of constantly inventing new names, of discovering new factual details substantially diminishes the value of his theories. He used to enjoy cataloguing his observations under new labels, as though by naming a

---

[1] The author assiduously attended Janet's lectures at the Collège de France during the years 1928–30.

thing we had solved the problem it sets us. Among these many labels there is one which runs, '*obsession and impulse of self-shame*', and which Janet explains as follows: 'It is not merely a question of remorse, strictly speaking, but of contempt and dissatisfaction felt by the subject for his own actions and moral faculties. The patient is pursued by the thought that everything he does, everything that he is and everything that belongs to him is bad': *Les Névroses*, p. 20. (Janet does not seem to have known that his diagnosis is simply a new edition of the *erreurs d'âme* so subtly described by Montaigne.) But Janet did not stop there. He took the term *obsession* to mean 'the exaggerated importance assumed by a given idea', a definition which could possibly apply to the *idée fixe* or, better still, to the *over-estimated idea* of modern psychiatry, and he christened another clinical syndrome '*the obsession of shame of one's own body*'. This discovery practically opened the way to the feelings of inferiority. But instead of attempting to synthesise, as Alfred Adler was to do later on, all the phenomena of negative auto-estimation which he had discovered, Janet seems to have felt only the need to subdivide them yet further, according to Cartesian principles. Thus he speaks of the subjects who are ashamed of their body, of the whole of it, 'so that their general obsession becomes subdivided into a multitude of minor deliria'. But this is the wrong road to take and only leads to an accumulation of minutiae; one cannot see the wood for the trees. All the same, Janet did find the common denominator for this group of phenomena, for he recognised that 'the essential thing of which all these patients complain is the unfinished, inadequate and incomplete character of all these psychological phenomena. I have named this fundamental feature the feeling of *incompleteness*' (*Obsessions et Psychasthénie*, vol. I, p. 264).

These phenomena, rightly observed but too superficially interpreted, led Janet to state his famous theory of *psychasthenia*, a term which was designed to put an end to the abuses connected with a so-called 'neurasthenia' and other analogous conceptions. 'Psychasthenia', he writes, 'is a form of mental depression characterised by a lowering of the psychological tension, by a diminution of the functions which enable the subject to perceive and act upon reality, by the substitution of inferior and exaggerated operations under the form of doubts, agitation, anguish, and by obsessive ideas which express these disorders and have their own characteristics.'

If we scrutinise these words we shall find, hidden behind the nominalism of an outdated terminology, the diagnosis of what to-day are called the feelings of inferiority. All the main points are there. Janet devoted a whole course of lectures at the Collège de France to *La Force et la Faiblesse psychologiques*, a subject which, if he had followed his ideas to their logical conclusion, should have led him to a theory very similar to Adler's. And yet in dealing with the problem of the feelings of economic and social inferiority he confines himself to a few superficial remarks on 'psychological wealth' in relation to 'pecuniary wealth'. ('Money changes people completely. . . . One is far less insane when one is rich. . . .') and pursues the subject no further.

'A distinguished anthropologist, M. Manouvrier,' he writes, 'once pointed to this problem in connection with the treatment of neuroses, and maintained that people's financial position had a considerable influence on their neurosis and modified its character. Sometimes it gives them an assurance and an air of intelligence which they do not deserve, sometimes it produces illness, timidity, scruples and inferiority. This is very important to note. Another foreign author, M. Adler of Vienna, has also taken up this question again. He has studied the early phases of neurosis and the influence of wealth on timidity, scruples and inferiority.'

This is an extraordinary simplification of Adler's ideas. And yet all the ideas of the Adlerian theory are present in germ in the work of Pierre Janet. Adler never denied the profit he derived from reading his works, and on several occasions mentions the name of Janet, or refers to the idea of incompleteness. When Janet states (without mentioning Pascal, whose ideas he is unwittingly reproducing) that what is significant in a sick person is not what he says, but his way of behaving and thinking, indeed the sum of the ideas that accompany his *petite tristesse*, he is not only speaking true, but he is adopting the Adlerian attitude to the patient.[1] He gives the name of *péjoration* to what H. W. Maier has called *catathymie* and Adler *Entwertungstendenz*, i.e. a tendency to devaluate things and persons. And when in *La Force et la Faiblesse*, p. 25, he speaks of *sur-estimation* and *sous-estimation* he is (and remains) at the threshold of a system of estimative psychology, such as was first elaborated by Adler, and then outlined in philosophical guise by Max Scheler and by José Ortega y Gasset. The same thing is true

---

[1] It would be interesting one day to write the history of psychiatry according to the attitude taken by the doctor towards his patient. That of Ferenczi was maternal; that of Freud, judiciary. Janet seems to be content with a kind of θαυμαζειν, an amused astonishment.

of Janet's descriptions of certain of his patients' feelings, such as the feeling of being encumbered, the feeling of one's body in space, the feeling of a very small space, or the feelings of elevation and depression.[1]

Thus Janet, conservative though he was in outlook, sceptical though he remained of his own observations, and disinclined though he was to revolutionise the psychiatry of his day, did nevertheless reach the threshold of the promised land. Unfortunately, it was not granted him to enter it. He hesitated to take the decisive step, alarmed no doubt at the revolutionary tendency of his own theories. The same thing was to happen later to Freud, who, after having outlined a theory of what might be called 'pure' psycho-analysis, i.e. an exclusively psychological and socio-psychological theory, took up a completely new mental orientation.

The task of quarrying the abandoned seam of *psychological determinism* (which many neo-psycho-analysts, such as Karen Horney, are now exploiting) has therefore devolved upon Adler. He was the first who (though he was ignorant of it) ventured to carry out an ancient postulate of Comte's, namely, to divide psychology into two definite parts, the 'inferior' and the 'superior', the first dealing only with what the founder of Positivism would have called problems of 'zoological origin' (we would say physiological origin), the other devoted to the study of inter-human relations, 'sociological in origin and alone adequate to carry out its noble task'.[2]

---

[1] Of course these phenomena are connected with the problem of the 'body image' which has been so well examined by Head, Pick and Schilder, and which M. Lhermitte has only recently incorporated into French psychiatry under the name of 'image of one's own body' (*image du propre corps*).

[2] Cf. my own study on the psychology of Alfred Adler and the teaching of Auguste Comte in the *Revue de philosophie positive*, 1930. Also, Lalande in his introduction to the work on Dumas, p. 39; 'One could thus', he writes, 'divide psychology, as Auguste Comte forecast, into two separate fragments; the first tending towards Biology, the other more connected with the normative sciences and thus tending to be part of Sociology'. See also Paul Schilder, *The Image and Appearance of the Human Body*, Psyche Monographs, 4, Kegan Paul, 1935.

CHAPTER IV

GENEVA STUDIES:
CLAPARÈDE, M. GANZ AND R. DE SAUSSURE

Iɴ the history of the psycho-analytical movement, Switzerland has from the first played the part of mediator between the German-speaking and the French-speaking specialists, as appears in the work of Maeder, Flournoy, Claparède and Charles Baudouin. But as regards the study of the feelings of inferiority, the contribution of the Geneva school has been very meagre and has consisted mainly in popularising Adler's results, without sufficient acknowledgment, this being particularly true of R. de Saussure. Claparède has been mainly concerned with classifying the various feelings of inferiority. Madeleine Ganz, in her thesis which won the Cellerier prize, is the author of the only fairly complete introduction to Adler's ideas. M. Pierre Bovet, in his excellent book *L'Instinct combatif*, is the first French writer to have drawn attention to the Adlerian theories on aggressiveness and the feelings of inferiority, but it is surprising that in his preface to Madeleine Ganz's book he should have taken Adler to task for despising those psychotechnical methods which were so fundamentally opposed to and so incompatible with the mental outlook of that great Viennese, with his deep knowledge of human nature.

The late Edouard Claparède, co-director with Pierre Bovet of the Institut Jean-Jacques Rousseau, devoted a special pamphlet to the study of the feelings of inferiority, considered especially from the educational angle.[1] In this pamphlet, which is a clear and succinct version of his own lecture, he looks for the 'causes of the feeling of inferiority, its consequences and its treatment'.

'Much has been said', he writes, 'in the last few years about the feeling of inferiority. Not that the thing itself is new. But it had not formerly been clearly perceived. Above all, people had not realised what part this feeling could play in the destiny of the individual, in the

---

[1] Cf. *Le Sentiment d'Infériorité chez l'Enfant*, a lecture delivered at Barcelona in 1928 the text of which was printed in the *Revue de Genève* in June 1930 and later in the first number of *Cahiers de Pédagogie Expérimentale et de Psychologie de l'Enfant*, Geneva, 1934.

determination of his character, and in the appearance of certain nervous disorders. Important for the science of psychology, it was no less so for the art of education. . . . An important question too, because it raises the delicate problem of the relation of the individual to society.'

Claparède admits that 'the feeling of inferiority has its origin in a failure on the part of the dominating tendency', a tendency derived from the innate instinct of expansion. But this is to confuse the effect with the cause. The feeling of inferiority accompanies the child from his birth; the tendency to dominate arises only from the inevitable diminution of his ego-feeling, of his 'sense of being'. The expansion of the ego which Claparède speaks of is already a consequence of the child's feelings of impotence, which come before anything else.

Claparède is right in the following admissions:

'This feeling is therefore natural in the child. In itself it is not injurious; on the contrary it is salutary, even though it gives rise to passing fits of crying. It stimulates the desire to "grow up", to be "like daddy", to imitate his elders. It motivates innumerable games in which the child imitates adults and their ways of behaving. It is therefore "the most valuable of the motive forces which cause the child to educate himself" (*Das nervöse Kind*, by Dr. Wexberg, Vienna and Leipzig, 1926, p. 33).[1] It gradually disappears as the personality of the child asserts itself.'

But our author immediately reminds us that this describes the ideal case.

'Unfortunately things do not always happen like this. Various causes —which I will group under three headings: unfavourable influence of the surroundings, real inferiority, some eccentric or ridiculous anomaly—may intensify the feeling of inferiority, fix it in the child's moral nature like a thorn in the flesh. Such a wound will then leave an indelible mark, a sensitive spot which will remain for life, and become the source of all kinds of defence reactions.'

All these observations of Claparède's are relevant to our problem.[2]

---

[1] An English translation of this work exists under the title of *Your Nervous Child*.

[2] Except on a minor point Claparède pays tribute to Adler and his school, indeed his lecture only summarises their results. 'The consequences of the feeling of inferiority', he writes, 'have been clearly brought to light during the last twenty years by Dr. Alfred Adler, a dissident disciple of Freud's. According to this author, this feeling—or rather this complex, for it operates on the subconscious— can give rise according to the case in question to the most diverse kinds of

The only criticism of them one can make is that they deal only with the individual aspect, which is but a partial aspect of this vast problem.

'Let us first examine the influence of the immediate surroundings. Here the originally "normal" feeling of inferiority is exasperated by the existing conditions.

'Thus it may be a case of conceited parents who, because they are ashamed of not having an exceptional child, are always comparing him to some more gifted cousin, to a more brilliant friend, and reproach him for not having reached their level. Or else elder brothers are always calling the youngest of the family a "baby", regarding him as a negligible quantity and all the more so (as a result of unconscious jealousy) if the younger child is more gifted than they are.'

It is undoubtedly a mistake to accept without comment the fact, frequently observed, that younger children are more gifted than their older brothers and sisters. The fact is due to the curious interactions of the feelings of inferiority in the brother and sister constellation, and has been very closely studied by the Adlerian school in connection with the Joseph and Benjamin bible story and with the popular tale of Tom Thumb. To quote from Claparède again:

'We may have a master scolding a pupil for his bad work and humiliating him before the whole class when the child is conscious of having done his best. Or the system of "places", in which one scholar will be relegated to the bottom of the class, a procedure which will embitter him and gradually destroy his self-confidence.

'... In a general way to require of a child more than he is able to give is to predispose him to a feeling of inferiority, for it is condemning him never to obtain a satisfactory result, never to reap the fruit of his effort.

behaviour, ranging from resignation to revolt, from timidity to despotism, from empty boasting to real talent, from neurosis to crime, from wickedness to a spirit of service, from cowardice to heroism, from aboulia to the most sublime use of the will.' Note that Claparède distinguishes between a feeling and a complex according as the affective phenomenon is conscious or unconscious. He seems to wish to make the reader believe that Adler admits the existence of the 'subconscious', and that the distinction was originally made by him. But this is not the case. Adler saw no essential difference between the conscious and the unconscious. The effects of the feeling of inferiority vary very little whether they are or are not conscious. It should be noted that another 'dissident' from the psycho-analytical school, W. Stekel, has declared, 'I do not believe in the unconscious' (*Das Unbewusste ist das Ungewusste*, he said) in *Die Technik der analytischen Psychotherapie*, ed. Huber, Switzerland, 1938.

Not only does he not satisfy others, but what is more serious, he does not satisfy himself. And the idea becomes ever more deeply rooted in his mind that he is below the normal level.'

Claparède then examines the cases of neglected school children on the one hand, and on the other those of spoiled or pampered children, and he devotes a chapter to the children belonging to the working class, who

'besides being in general less robust, less well nourished, often meet with rough treatment in their families. In addition to this, in the running of the home they are given the tasks and responsibilities of adults without enjoying adult position or privileges. They have a vague feeling of being exploited; also when they compare themselves to their wealthier contemporaries they feel acutely the inferiority of their condition.'

It is a pity that the excellent theoretician of *Comment diagnostiquer les aptitudes chez les écoliers* should not have taken account of the differences in mental age of working-class children, differences which begin with a real linguistic inferiority. These problems have been elucidated not only by skilled Adlerian observers of proletarian children, such as Rühle and Kanitz, but also and chiefly by the school of Charlotte Bühler and Hildegard Hetzer of Vienna. Claparède, faithfully following the Adlerian classifications which are only thinly disguised in his text, then deals with the children suffering from a genuine inferiority, whether organic or psychological, and finally turns to the case of inferiority which we call social or *situational*.

'Finally, in the absence of any real inferiority, an odd or unusual feature may saddle the child with an ironic nickname which will stick to him all his life. Very red hair ("Ginger") or very fair ("Blondie"), a streak of white hair, a naevus on the cheek, a sixth finger on one hand, or simply being too short or too tall, too fat or too thin, or extremely plain. . . .'

In reviewing the different kinds of compensations (we shall deal with these again in a later chapter) Claparède has some very wise things to say about the psycho-pedagogy of the feeling of inferiority. He is in agreement with Adler in insisting that 'the pedagogy of the feeling of inferiority cannot be distinguished from pedagogy in general'.

'A perfect education, faultless teachers penetrated with the *primo non nocere* of the old medicine, school fellows brought up in a healthy social atmosphere—in such conditions there would be nothing conducive to the breeding of the inferiority complex.'

Education must therefore be (1) prophylactic and (2) curative. Unfortunately complexes are often created in children by the defects both of teachers and methods. Some practical advice as well as some remarkable theoretical observations bring to an end this excellent exposition, which one could criticise only on the ground that it is too deliberately succinct and too schematic.

Another Geneva author, M. Charles Baudouin, has had a good deal to say on our subject in *L'Ame enfantine et la Psychanalyse*[1] (1931), in his obituary article on Alfred Adler, published in his valiant little review *Action et Pensée*, and in other works.

Baudouin has tried to reconcile the views of Adler and Freud, while simultaneously retaining treatment by suggestion (incidentally he has reduced hetero-suggestion to auto-suggestion). In a number of his works he has dealt with the problem of the feelings of inferiority. It is to him that we owe the expression 'Cain complex' to express the jealous hostility of the elder child towards his younger brother. (Camargo, the Spanish judge, in a vast work on psycho-analysis, *La Psicoandlisis*, ed. Javier Morata, Madrid, has used the same term in a slightly different sense.) Baudouin is the most clear-sighted of the French-speaking interpreters of Adler's ideas. 'The desire for superiority,' he writes, 'and the feeling of inferiority are part of a single whole and the former, as Adler's analyses have shown, is mainly a reaction against the latter.' In another equally interesting work, *La Psychanalyse de l'Art*,[2] he has tried to bring Freud's idea of the 'castration complex' into harmony with Adler's ideas on the feelings of inferiority. This is a very remarkable attempt and in no wise consists in the one notion being reduced to or absorbed into the other, as has been the case with the 'pure' representatives of the two schools.

'In my opinion', he writes, 'the study of complexes *as such* should become the main object of psycho-analysis. The question as to what is the most important component of the complex is of secondary importance, though it is the bone of contention between the rival schools of thought. If there is a complex at all, it has by definition several components; the complex only exists in virtue of this plurality. Thus in

[1] Translated into English as *The Mind of the Child: a Psycho-analytical Study*, by Eden and Cedar Paul; Allen and Unwin, 1933.

[2] *Psycho-Analysis and Aesthetics*, translated into English by Eden and Cedar Paul; Dodd, Mead & Co., New York, 1924.

connection with the mutilation complex the argument turns on whether all the inferiority fantasies connected with it are merely disguised castration complexes, or whether, on the contrary, castration is not a *modus dicendi*, a concrete means of expressing the abstract idea of inferiority. The question is not in any sense fundamental and, moreover, it is badly put. The complex consists in the grouping of these disparate elements, and not in the representation of one by the others. That is why it is always better to designate the complex by a synthetic term which will reflect the plurality of the components. Thus the term "mutilation" strikes me as preferable to the purely sexual term of castration and to the highly abstract term of *inferiority*.'

The slight change of meaning due to a change in the terms— mutilation instead of castration—can be very useful. Recently the term 'intrusion complex' has been suggested to describe the general attitude arising from the situation of the second-born child. If, however, we want a term that will cover at a glance the most varied feelings arising from the 'diminution of the self', we shall be hard put to it to find a better one than 'inferiority'. We have suggested the name *Gulliver complex* to designate the complex of inferiority and of superiority. But the word has not made its mark in literature, and would be incomprehensible to the general public. *Feeling of inferiority* still seems to us the easier to handle, no doubt because it has a fairly long past. The 'mutilation complex' is, after all, too partial an aspect. At the best it can be regarded as one variety—among many others—of the injuries affecting the estimative feeling of the ego.

Similarly it seems excessive to reduce all conscious feelings of inferiority to an unconscious feeling of guilt, as does Baudouin in *L'Ame Enfantine*, or to suppose that the clumsy search for an illusory security is always 'a search for maternal protection'. But Baudouin has seen very clearly that anything, absolutely anything, can become the starting-point in the formation of a feeling of inferiority; it all depends on the subject's 'opinion'.

'If a boy has, on medical or hygienic grounds, to be circumcised, he feels this to be equivalent to castration; yet if it should happen that a little Jew is not circumcised, as are all his co-religionists, analysis has again and again shown that the fact of being uncircumcised is then interpreted as a mutilation' (*The Mind of the Child*, p. 121).

But is not this an obvious argument against the whole fallacious conception of the 'mutilation complex' in the Freudian sense? The relative nature of the feeling of inferiority and its complete independence of organic inferiorities, whether functional or real, appears in other interesting and suggestive passages.

'The feeling of inferiority is mixed up with the knowledge that such and such an organ is below *par*, so that the child feels humiliated. Adler has shown that the desire to be superior is rooted in the knowledge of some physical lack, and that every child tries to compensate itself for some very definite inferiority of its person. If it stutters it will dream of being a fine public speaker (compensation), and if it happens to be Demosthenes it will become a great orator (over-compensation).

'Curiously enough, the organic inferiority which humiliates and tortures a child is not always the one most obvious to those around it. Often it is some trifling defect, such as too long or too stubby a nose, ears sticking out, or what-not, that the child feels to be intolerable. Blanchard (in *The Care of the Adolescent Girl*, p. 68) tells us of a girl with a strongly developed sense of inferiority and a morbid desire for admiration, etc., caused by a negligible facial disfigurement in the form of a peculiar birthmark. If one asks for associations connected with the particular sore point of each patient, one often finds that the sentiment a child has in regard to the failing in question is actually symbolical of its observation of its own genital organs' (*The Mind of the Child*, p. 119).

This last observation could easily be explained without introducing Freudian theories, by the importance a child attaches to belonging to one or the other sex. On this point Baudouin has made a very valuable contribution in carrying out the enquiry begun by Pipal, which consisted in asking children 'Do you like being a boy or would you rather have been a girl and if so, why?' All these are valuable contributions to the study of inferiority feelings in children.

Apart from Edouard Claparède, the only French-speaking author who has devoted a special study to our subject is R. de Saussure.[1] In the article from which we are transcribing certain passages, the most valuable elements are drawn from the books the author has read and of which he makes no mention. We shall select only those passages in which the issues tend to be confused.

'Perfection is not of this world,' writes de Saussure. 'We all have

[1] 'Les Sentiments d'Infériorité,' R. de Saussure, in *Annales Médico-psychologiques*, xv, 93rd year. The periodical in question is a popular and not a scientific publication.

some physical defect or some gap in our qualifications which we regret. An accident may in the course of our life have robbed us of a finger, caused us to limp, or disfigured us with a scar.

'The human character reacts in different ways to those imperfections. Some submit quite simply to having too long or too short a nose, while others will be tormented all their lives because their profile is not that of an Adonis. Some are content to do conscientiously the work for which they are fitted, while others suffer acutely because they are not men of genius, not universally recognised for some important discovery or brilliant exploit. Some again are proud to have been born peasants or workers, while others believe themselves to be despised because they are not of noble birth.'

Rather a jumble of themes! It would be interesting to know the causes that lead some to accept their misfortune calmly and others to suffer through it. One would have thought even the psychiatrist, who takes no account of the social aspect of physical ills and is content merely to state them, would have felt the need to seek for the causes of these differences. M. de Saussure modestly confines himself to the therapeutic problem.

'At first sight it would seem an easy task to induce these dissatisfied people, of whom we have been speaking, to accept what cannot be changed. [Unfortunately there are too many 'non-conformists'!] These folk cling to an attitude which brings them only bitterness and disappointment. This, because the inferiority from which they are suffering has aroused in them a conflict, a conflict of *amour-propre* which might be expressed in the words, "I shall never be any good at anything because I am not clever". But at the same time as they reason in this way, another part of them is arguing, "I'm not such a fool as people think. One day I'll show them what I can do". And then this type of subject begins to denigrate those whose intelligence he envies.'

This state of mind is generally described in psychiatric works as resentment (*ressentiment*) or a *catathymic* attitude; it is a consequence of inferiority feelings and not, as M. de Saussure thinks, identical with them. He is wrong, moreover, to identify the *feeling* of inferiority with the consciousness of it, though he admits the ambivalent nature of this consciousness. 'One part of them' is in opposition to another part, and it seems that they are perfectly well aware of this. M. de Saussure is fortunate to have chanced upon patients who think *a priori* in the

Freudian categories with which his own mind is so deeply impreg-
nated. If the inferiority syndrome were so easy to unearth in patients,
any child could make a psychiatric diagnosis. In that case, moreover,
should not M. de Saussure's essay have been entitled 'The Consciousness of Inferiority'?

'Similarly, the young girl who thinks herself hopelessly plain does
not believe this deep down, and seizes on a hundred and one reasons for
reassuring herself and running down other girls, indulging in innumerable daydreams of success. But no sooner has she finished reassuring
herself than once again doubt assails her and she imagines herself the
most hideous of God's creatures.'

But is not the effect taken for the cause in this very commonplace
example? The imputed ambivalence does not exist in such a case;
rather are we in the presence of a vicious circle characterised by a single
fundamental feeling, that of being ugly. The opposite feeling which
appears from time to time is only its compensation. Adler has shown
that the imputation of ambivalence to feelings rests on a false perspective. The ambivalence is only apparent, for of the two feelings one is
always definitely stronger than the other, which only derives from
the first and serves to mask it or compensate for it. Ambivalence
is an *arrangement* one makes so as not to decide. M. de Saussure
continues:

'From what has been said we can distinguish two very different
attitudes. (1) People who have the feeling of a real inferiority, who
accept it and remedy it as far as possible. (2) People who have a feeling
of inferiority based on an inferiority which may or may not be real,
but in whom a whole part of the personality does not accept this feeling. When in mental therapy someone is said to be suffering from
inferiority feelings, it is to the second group of persons that allusion is
being made.'

But this is rather a narrow and arbitrary viewpoint. Are the inferiority feelings which fail to become fully conscious, then, of no interest to
mental therapy? A little patient mentioned by Baudouin is incapable of
writing a capital 'C', the initial of his name, Charles, although he can
write all the other letters extremely well. Is he to be regarded as conscious of the inferiority feeling which is the cause of this little *acte
manqué*? M. de Saussure thinks that inferiority feelings are indistinguishable from obsessional symptoms. 'At bottom', he says, 'these

folk are the prey of an obsessional doubt—"Am I or am I not stupid?" "Am I or am I not ugly?"' His choice of examples, moreover, is significant; stupidity, ugliness, etc., are reckoned by him as genuine inferiorities, and it would seem that he is most at home, that his mind moves most easily, among such petty bourgeois categories.

'If we examine more closely how this attitude is composed we shall find that it contains two separate conflicts. (1) A conflict of pride; the subject refuses to accept the moral or physical defect observed by another part of him. (2) A conflict of jealousy; the subject envies everyone who is not oppressed by similar feelings and everyone who is free of the inferiority from which he suffers.'

But here again there is confusion between resentment and the feeling of inferiority which precedes it, just as it precedes jealousy, envy, etc., without being identical with them. All these phenomena derive from the malady of inferiority, and our author himself notes 'a certain latent aggressiveness, a certain need for decrying others, in persons afflicted with feelings of inferiority'.

Passing on to the origin of these feelings, our author states that 'Every individual who has feelings of inferiority has suffered from them since his childhood.' This is true only if we assume, with the authors whom M. de Saussure follows very closely but does not mention, that feelings of inferiority are present from birth. Otherwise it might easily be supposed that an individual is not affected by the trouble we are speaking of till the onset of puberty or as a result of painful experiences in adult life which undermine his self-confidence or his pride.

In view of this, the following statement is rather superficial, 'As the subject grows older these feelings have only increased or decreased in importance according to the case in question. We must also note that although these feelings are abnormal they are extremely common and this must mean that the conditions which give rise to them are very widespread.'

It is a pity that the author has not had the courage to pursue this thought to its logical conclusion, and to ask himself what are these 'very widespread' conditions. He would then have been led to the heart of the problem, which is inherent in the structure of present-day society. But as all his sympathies go to the good 'conformists' who 'accept and correct' their inferiorities as best they may, he confines himself to generalities ('very widespread', 'extremely common'). 'As these feelings always arise in childhood', our author continues, 'it is in this period that we must look for the causes which occasion them.' But surely this is in flat contradiction with what was said above about 'accidents in the course of our life which may have robbed us of a finger', etc. For a personal disciple of Freud's, M. de Saussure is singularly lacking in consistency.

'The first of these causes is due to the fact that, as Piaget has shown in his remarkable studies, the child is ignorant of the logic of relations. To him an object is not heavier or less heavy in relation to another. It is heavy or light. In the same way, a person is not more or less intelligent or pretty, but simply intelligent or stupid, pretty or ugly.

(But the child long before having any idea of intelligence or ugliness can suffer and does indeed suffer from many feelings of insufficiency and inferiority.)

'This explains why in a family where there are several children and one of them is considered by the parents to be less gifted, less attractive, more difficult than the others, then the child on whom this judgment is passed by the parents (whether they express it or merely feel it) will feel himself to be stupid, ugly or disagreeable in an absolute sense. But at the same time his ego or, if you prefer, his pride will kick against this judgment. At this age, however, parents are regarded as omniscient and all-powerful, and the child accepts their judgments as absolute. An inner battle will therefore take place in the child between the parent's judgments and his own.'

But this is to take too simple, too static a view of the child's inner life and of his consciousness of relations. If our author had reflected more carefully about the cases which must have come his way or if he had paid more attention to his authors, he would know that a great many children suffer from feelings of inferiority precisely because they are their parents' favourites, and know that a lot is expected of them—especially in a social class where it matters that a child should be 'gifted' and 'work well at school'. The purely dialectical notion of inferiority feeling and, as compensation, the complicated relations of valuation obtaining between parents and child, brothers and sisters, to say nothing of the servants, are factors which do not seem to have occurred to M. de Saussure.

'This conflict', he continues, 'can be resolved in three different ways.' (Why exactly three? For the sake of simplicity?) '1. The child will repress the judgment passed by the parents, the feeling of inferiority will remain in his unconscious, but he will compensate it by an opposite trait of character. Thus, instead of consciously accepting the idea of her plainness, the little girl will repress it, will confidently express herself in an exaggerated coquetry. She does not consciously suffer from her inferiority, but her coquetry and somewhat arrogant self-confidence will be continually fed by the repressed feeling of inferiority which persists in the unconscious.'

All this is too complicated, too far-fetched. How can one consciously compensate for a lack of which one is not conscious? And must not the contents of the Unconscious (for once we may grant M. de Saussure the use of this denizen of the Freudian mythology) have been previously present in consciousness? For if not, then we are dealing with the Pre-conscious. Moreover, if we bring the feeling of inferiority into consciousness, will the arrogance and vanity disappear?

'3. The child tries to repress the judgment passed by the parents and only partly succeeds in the attempt. He accepts it in spite of himself, and exactly the same thing happens as with a patient suffering from an obsession. It is in this case that the feelings of inferiority persist.'

But, we will ask, do they really persist? The parents have realised with dismay that their little girl is unattractive, difficult, etc., and they will certainly not fail to notice the arrogance and excessive vanity of their darling child. They will therefore pass a fresh judgment of condemnation upon her. Will not this call forth new and stronger feelings of inferiority? Thus, if we accept M. de Saussure's ideas, even if we enter into his game, we cannot possibly admit that the feelings of inferiority are of a static character. Whenever we are dealing with feelings of inferiority we are in the presence of a dialectical process, of action and counter-action, which takes the form of a vicious spiral.

'In the long run the child succeeds in repressing the conflict, but two traits of character subsist which are in a sense the legacy of this early torment. These are a feeling of inferiority towards other people, a dissatisfaction with everything one possesses, accompanied by a devouring envy of what belongs to others. Thus the feelings of inferiority are not an isolated trait of character, they are associated with a whole attitude to life.'

Once again the author is drawing a picture of resentment, forgetting that this is only one of the many derivatives of the feelings of inferiority, which feelings he has not succeeded in separating from their effects.

'We have established the first cause of the feelings of inferiority;

66

here is the second. Every child, in order to adapt himself to the external world, uses two completely different methods; on the one hand he uses the ideas and commands laid upon him by his parents, on the other he experiments with his own ideas.' (This distinction strikes us as purely arbitrary. How can a child distinguish its own ideas from those of its environment, and is not the conception of 'ideas' an outmoded one?) 'The result is a dual adaptation, that which takes place in function of the parents and that which is achieved by the child itself. Hence the child acquires two kinds of conduct, which are often in opposition to each other, the conduct of óbedience and the conduct of experience.'

At this point M. de Saussure speaks of that 'attitude of hesitation' which was long ago so well described by Adler and his disciples. But is that attitude really due to the conflict between two kinds of behaviour which, in our view, are not really distinct? According to the author, the children who learn the two conducts aright 'become independent in their judgments. . . . They do not suffer from feelings of inferiority, because they are indifferent to what others think of them.' But do not the most hardened egoists who have never learned these ways of behaviour flaunt the opinion of others? And what of the *idiots* (the Greek origin of the word emphasises their 'particularity') who live entirely wrapped up in themselves without a thought for the opinion of others? To be unconcerned with the opinion of others may be a sign of great objectivity, but also one of excessive subjectivity. And did not the author tell us earlier that it was the subject's own personal judgment of his deficiencies which determined his feelings of inferiority? In spite of his apparent tendency to simplification, M. de Saussure's exposition becomes increasingly confused.

'In view of this dual attitude to life (obedience and experience) in bringing up children, the adult must take good care: (1) Gradually to replace the behaviour of obedience by the behaviour of experience; (2) Not to impose all sorts of commands which reflect the desires of the adult rather than the needs of the child; (3) Not to indulge in negative judgments which the child takes literally and which may destroy his self-confidence for life.'

Surely it was hardly necessary to have oneself analysed personally by Freud and then to dabble in Adlerian psychology in order to come to such an obvious conclusion. I intend to publish elsewhere a study by Adler's brilliant pupil, Dr. Alice Friedmann, in which she advises the reader as to what not to say to children. It contains a whole list of sentences, not of blame but of praise, for it has been shown that praise, and especially flattery, engender feelings of inferiority no less than do blame or criticism. But to return to M. de Saussure.

'The more a child is expected to obey', he says, 'and the less he has opportunities of experimenting, the more he will regard his parents as infallible. He will then become more sensitive than ever to their judgments. He will crave for their consent and, lacking it, will get into a state of anguish which in the long run will produce feelings of inferiority. Once these have developed the child is involved in a vicious circle, for the more inferior he feels, the more he will need his parents' reassurance, and consequently the more dependent he will become on their approval instead of progressing towards personal autonomy.'

This, on the whole, is sound, if rather too schematic in treatment. The vicious circle will begin much earlier, and the feeling of inferiority is very likely at the root of the first anguish ever felt. Nor can we be sure that the child who is made to obey his parents and realises on a particular occasion that they are in the wrong will regard them as infallible! But the more he realises their injustice, the greater will be his feelings of inferiority, for he will see that they are supported not by reason but by superior physical strength alone. Again, our author has only seen one side of the question, and his treatment barely escapes the charge of superficiality.

'A third factor which often plays a very important part is . . . the element of jealousy. In a large family it may easily happen that one child, less gifted and attractive than the others, gradually becomes the target of criticism or receives less attention than the others. This difference in affection on the part of the parents will develop all the greater a craving for love in the child. Feeling cut off, he will be afraid to respond to any affection from his own people and will allow the unsatisfied longing to grow within him. This need will make him more sensitive than ever to criticism. The situation thus created will prepare the ground for feelings of inferiority, and these will finally ripen when the child realises that his brothers and sisters are more cherished than he is. In the end he will think that it is because of his personal defects that he is left out in the cold, but this realisation, instead of filling the gap, will only depress him further. In many people the early conflict of jealousy is finally repressed and all that remains in consciousness is the misery of feelings of inferiority.'

One would like to give one's full assent to this eloquent passage, but alas, it is not possible. In point of fact the mere arrival of a younger brother or sister, who cannot therefore be more loved than he is, is enough to produce feelings of inferiority in the child, from which infantile jealousy will result later. One must not put the cart before the horse. The mere presence of a brother or sister will arouse these feelings in a child even if there is no marked difference in affection on the part of the parents. M. de Saussure's treatment is too logical and schematic, and he does not see that even the favourite child can be tortured by feelings of inferiority and by 'jealousy', trembling all the time lest he lose his privileged position in the constellation of brothers and sisters. It is not jealousy that prepares the ground for feelings of inferiority, but, on the contrary, those are themselves the breeding-ground of the neurosis.

But let us now pass on to the problem of the only child.

'In families where there is only one child', writes M. de Saussure, 'jealousy often arises between mother and daughter or between father and son. The little girl thinks that her father loves only her mother, the son imagines that his mother loves no one but his father.' (Curious that the author should not have mentioned the Oedipus complex at this point.) 'Or else a second child is born four or five years after the first; the mother is obliged to give more attention to the baby and this coincides with the time when the elder child must go to school. He becomes jealous and interprets the feeling of not being loved as due to the fact that he is inferior to his brother or sister, and begins to experience feelings of inferiority.'

It is a pity that the author did not immediately add that *every* first-born child experiences a similar little crisis on the arrival of a new baby. It is, moreover, rather a bold assumption to say that the child 'interprets' his feeling of being unloved. What he experiences is something vague, confused and almost instinctive, for if he could interpret it, he would reach the correct and logical conclusion which would relieve his distress, namely, that the smaller child necessarily has more need of maternal care than he has.

'Jealousy, the need for parental approval, absence of the logic of relations' (it would be better to say tendentious apperception and the need to make his worth felt), 'such are the three important factors which we must regard as determining the feelings of inferiority. But to these must be added the feelings of guilt. . . .' These are produced 'chiefly in connection with acts of disobedience of a sexual order. As this is a subject on which he rarely talks with his companions and still less with his parents, the child feels that he is alone in sinning in this field and there is a resulting increase in his feelings of inferiority.'

Finally, according to de Saussure, the child inevitably discovers the difference between the two sexes. But we would point out here that what the child first discovers is the respective social standing of the two sexes, while not necessarily being aware of the anatomical features which differentiate them. Children who have no brothers or sisters or who have not chanced to see other children of the opposite sex naked in their bath or elsewhere, will surely be none the less aware of the difference in social status between the two sexes. M. de Saussure goes on to tell us that at a certain age, from three to five:

'Children regard boys alone as endowed with sex. Little girls often regard this privilege with the greatest envy. They are consequently the more strongly convinced that they lack something in themselves. Sometimes they do not realise that all little girls are made in the same way and imagine that they alone are deprived of this fascinating organ. A great many little girls quite naturally grow out of these childish ideas, but in a large number this early conception of sex remains more or less fixed. Emotionally they remain oppressed, overshadowed by a certain feeling of incompleteness. This creates or reinforces the feelings of inferiority which are all the more lasting because the situation which occasions them is at bottom one of jealousy of the girl towards the boy. This constellation of feelings has been named the feeling of castration.'

This is simply a popular and simplified exposition of Freud's doctrine of the castration complex, which, as we know, is advanced by him as the explanation of *all* feelings of inferiority. It is a tempting theory, but it does not always correspond with the facts. In support of this claim we give the following short case histories taken from our own clinical observations.

Nuria S., four years old, who has a younger sister of four months, having seen little boys making water in the park, has become violently jealous of them. She begs her mother to 'put a worm on her' like boys have. The story more or less follows the Freudian schema.

But Asuncion B., ten years old, who has a brother of thirteen, has never shown the least jealousy of him, let alone jealousy on sexual grounds. Her brother, on the other hand, has shown violent and sullen jealousy towards his sister from the day of her birth, on which occasion

70

he cut his head by banging it against the balcony railing. The girl, a remarkably intelligent child, has always accepted as quite natural the fact that her brother should be bigger and stronger and the parents' favourite. She has therefore never felt any envy or jealousy on the subject, only a submissive sympathy. She does not seem to be aware of the anatomical difference between the sexes and is consequently not afflicted with a 'castration complex'.

We could multiply these examples. In many girls the longing to be a boy and not to belong to the weaker sex appears only on the occasion of their first menstrual period. Till then the fact of being a girl presented no problems to them. Here is one example.

Maria G., a precocious little Spanish girl, had her first period at the age of eleven. The event upset her greatly and the following night she dreamed that she was standing at the door of a house, her hands in her pockets, passively watching other little girls at play. She could not join in their games because she was no longer 'a little girl'. Having been told that all women were subjected to this natural law she had asked her mother whether boys suffered from the same 'illness'. On being told that they did not, she experienced *for the first time in her life* regret at not being a man but a woman.

This case shows first of all regret for the state of early childhood which the young Maria G. has just outgrown. Henceforth she is a 'real' woman and experiences feelings of inferiority towards her former companions. She would like to become a little girl again so as to play with them. But secondly there is born in her 'the masculine protest'. We could multiply examples to show how isolated are the cases fitting the Freudian interpretation and how little it can be considered as the norm. But let us return to our author:

'What is curious', he writes, 'is that analogous feelings can occur in boys'. (Not in the least curious really once one has realised that every difference, whether a possession or a lack, can engender feelings of inferiority.) 'Some of them, when at the age of three or four they become aware of the anatomical difference, imagine that they have an abnormal excrescence, others think that they may lose this organ. These beliefs are often reinforced by foolish threats on the part of the parents, who think that they can stop onanistic habits by telling the child that his organ will be cut off. We notice then that boys who are afraid of a possible castration react in the same way as little girls who believe themselves to be castrated, and they develop marked feelings of inferiority on this subject. In the adult these childish conflicts are repressed, but as in all cases of repressed conflicts, they leave character traits which in this case appear as inveterate feelings of inferiority.'

And M. de Saussure ends his study with certain prophylactic measures logically based on his previous analysis. At times his conclusions show too facile an optimism.

'A man appears to have lost all faith in himself. Quite naturally we try to restore his self-confidence by suggestion and persuasion. But this is the wrong method. It is like putting a plaster on a wooden leg or filling a tooth without first removing the decay that was eating into it. To cure such cases the person's whole character must be worked up afresh. The traces left by too much obedient conduct must be run to earth and the subject brought to a more personal mode of life; he must learn a conduct based on his own experiences. As the subject ceases to be dependent upon the opinion and judgments of others and learns to face up to himself, with all his qualities and all his defects, his feelings of inferiority will gradually disappear. To-day there are a great many people afflicted with feelings of inferiority, but a big step forward will have been made for the mental health of our race if we can say exactly to what pedagogic mistakes these feelings are due. Let us hope that the generations to come will have more confidence in themselves and will thus go forward from progress to progress in the moral, intellectual and social fields.'

This cheap optimism, based on an old-fashioned belief in progress, does not convince. It fails entirely to look the difficulties squarely in the face and takes no account of the thousand and one factors which conspire to *inferiorise* modern man in his present-day struggle. The study, which we have partly transcribed in this chapter—for it is, after all, the work of one of the most prominent of the French-speaking psychoanalysts—is, when all is said and done, only a feeble rehash of the studies carried out in Vienna and elsewhere. Just as in the realm of Freudian psycho-analysis the work of Laforgue failed to enlist the support of his colleagues abroad, so the somewhat ill-digested Adlerian conceptions of M. de Saussure stand little chance of raising the standard of French research to the level reached in other countries.

Having passed in review all that has been accomplished by French-speaking authors, we are now in a position to approach the fountain-head of all the work that has been mentioned on the subject of the feelings of inferiority. If Pierre Janet was the forerunner of the theory whose history we are about to trace, the Swiss authors may be regarded as having done the work of popularising it.

CHAPTER V

ALFRED ADLER AND HIS COMPARATIVE
PSYCHOLOGY OF INDIVIDUALS

IN Levin D. Schucking's work *The Sociology of Literary Taste* (Kegan Paul) we possess an able, if incomplete, study of the changes of fashion in the domain of literature. But no one so far has attempted to give an account of the formation and development of taste in psychological matters. And yet psychology is a popular science nowadays, especially in America, and, by ricochet, throughout the world. The cult has had its repercussion on literary fashion. Hence the vogue for Kafka and Proust in the United States, with the result that these authors' works, somewhat neglected during the last twenty years, are now being displayed in all the European bookstalls. The psychology of Adler has undergone a similar revival, all the more salutary as it was still far from being appreciated at its true worth.

The conception of 'feelings of inferiority' is now inseparably connected with the name of Alfred Adler, and we shall have, therefore, to deal at some length with the body of his theories. His contribution to sociology[1] will be the subject of a later work, which will also touch upon his 'personal equation' and the social factors which contributed to the formation of his ideas. We shall follow in this the lines laid down by the late Professor Karl Mannheim in his theory of the sociology of knowledge.

In this volume sociological factors will only be lightly touched upon, but we must nevertheless attempt to throw some light upon the scientific background against which Adler's ideas on the feelings of inferiority took shape.

At the beginning of the present century these ideas were already, so to speak, in the air. If we look through any Central European review on psychology or sex we shall find at this period 'a great fear' on every page. Everywhere the same lament is raised—'Humanity is *degenera-*

---

[1] A first instalment has appeared under the title *La Psicologia Adleriana et la Sociologia* in the *Revista Internacional de Sociologia*, Vol. VI, No. 24, May 1949, Madrid.

ting!' The idea of degeneracy[1] was, no doubt, derived from the ideas of Darwin and Spencer on evolution, but it also gave an echo to the dissatisfaction felt at this period in an ultra-urbanised civilisation. Everywhere 'degenerates' began to crop up—*Minderwertige*, as the Germans called them, i.e. persons of *minus* biological value. This minus-value gave the medical men food for thought, and their concern was being increasingly shared by the general public.

At the same time, the university professors were turning their attention not only to pathological psychology but to the minor defects of ordinary thought called 'inhibitions'. The studies of the Hungarian writer, Paul Ranschburg, on this subject created a sensation, and where to-day we speak of the 'inferiority complex', the talk then was all of 'inhibition' and 'inhibited persons'.

This period also witnessed a revolt against the psychological atomism which was superseded by the psychology of Acts leading to the more complex psychology of Function. In his *Gestaltqualität*, Ehrenfels discovered a whole new psychology of Form. In German-speaking countries, the *Ganzheitsbetrachtung* of William Stern broke fresh ground and found brilliant confirmation in the Vitalism of Hans Driesch. The study of sex inevitably led to a deeper appreciation of the psychic factors involved, partly through the influence of Freud, but also independently of him. Thus Näcke, though he contributes to the *Jahrbücher für sexuelle Zwischenstufen* edited by the materialist Magnus Hirschfeld, came to the conclusion that human sexuality cannot be understood without taking account of psychic factors. Adler himself started from a naturalistic standpoint in his studies of the Organic Inferiority in 1907, since this conception was already present in medical science. Independently of this, Professor Carl Pelmann's sensational work *Die Psychischen Grenzzustände*, Bonn, was already in its second edition in 1910. In it, he wrote of conditions which he regarded as taking place at the borderline between body and mind. Like Adler he can, therefore, be regarded as one of the forgotten forerunners of the psycho-somatic therapy of to-day. He circumscribes with great eloquence the term 'mental minus-value' (*geistige Minderwertigkeit*). The term 'mental' need not mislead us, for in the technical vocabulary of this period the word is equivalent to 'moral' or 'psychological'; to-day

---

[1] This problem, treated later by Artur Holub in one of the *Beihefte zur Int. Zeitschr. f. Individualpsychologie*, is still alive to-day.

Cf. Alberto Seguin in "A Note on the Concept of Cure" in *Psychosomatic Medicine*, 1949, v, 120.

we should say 'psycho-genetic'. The notion of mental degenerates was adopted by the psychology of this time, and psychogenetic factors began to be taken into consideration in addition to those of a purely hereditary, biological, or somatic character. In *Sexual-Probleme*, 1910, one of Pelmann's critics, the sexologist Max Marcuse, noted the preponderant influence exercised on our civilisation by the French *Minderwertige, les dégénérés supérieurs*. This was the same path along which Lombroso was travelling, and it led to the present *Pathography* of Lange-Eichbaum.[1]

The final stage had yet to be reached. Once Freud had crossed the Rubicon with the help of his idea of psychological determinism, it only needed a thinker of courage and genius to take the decisive step forward. It was at this point that Alfred Adler appeared on the scene and rescued the idea of *Minderwertigkeit* by incorporating it into a new theory of striking simplicity. Thus Adler's ideas are in no way a *creatio ex nihilo* (such a thing does not exist in the evolution of ideas). He is the author of a new and creative synthesis gathering the many converging rivulets into one mighty stream. Adler's ideas on *Minderwertigkeit* and on mental degeneracy (wrongly so-called) combine logically, naturally, one might almost say organically, in the formation of a new and extremely original theory.

The war of 1914 was a severe setback to the diffusion of Adler's ideas, which for the time being merely followed in the wake of the Freudian theories.

In spite of the marked hostility of Professor McDougall, England was, however, one of the countries where from the start Adler's ideas met with a certain success. The novelist Phyllis Bottome was one of his best-known sponsors, and contributed an interesting biography, *Alfred Adler, the Man and his Work* (Putnam), which very usefully supplements that of Hertha Orgler. We may mention in passing that Adler came into contact with General Smuts, who contributed to his review *Internationale Zeitschrift für Individualpsychologie*. The great South African discovered a close affinity between his philosophy of *Holism* and Adler's psychology. In America, Morton Prince helped appreciably to spread the Adlerian teaching. Adler made his first visit to the United States in 1926, where his daily lectures at Columbia University were heard by over three thousand persons. He then went to Long Island Medical College, of which he was professor till his untimely death in 1937 at Aberdeen, where he was delivering a course of summer lectures.

[1] *The Problem of Genius*, by Lange-Eichbaum (Kegan Paul, 1931).

ALFRED ADLER

During his sojourn in America he edited the *International Journal of Individual Psychology* (1934–37) in Chicago, where a large group of his disciples is still in existence.[1]

In France, on the other hand, where the term alone *sentiment d'infériorité* (translated from *Minderwertigkeitsgefühl*) ought to have aroused echoes of Montaigne, Vauvenargues, Stendhal, and the contemporary Pierre Janet, the reception of Adler's ideas was less than mediocre. The result is that his theories are in the main unknown in France. The two lectures he gave in Paris in 1926 and again in 1937, barely ten days before his death,[2] attracted only the specialists. The only work of his that has been translated into French is *Über den nervösen Charakter*, and then under the completely erroneous title of *Le Tempérament nerveux*, which in a sense contradicts the fundamental thesis of the book.[3] The psycho-analysts were the first to speak of him[4]; among the psychologists, Pierre Janet, among the writers, Paul Morand, spoke of an 'inferiority complex imported from America', but without knowing the name of Adler. Professor Wallon would quote him sometimes in his lectures on Vocational Guidance. Dr. Gilbert-Robin spread his ideas in a more popular field. I myself with the collaboration of Mlle. Rose Pfeiffer conducted, from 1929 to 1930, a circle of Adlerian studies in Paris which organised lectures among the various groups of students at the Sorbonne; I also published a number of articles and tried to interest publishers in my master's work. Berthold Friedl continued the good

[1] This group is under the leadership of Dr. Rudolf Dreikurs, who directs the International Individual Psychology Association Inc. and publishes the *Individual Psychology Bulletin*.

[2] The first of these, in 1926, was given before a very small gathering at the Sorbonne of the *Groupe d'études philosophiques et scientifiques*. The second was at the Centre Laennec and is mentioned by Miss Phyllis Bottome in her biography. It was attended by Fathers Riquet and Bruno, by Prof. Lhermitte, Drs. Hazemann and Okencycz, and by M. Jacques Maritain. In 1928 Adler held a meeting in Dr. Allendy's house.

[3] After a completely unusable translation had been made in 1926 by one of Dr. Allendy's patients the book was translated by Dr. Roussel, but contains many errors which were noted by M. Plottke in the Adlerian bulletin *Courage*. A second edition, almost unchanged, was brought out in 1948 by the same firm, Payot, which is also publishing *La Connaissance de l'Homme*.

[4] Dr. R. Laforgue and Dr. Allendy in *La Psychanalyse et les Névroses*, Payot, Paris, 1924, which shows in many places the influence which Adler had on the development of Freud's theories and mentions Adler's secession from Freud in 1910 and the foundation of the *Centralblatt für Psychoanalyse* in opposition to Freud. In 1913 there were eight different groups of psycho-analysts.

work in student circles, and the name of Adler and his ideas appeared more and more frequently in reviews and newspapers. André Maurois seems to have met Adler in America and read his books, as may be seen from some of his novels; when an enquiry was conducted as to 'what books to translate', he recommended all the works of the Viennese master. Intelligent specialists like Dr. Ombredanne have taken careful note of Adlerian results, not to mention the man who has done most to introduce modern ideas on psychology in France, Dr. René Allendy, the indefatigable and inspiring director of the Groupe d'Études Philosophiques et Scientifiques pour l'Examen des Tendances Nouvelles. For a long time this was the only place where foreign specialists could establish contact with the educated public in Paris. In 1933 Manes Sperber began to present the Adlerian ideas in Paris, but in an expanded form of his own, against a background of a distinctly political character. A few years later a pupil and friend whom Adler valued very highly, perhaps beyond his deserts, Dr. Alexandre Neuer, organised a feminine association of Adlerian 'initiates'. Another personal friend, Herr Schlesinger, proved a zealous and skilful propagandist in the paper *Vendredi*, while Mr. Paul Plottke, a young German professor in exile, who later served in H.M. Forces in Africa and Italy as psychologist and is now established in England, brought out roneographed bulletins on Adlerian psychology in German and in French.

Thus Adler's ideas have not penetrated into France to anything like the same extent as have Freud's. There has never been a real Adlerian movement comparable to the Freudian movement. The latter was enormously helped by the interest aroused by psycho-analytical ideas in certain artistic and literary circles, especially those of Surrealism, and one can safely say that without the moral and financial support of a princess of the blood royal Freud's ideas would certainly have met with far more resistance. The Adlerian psychology, handicapped by an ill-chosen name and by the unwillingness on the part of its followers to use it as an artistic and literary stimulus, was therefore infinitely less of a social and literary success in France than in Germany, Austria, Hungary, Spain or America.

In Hungary I was one of the founders of the Magyar Individual-psychologiai Társaság, with Professor Stephen de Màday as president. This society survived the disasters of the political reaction caused by Hitler's influence, and thanks to the ability of Professor de Máday it continued its good work even throughout the last war.

In 1929 I lectured in Madrid and Barcelona on 'Post-Freudian

Psychology: Alfred Adler'. As Ortega y Gasset was interested in Adlerian ideas, *Menschenkenntnis* ("Understanding Human Nature") was immediately translated into Spanish and is now in its third edition. In 1931 I took up my residence in Spain, lecturing and publishing many papers on Adlerian psychology. In 1934 I translated *What Life Should Mean to You*, which became the psychological best-seller in Spain, running to four editions. Then *The Problem of Homosexuality*: the first edition of the present book was published in 1936; two 'private' editions appeared in Chile (1937) and in the Argentine (1942); and the second legal edition (1944) has been out of print for a few years. Dr. Ramón Sarró, author of the preface to that edition, remarked in his preface to the third edition of *What Life Should Mean to You* that of the big three—Freud, Adler and Jung—Adler's psychology seemed to him the best suited to the Spanish character. When, in 1936, Adler was planning a lecture tour in Spain, the Madrid teachers wanted to invite him to a banquet at which 10,000 guests were to be present.

Individualpsychologie in der Schule was the first of his books to be translated into Spanish; it is now in its third edition, in Buenos Aires, as the publisher emigrated to Argentina. A book called *Guiando el Niño* (Guiding the Child) has also appeared recently in Buenos Aires. It contains a selection of articles originally published in Adlerian reviews. The editor, Señor Bernstein, is occasionally at fault in his method of introducing Adler's ideas to Spanish-speaking countries.

In general, Adler's idea met with varied and contradictory fortunes. Sometimes it was held up as a kind of revelation, sometimes dismissed as a commonplace, a 'psychology for schoolmasters'—which is true enough, but in no derogatory sense. Some writers, such as E. Utitz in his *Charakterologie*, look upon Adler as a modern Christian Wolff, Freud being the corresponding Leibnitz. Others regard it as Adler's merit to have made it possible for the first time to discuss openly the results of psycho-analysis by freeing these of their somewhat stifling pansexualist aura. Some again saw in Adlerism a useful complement to the economic theories of Karl Marx, while others were to find in it the first attempt to free man from the network of scientific determinism, thus restoring his freedom of will in spite of an inexorable biological heredity. As a matter of fact, none of these views is completely false. They are due to the many-sided character of Adler's work, where psycho-therapy, pedagogy, medicine, social improvement mingle with 'hints for the conquest of happiness' and 'a quick and infallible method for the Conquest of Health'. Nearest the truth are those who see in it a way of interpreting the problems of the modern world regarded as family conflicts on a gigantic scale. Like Freud, Adler starts from the analysis of neuroses rooted in family life, in *libido* and *destrudo*, in Eros and Thanatos; but he is the first to offer a psychology that will enable one to evaluate oneself and others. 'Among all the schools and trends of modern psychology,' says Sperber, 'Adler's was the only one to give to the purely psychological problems of power and valence (*Geltung*) the position they deserve, i.e. one of cardinal importance.' The Americans speak of 'feeling important', and this is also one aspect of the German *Geltung*.

But the circumstances in which this psychology first arose were peculiarly unfavourable, and were to lead to errors and confusions from which neither Adler nor his followers remained exempt. From the start their pitch was queered by factors of purely social and historic order, and for a long time their teaching appeared in a wrong perspective.

It is a hard fate to live in the shadow of a great personality possessed of powerful ideas, and yet it is by no means certain that Adler ever harboured this as a grudge against Freud, as the latter maintains in his autobiography, *My Life in Psycho-Analysis*. What is certain is that in 1907 Adler discovered the precious vein from which he was laboriously to quarry all his theories during the next twenty years, and that although he did not realise it himself, his work was thwarted by the presence of Freud in Vienna. Freud was fifteen years his senior, exercised a powerful influence in intellectual circles, and enjoyed the reputation of being the creator of psycho-analysis. Adler himself felt his personal charm; he was his collaborator, but he was not his pupil.[1] It may be that without Freud Adler would not have carried his ideas in the direction he chose, but it is no less certain that his thought was something very different from a mere 'imitation by opposition' (Tarde) of psycho-analysis. And yet that is what the world believed, and what it still believes, thus placing Adler on the same footing as men like Jung, Stekel, Rank or Bjerre. Thus, in his work as in his life, he is overshadowed by the mighty figure of Freud.

[1] Adler has always protested against the allegation of having been a pupil of Freud's, and has made this clear in *What Life Should Mean to You*. In a little book which its author regards as a youthful indiscretion, M. Manes Sperber refers to a story current in Vienna, of how Freud was howled down by the Medical Society of Vienna, to whom he had exposed his theories in a first lecture. Adler took up his defence, and the next day received an invitation to found with him a new Society of Medical Psychology.

The influence of a master from whom one wants to liberate oneself can sometimes be fatal. Had it not been for Hegel's idealism, Marx might have christened his own philosophy historical realism, instead of materialism, a term which has completely misrepresented his true thought and even more so that of his votaries.

It has been thought that the Adlerian and the Freudian systems resemble each other like two brothers; it has been thought that both have sprung from the same *social need*—collective nervosity, disproportionate neglect of the science of man as compared to the technical and natural sciences—which is true. But it has also been claimed that both arise from, or are part of the same spiritual tendency, the same mental approach, the same historical line in the development of ideas —which is not true at all. 'The Comparative Psychology of Individuals', i.e. of the individual as an undivided unity (*in-dividuum*) is not a form of psycho-analysis. True, it may have regarded itself as such at one time, and this error arose because the Adlerians themselves thought that the necessity of their historic 'moment' should make them offer dialectical battle to the ideas of Freud. The results achieved by Adler and his school are something of a different order from that attaching to the 'Psycho-analytical Revolution'. And this is true in spite of all appearances, in spite of the mutual imprecations of both sides, in spite of the hatred which continues after both the masters are dead.[1]

Far too much importance has been given to the various differences between Adler and Freud. It has been said that the latter wanted merely to be the 'retrospective historian' of the psychic development of the individual, while the former was 'turned towards the future'; that Psycho-analysis looked for the *causes* of nervous symptoms, while Individual Psychology attributed them to *goals*, to characteristic pieces in a teleological puzzle. Actually this argument is merely 'popular' since the idea of *final cause* bridges the gap in question. That Freud sees in the dream the *via regia* leading to the heart of the unconscious, whereas for Adler it is merely *auch ein Symptom*, one more symptom amongst so many others. It has also been said that Freud atomises the personality with his conception of partial and more or less autonomous impulses, whereas for Adler only the integral man, only the 'psycho-physical unit' exists; that Freud is a 'pansexualist' whereas for Adler the sexual

[1] Cf. in the *American Journal of Sociology*, 1939, a rather frivolous article by Wittels (Jr.) against the Neo-Adlerism of many psycho-analysts.

problem is at the most a *primus inter pares*.[1] I know all these arguments, because for years I have myself repeated them *ad nauseam*. They are not false, certainly not; but to repeat them indefinitely, to elaborate them, to add to them is—futile. The real difference is elsewhere; it lies much deeper. It is axiomatic, for it resides in a difference of fundamental inspiration, of *Weltanschauung*. Here again we have been met with a host of arguments: Adler, at any rate to begin with, was a moderate Socialist, thus in the opposite camp to Freud, a 'bloated bourgeois'; again, the psycho-analyst has his patient lying on a sofa in a darkened room and takes up his position behind him, as though he wanted to shove himself into his unconscious, whereas the Adlerian engages in a talk as between equals, expressing by this attitude a complete difference of conceptions. We may add that Freud was an *Ausläufer*, a last representative of the liberal epoch marked by disorder and anarchy, in which the liberty of all was to create a general harmony, even *in sexualibus*, whereas Adler is the herald of a new era of Order, since according to him 'sexuality cannot be regarded as a private matter'. His supreme postulate was the Community (*Gemeinschaft*), and he regarded events in the lives of individuals as having no meaning except as participating in a collective whole.

But the differences spring from a deeper source. All the points we have mentioned are only symptoms, only derivative results. In reality Freud's system is a physiology that does not dare to call itself so. The master himself admitted that he was only dealing with a 'provisional science, pending the advent of a more perfect physiology'. This important point has, with the exception of Gerö, been ignored or forgotten by all the writers on the subject, especially by the new brand of Catholic psycho-analyst, headed by Mme. Maryse Choisy. Freud's system is the final consequence of the Darwinian Theory of Evolution (the Jungian version being pure mythology and the starting-point of the curious literary psycho-analysis very much in fashion in France—witness the curious Gaston Bachelard). Adler was the first to revive the true concrete *Characterology*, which had been castigated by Humboldt almost as soon as it appeared, and then committed to oblivion. The Adlerian psychology is not a science, it is not even a psychology in the usual sense of the word. It is more than that, it is a 'science', only with certain reservations and in a new sense. At the most it is an *ideographic* and not a *nomothetic* science, for the luminous phrase which Pierre Abraham

[1] Cf. my study 'Alfred Adler, der Sexualpsychologe' in *Zeitsch. f. Sex. Wissenschaft und Sexualpolitik*, Berlin, 1936.

wrote as a heading in his book, *Figures*, could also be made to serve here—'Apart from the general, no science; apart from the individual, no truth.'

Adler was always very much concerned to retain the strictly scientific character of his 'Psychology of the Individual'. But at the same time he always maintained that his Individual Psychology was *an art*, and on his lips the word assumed the same meaning as when one speaks, for example, of the Hippocratic *art*. The Greek τέχνη means art; just as medicine is a technique based on science, or on several sciences, without being itself a science, so much the same could be said of the Adlerian method. Psycho-analysis, on the other hand, though born under the impulse of certain results in the field of psycho-therapy, is a theory, whereas the Adlerian system is merely a corollary to practice. The Adlerian 'discoveries' can be 'theorised' after the event, as it were, and that is the task which we have set ourselves at the moment. But is it not significant that Adler was never able to construct a 'theory'? That was the task which, from the first, fell to his disciples, and one of which, let us admit it, they have not acquitted themselves too well. One cannot accept Freud's ideas without *ipso facto* adopting a definitely materialistic and mechanistic ideology. But one can be an Adlerian and remain what one was, go on thinking what one thought before, just as one can be a doctor and still be either a Catholic or a Communist. And when men like Rühle or Sperber have to 'enlarge' the Adlerian theory till it has become a Marxist tool, they have been no more successful than a writer like Rudolf Allers, Professor at the Catholic University of Washington, who claims to have incorporated the whole Adlerian system into his own Thomistic system of thought. (*The Psychology of Character*, Sheed & Ward, 1939, and *The Successful Error, a Critical Study of Freudian Psycho-analysis*, 1943.)

Freud was a man of science, Adler an educator. The fact that both were doctors was an accident due to their 'moment', to their 'milieu', and not to their 'dominant faculty' (Taine's *faculté maîtresse*). They do not speak the same language. The words may often be the same, but they are used in a totally different sense. There is neither identity nor opposition. Not only are their points of view utterly different, but the two men are not, in spite of appearances, talking of the same thing. With the tenacity of a Sherlock Holmes and the searching eye of a Public Prosecutor, Freud has brought forward a gigantic indictment of humanity. Whatever is obvious, whatever is clearly there, is only façade (as he says in connection with our 'earliest memories'), a façade designed to cover something hidden. Whatever is manifest is only the symbol of what is latent. The descriptive geography of the human psyche does not satisfy him, he wants to write its geology, its geodesy. His psychology therefore becomes a *Tiefenpsychologie*, a 'depth psychology'. For a very long time this term was used to denote both systems, the Freudian and the Adlerian. This was a mistake. Regarded as 'depth psychology'[1] the Adlerian method would appear very superficial. Jung's is the only system that really deserves the name.[2]

Oceanography is certainly a noble science, but woe to the sailor who relies on it alone to cross the ocean! Adler never wanted to give men more than a practical treatise on how to sail most successfully, given the means at his disposal, through the troubled waters of life. If he does plumb the depths of the unconscious—which he does not at all regard as an inferno to which all the worst in man has been relegated—he does so only the better to find the course which the ship must steer.

Adler took as his starting-point a paradox of biology, viz. the faculty of compensation for defective or inadequate organs. From this he travelled step by step towards the ambitious aim of creating with psychology a Scientific Knowledge of Man. For him, psychology was not the research carried on in laboratories designed to impress us with a bewildering array of figures; he distrusted tests as heartily as he distrusted the 'infinitesimal analysis of the ego' which Freud carried to such lengths. A knowledge of the soul and of human conduct, worked out on a human scale, inspired simply by good sense and accessible to the man in the street—such was his aim. A doctor of sick souls, his chief concern was to heal. And since to heal is not so much a science as an art, Adler, whose penetrating spirit was devoid of all philosophical or metaphysical preoccupation, dreamed of a psychology which would be at once a science and an art. He gave intuition its due, although this

---

[1] In February 1930, I gave a lecture to the *Groupe d'études philosophiques et scientifiques* at the Sorbonne and I named it 'La Psychologie profonde: Freud et Adler.'

[2] The latest variant of the psycho-analysis professed by Jung is a significant apotheosis of human servitude. According to him every Ego is only the point of an iceberg which emerges from the vast sea of the Collective Unconscious. It is not we who have dreams but the dreams which have us! This leads to a panpsychism as ridiculous as it is picturesque. The theme of passivity, so dear to the ideologists of totalitarian regimes, is predominant in Jung's work. What was 'sociological blindness' in the case of Freud, becomes pure political reaction in his disciple, whose latest books almost make us forget his brilliant beginnings. True, he has since rectified this.

inevitably shocked those who rather stupidly regarded the empirical data of natural science as alone of any positive value. He has been reproached with his distrust for psychological apparatus, his scorn for the battery of tests, his general dislike of psycho-technique or psychometry. But since in experimental psychology practically everything can become a test, so Adler's 'test' was *a determinate situation in life*. He could open a 'human document' at any page; the least fragment of autobiography was enough for him to tell us with almost unerring vision the essential points of the subject's *style of life*. His enormous practical knowledge of men enabled him to skip the earlier stages of interpretation and to dispense with 'profiles' and 'psychological batteries'. Where there was only one in 1929 there are no less than five professors teaching the statistical method at the *Institut de Psychologie* at the Sorbonne to-day, and yet we know how frail is this method of tests, based as it is on a misconception of social facts and involving a veritable *petitio principii*.[1]

Adler, who at the outset would eagerly embrace any idea or tendency faintly resembling his own, was fortunately preserved from following the methods then in vogue—psycho-analysis and psycho-technique. He was prevented from doing so by the discovery of the physiological and psychological relativity residing in the law of compensation and over-compensation. His thought was not 'evolved'; it was contained in embryo in his first work, the *Studie über Minderwertigkeit der Organen*,[2] first published in 1907 and reprinted twenty years later without the author having to change a single word in it. It is in this book, moreover, that we shall find the starting-point of his theories and of all our present knowledge on the subject of the feelings of inferiority.

[1] The 'critical theory' advocated by M. Horkheimer and his school in *Zeitschrift für Sozialforschung* (Alcan, Paris) adds to the arguments against the system of tests. In Vol. VII, 3, 1938, of this journal, M. T.-W. Adorno severely criticises musical tests (*Über dem Fetischcharakter in der Musik*). Since nowadays individuals are no longer 'themselves' it is impossible to influence them and idle to ask them for their impressions—especially of jazz music. To use such positivistic methods in the Social Sciences is to be guilty of intellectual sabotage. It is hopeless to try and provoke completely unprejudiced reactions in subjects. Man's present social position, the fact that he is only a cog in the economic and political machine, prevents him from reacting freely. It is better therefore to *deduce* these reactions and to complete these deductions with empirical data taken from the subject. These observations only apply to musical reactions but will at a not very distant date be the starting point of a new orientation in experimental psychology.

[2] Translated as *Study of Organ Inferiority and its Physical Compensation*, by S. E. Jelliffe, New York, 1917.

Inferiority, a term long used in medicine and in jurisprudence, is a notion that has come to us from Darwinism. In human beings the existence of organic inferiorities can really only be noted at the moment of birth or during childhood. All the organs may suffer from a complete or partial deficiency, or inferiority; the sensory organs, the digestive system, the organs of respiration, the circulation of the blood, the glandular, urinary or genital systems, the nervous system. The fate of an 'inferior' organ will always vary according to the individual. Under the impact of external stimuli the instinct of self-preservation will drive the individual afflicted with a deficiency to level things up, to compensate for his inferiority. From an extensive study of persons and families showing organic deficiencies of all kinds, Adler concludes that the levelling process generally goes through the following stages: vital incapacity, morphological or functional anomalies; inability to resist and predisposition to certain definite illnesses; compensation through the organ itself; compensation through another organ; compensation by 'psychic superstructure'; organic or, alternatively, psychological over-compensation. The central nervous system takes part in a general way in any partial compensation, beginning with an increase of growth or of function (e.g. the one-armed man's arm which assumes athletic proportions). The inferior organ takes longer to function properly than the perfect organ. Adler was therefore able to state that to overcome an inferiority presupposes increased cerebral activity, a cerebral compensation. The next step seemed to be the assumption that every defective organ called forth the creation of a 'psychic superstructure', and that the individual in question will be 'more gifted' than if his organ had been perfectly constituted from the first. Thus it might well be, thought Adler, that an inadequate digestive system might acquire higher working capacity than a normal one. But at the same time, since the starting point of the compensation is in the digestive organs, the psychic superstructure founded on the deficiency would logically be stronger than anything else and attract all the other psychic complexes around it. In such a case anything connected with digestion or nutrition will have a special psychic 'value' or 'accent'. The nutritive instinct will therefore predominate in the subject, with greediness and avidity in its wake; but it may also produce greed, avarice, covetousness and possessiveness generally on the moral plane. Such a process (which is only one example, for compensations take place analogously in the case of inferiority of any organ) would seem to favour the formation in the individual of *psychic axes* closely dependent upon *one* or *several* inferior organs. These 'psychic axes' manifest themselves in the subject's whole psychological set-up, in his dreams, in the choice of his profession, etc. The defective organ then indulges in regular exercises—rather like an athlete training for a contest, and having overcome its difficulties, it is rewarded by the pleasure that henceforth accompanies its activity. Hence the special attitude of the subject towards this functional pleasure brought with such effort, as indeed towards all pleasure and towards sexual pleasure in particular. In a word, Adler has found the concrete point where purely physical or physiological facts are transformed into psychic facts. The discovery is of capital importance and was not exploited as it should have been. For very soon Adler was to discover that it was not so much the organic inferiority as its psychic superstructure which released the compensation. Similarly the compensations vary qualitatively and quantitatively in response to an imponderable element—a vague, confused and ill-defined feeling of insufficiency. Having started from purely biological work on the heredity of certain organs, especially those of the visual organ, in which he was a specialist, Adler now turned to the study of inferiorities *in natura vili*, i.e. in children without, however, going into the problem of *Kinderfehler*. Thus, from being a child doctor he became, in pursuing the paradoxical destiny of organic inferiorities, a nerve doctor and a psychiatrist. The *psychic axes*, which were the result of the compensation or over-compensation for inadequate organs, had thus been discovered. But the word 'psychic' presupposes an opposition to 'somatic'. Adler, however, had gradually become convinced that body and soul were so closely connected as to constitute a single undivided unity and that even purely imaginary inferiorities, or such as existed only in virtue of some social convention (such as being left-handed, having red hair, etc.), would call forth compensations without the presence of any organic inferiority properly so called. Thus the *psychic axes*, which at first were landmarks for the exploration of the personality, became directing lines of behaviour —the meridians, as it were, of the subject's life.

But man does not live in a vacuum. Organism presupposes environment,[1] the one cannot exist without the other. The human person

[1] It cannot be sufficiently emphasised how profound was Adler's influence in introducing into German biological and medical science *the integral conception of man* (*Ganzheitsbetrachtung*). Adler discerned the dialectical process between organism and environment which men of science are only now beginning to formulate. Thus in Kurt Goldstein's remarkable work, *Der Aufbau des Organismus*, The

receives a host of stimuli from the external world and this amorphous mass becomes ordered along certain 'axes' or 'directing lines' which we may call tendencies. But Adler was not content with what the manuals of psychology called 'directed attention'. He saw at once that memory itself did not escape from this *law of tendencies*. Memories are in a sense like metal filings lying on a piece of cardboard. If a magnet is placed above them they will dispose themselves along symmetrical magnetic lines. The magnetic pole which determines the directing lines of character is the *ideal aim* pursued by the subject; its opposite pole is the *earliest childhood recollection*. Man's whole being tends, whether he knows it or not (and more often he does not know it), towards a fictitious goal of superiority. We are set in motion, not by our innate dispositions, but by the position in which we stand in relation to this goal. Each of our actions indicates our position in this continual voyage which starts from inferiority and moves towards superiority—a position of struggle or an attitude of hesitation and indecision. There is a whole 'dialect of the organs', including a 'sexual jargon' which, to the astute observer, will indicate the kinetic law of each. For in Adler's view there was nothing static in man, everything was in motion, and no one psychic process could be taken as expressing the whole human being. What does it matter what we bring with us into the world at birth? What we do with it, that alone is important. It would therefore be useless to make out a list of our innate dispositions—(*Besitzes-psychologie*—the psychology of possession). The Adlerian psychology aims quite consciously at the utilisation of what we have—(*Gebrauchs-psychologie*—the psychology of use). Hence the *heuristic* principle which is of primary importance in the Adlerian psychology. It tells us not to lose ourselves in questions of detail, such as how the eye or the ear functions, how dreams are produced, etc. These theoretical matters can be left to the academic psychologists. What matters to the Adlerian psychologists is what the eye wants to see, what the ear wants to hear, the *tendency* which the dream reveals, the function of the dream—whether it encourages or discourages.

Later on, a new term replaced the 'directing lines', which had themselves replaced the 'psychic axes'. Not that the facts observed by Adler

Hague, 1935, we read sentences like the following: 'By the mere act of dividing the world into two (subject and environment) we are assuming the presence of a determinate organism. How then could the latter be determined only by the environment? The world becomes environment only when it already contains an ordered organism.'

had changed, nor his methods of interpretation and cure; only the theoretical conception had altered. The new term was *style of life*. The importance of this change in terminology must not be over-estimated. It certainly marks a new stage in the emancipation of Adler's thought from the ultra-naturalistic ideas in which he had been educated and which had gone to form his first terminology. But it should be noted that this emancipation was never complete. Nevertheless, to talk of a 'style of life' expresses a definitely *personalist* point of view and an approach to the idea of life as being man's continual creation.

According to Adler, the *style of life* is established in early childhood, generally between the third and fifth year. In his analyses of 'The Neurotic's Conception of the World' or of the 'Soul of the Criminal' in the *Internationale Zeitschrift für Individual Psychologie* of Vienna and in the *International Journal of Individual Psychology* of Chicago, he claimed that the neurosis or delinquency *invariably* mirrored a situation in childhood when the neurotic or the criminal was taking his first steps in life. This is particularly true of criminals. 'It is sufficient', he writes, 'to ask them for their earliest memory, the oldest impressions which have lasted since their childhood. They will answer something like this. "I was helping to clean some clothes: and it was then I noticed a coin and I took it. I was six." Or else, "When I was five I saw a railway carriage catch fire. It was full of children's balloons that were being thrown out: I took as many as I could." Or again, "My mother was in the habit of leaving money lying about; every week I used to take a little."'

It would seem, then, that in affirming that the style of life is established in early childhood, Adler is basing his deduction on such early memories, or mirrors of the adult's style of life. But in this I am of the opinion that Adler is guilty of a *petitio principii*, or that he has been the victim at any rate of an error in perspective. The idea that our subsequent fate is cast in childhood 'between the third and fifth year' is nothing but a legacy from Freud, in spite of the fact that Adler understood the supposed Oedipus Complex in a completely different sense from Freud's. The Freudian idea that with the establishment of the Oedipus Complex the fate of our *libido* and consequently of the whole of our life is cast, was the logical outcome of the author's belief in Evolution. But such an idea appears out of place in the Adlerian system and does not conform to its general spirit. Had not Adler himself shown us that the earliest memory, far from being a manifest façade hiding an older and latent memory, was most often germane to the present situation, or simply expressed that same *style of life*, of which, like the dream, it was only a consequence? It was he, too, who had shown us that these earliest memories were very often not authentic, that they were often 'arranged' in favour of the subject's preoccupations at the time, that they were 'false recognitions' purely in function of the *present* goal. I have studied this question myself in several hundred subjects, and I can state that very often a change in the style of life will automatically arouse a fresh 'earliest recollection' which will be in conformity with the new situation.

Very often, too, a number of earliest memories subsist without our being able to say which of them is the oldest. We shall therefore name sometimes one, sometimes another as such, and this not by a chance caprice but in virtue of the magnetic attraction exercised by the *present situation* on the confused mass of mnemonic material. But, it will be asked, if according to Adler's own results the earliest memory is 'arranged' in virtue of the existing style of life or of the present situation, how can it be claimed that these same memories point to the precocious but definitive establishment of this very style of life? Adler used to say that to cure a patient consisted in changing his style of life. But could one change it if it dated from early childhood? It was all very well for the psycho-analysts to say that even in the case of an unfavourable Oedipus constellation (e.g. fixation on the parent of the same sex, leading to homosexuality in the adult) the normal form of the complex could always be 'diluted'. The Adlerian psychology (except in the case of the dissident Künkel) did not recognise the idea of affective transference. So all Adler could do was to appeal to commonsense, to the 'community feeling' which he believed to exist *a priori* in the depths of every human soul. He attacked the psycho-analysts' assumption that the child is a fundamentally selfish little creature; this he regarded as an error in perspective. Since man, from the dawn of his existence on this globe, has always lived and always will live in a society, it is impossible that this fact should not have made a deep mark upon the species and implanted in it a profound sense of community which is expressed in the mother-child relationship. The baby's relationship to its mother is not at all, as some have dared to maintain, a 'parasitical' one. The mother with her breasts full of milk, and the functional changes brought about in her organism by motherhood, needs the child just as much as the child needs her.

Let us try to sum up the Adlerian theory very briefly in its final form and with its ultimate implications. Every human being lives in accordance with a certain style of life which is peculiar to him. This style of life is marked through and through with the goal of superiority, real or fictitious, towards which tend all the great directing lines of the subject's behaviour. Everyone tends to assert his own worth (*Geltung*) to avoid situations of inferiority, and aspires to situations of superiority.

The stupid assertion has been made, and how often repeated, that Adler 'deified Nietzsche's Will to Power', that he proclaimed and extolled Hobbes' *libido dominandi* (cf. Ernest Seillière). Some of Adler's early writings lend a certain colour to this erroneous interpretation. In them he speaks of a *Streben nach Macht* and lays undue stress on the importance of the 'aggressive impulses' in neurosis and in life in general.[1] But the more he deepened and elaborated the results he drew from the analysis of thousands of subjects, the further he moved from this terminology. 'People confuse my psychology with that of my patients', he would say jokingly. For in his view the most powerful motive in every human action was not, as Nietzsche claimed, *power*, but *superiority*, whether fictitious or real. That superiority which lurks even in the soul of the masochist, for he is seeking it in the very extremity of the humiliation to which he subjects himself. To show one's worth, to feel important—that is the secret of the human soul. And here we can borrow a term from chemistry, that of *valence*, so as to distinguish clearly between real and objective worth (the German *Wert*), and this *Geltung* or *Geltungsstreben*, which is a deeply implanted and purely subjective tendency to show or display our worth. Thus the Will to Power would be only one form among a thousand others of this tendency towards valency; one of a theoretically infinite number of variants of the same theme.

But according to Adler this tendency to show our worth is not a primordial factor in human nature. It arises as compensation for a painful and sometimes burning feeling of a *lack*, of a *minus*, the Feeling of Inferiority, the *Minderwertigkeitsgefühl*. Man, owing to his greater differentiation as compared to the higher mammals and even to his cousin, the ape, has become, in a sense, an inferior species. He is an animal whose birth is premature. According to biologists he ought not to see the light until he has reached the weaning stage. This is what has forced

[1] Here again this might be regarded as an 'imitation by opposition' of Freud, who used to deduce the aggressive tendency from the repression of impulses. Aggressiveness was the fashion in Vienna at this time. Adler himself said, 'Melancholy is an aggression directed against the environment'. But the more his own thought developed, the less he spoke of the 'aggressive impulse' (*Agressionstrieb*).

him to live in society, for only union makes for strength. Society or, in Adlerian terminology, the Community (*Gemeinschaft*) is the primordial fact. It is prior to the individual, and in the latter there exists from the first a strong impulse towards communal solidarity. In this view, man is fundamentally altruistic and not, as so many psychologists seem to think, fundamentally egoistic. The sense of community is as natural to him as breathing. But alas, the feeling of his own insufficiency breaks in upon his spirit of solidarity and collaboration, and at each blow suffered by his self-esteem this spirit will lose strength. Hence all the many deviations from the 'straight' path. Here we have a man or woman showing nervous symptoms, another will succumb to psychosis, another to crime; yet another will compensate his feelings of insufficiency by a definite sexual perversion, while another will seek for a return to community by the path (somewhat problematic in Adler's view) of art. Mental hygiene would therefore require that the patient should adapt himself to the community. But what is this community? What is this mysterious entity? Adler has refused to define it. Every psychic deviation is an error which brings about inevitable retribution; it is a diseased state of our feeling of community, of our *common sense*. In *What Life Should Mean to You*, in the important chapter that bears the title of the book, we read, 'The Community Feeling means above all the urge towards a form of community conceived as eternal, such as one might imagine humanity to be if it had already achieved perfection. I am not thinking of any *existing* community or society, nor of any religious or political group. I am simply pointing out that the most suitable human ideal is the perfect community, which would contain the whole of humanity and thus mark the final stage of Evolution.'

At this point Adler ventures into Utopian regions which are far removed from the field of serious sociological observation. We do not wish to follow him in these metaphysical speculations, though he is the first to recognise that they do not admit of proof. In his view, 'Community' is to be regarded as 'absolute truth', as the 'absolute imperative'; but the notion has unfortunately remained completely vague and undefined. Religion is a community, and so is a political group, the relationship between mother and child, between the members of the same family or of the same nation. All these are 'communities', but Adler has neglected to set them out in any kind of hierarchy. He does not argue about the notion, just as a Christian does not argue about his God, and it is not difficult to see in Adler's thought the mark of a religious and metaphysical mind, though expressed in purely secular form. The community takes the place of the divinity; the feeling of inferiority that of evil or sin, and altruism or solidarity that of virtue. The schema is that of all Christian moralists and recalls in a curious way the doctrine of Mandeville, which we expounded in an earlier chapter.

Thus, in the Adlerian system, the feeling of inferiority seems to acquire the role of prime mover. It is the pivot around which all psychic movement revolves, the force that conditions all our actions, even our thoughts, our talent, our happiness or our unhappiness. And just as Mandeville admitted that, paradoxical as it may seem, the vices of individuals tended to the public advantage, so Adler drew attention mainly to the useful, the *socially* useful side of many feelings of insufficiency and minus-value.

In his patient study of the feeling of inferiority and in his far-seeing interpretation of it, Adler will long remain unequalled. In his hands it has become the pillar supporting the whole edifice of this system, whether in its practical or theoretical aspect, and almost acquires the rank and dignity of a metaphysical principle.

But the dictum that everything in our life arises from our feelings of inferiority has no sense unless we can specify in each concrete case *which* feelings of inferiority are involved. Every feeling of inferiority must be specific, for it is a feeling belonging to the ego and this ego will be condemned for this feeling by the logic of human relations, just as the sinner is condemned by God for *his* particular sin. Adler has not set out a panorama of the different degrees and kinds of feelings of inferiority as the moralists and theologians have done in connection with the vices. He seems to have flung the lot into a terrific *olla podrida* without any discrimination whatsoever. Some French-speaking writers like Claparède and de Saussure have tried to give us a classification of the feelings of inferiority, but the classification is useless for it is purely external and superficial. Another Swiss writer,[1] this time writing in German, Häberlin, has given us a different classification, based entirely on Christian morality. For ourselves, our object being to understand each particular case and to curtail its analysis, we have favoured the use of diagrams or 'profiles' so as to discover without undue loss of time the weak points in each subject's self-esteem. Such is also the aim of the American methods which use a detailed questionnaire. Naturally, all these methods are very unsatisfactory, not so much through their lack

[1] Also, recently, the late Birnbaum in *Zeitschr. f. Ind. Psych.*, Vienna, 1948.

of elasticity as (Schachtel has recently shown this very clearly)[1] by the inadequacy of their theoretical foundation.

As soon as Adler had presented his system, a violent argument took place concerning his ideas. It was only natural that this discussion should centre around the main idea of 'The Psychology of the Individual', viz. the feeling of inferiority.

We shall now examine what this, 'the most important' of Adler's discoveries, became in the hands of his disciples. We shall begin with one who was the most representative, who also had his day of popularity, Fritz Künkel. We may note in passing that a number of other Adlerian conceptions were discovered about the same time by other thinkers, such, e.g., as the 'integral conception of the person', the theory of 'organic insufficiencies' and their compensations, etc. These have all made headway in medicine,[2] but we must confine ourselves to the purely psychological aspect of the problem of inferiorities. Paradoxically enough, the disciple of Adler whom we are going to discuss, though formerly a very close friend, was eventually disowned by the master. This has not prevented Fritz Künkel from practising Adlerian psychology, while passing over in discreet silence the name of him without whom his innumerable books would never have seen the light of day.

[1] Cf. Schachtel, *Zum Begriff und zur Diagnose der Persönlichkeit* in 'Personality Tests' in *Zeitschrift für Sozialforschung*, VI, 1937, Alcan.

[1] A. Holub, *Die Lehre von der Organminderwertigkeit*, Leipzig, 1931. Also, Hans Fleckenstein, *Krankheit und Persönlichkeit*, Freiburg i.B., 1941, of which there exists a Spanish translation.

CHAPTER VI

FRITZ KÜNKEL'S TREATMENT OF THE
FEELING OF INFERIORITY

KÜNKEL did not substantially alter the broad Adlerian schemas describing the psychic events in man and showing how his movement through life is determined. Nevertheless, like all disciples, he modified the details, either by over-emphasising one aspect of Adler's theory, by following his own particular Protestant bent, or by stressing his own political conviction. This was of a curious character and was marked by a profound nostalgia for the 'feudal' (sic) spirit, which he hoped to re-establish by means of education.

Künkel was the first to try to represent the feelings of inferiority graphically by means of a scale of measurement which recalls that of a thermometer. The feeling of one's own worth or value varies from 0 to −100 or to +100. A 'bad experience' in infancy, a 'betrayal' on the part of the parents, such e.g. as having been left alone in a room in spite of the screaming intended to attract them, or any other 'pedagogic mistake', will provoke feelings of inferiority. The feeling of self-value will drop to, say, −20. But this immediately calls forth a compensation. The child will now aspire to a superiority, not of symmetrical value, i.e. +20, but one beyond that, of +30 or +40. 'Whoever feels himself to be at −100', writes Künkel in one of his later works, 'will aspire to +100; he can no longer content himself with 0, i.e. with objectivity and quiet work'. After experiencing such 'betrayals' on the part of his *entourage*, the child will lose faith in other people and consequently in himself and in the supra-personal order of life. Any discouragement affecting not merely the subject's external qualities or faculties but his 'central vitality' will lead immediately to feelings of inferiority and consequently to a tendency to self-assertion. Whoever loses confidence 'in life' becomes *ichhaft*, a term related to, but not identical with, *egoism* or *egocentricity*. This term, which translated literally means 'I-ish', or *egotic*, is opposed to *wirhaft*, 'we-ish', just as egoistic is opposed to altruistic. The altruist is one who does something for a *thou*; to be *wirhaft* is to seek the good of 'us', of a community of which one is a part. *Ichhaftigkeit* is a character trait in virtue of which all values are judged from the standpoint of an Ego and are in the last event postulated *for* this Ego. An egotic person is always seeking to compensate a −100 position by aspiring to a +100, by being 'on top' (*Obensein*). But this egocentricity leads him into a vicious circle, for there is an inexorable law which requires that an egotic tendency should be constantly fortified. The more the Ego wants to be 'on top', the more it will dread falling down, the more liable it will be to defeats, the more it will strive to shelter from then and the more insupportable will the idea of failure, or even of a setback become. 'The feeling of inferiority and the tendency to assert one's own worth mutually reinforce each other'. Moreover, to be egotic distorts the whole of man's instinctive life. 'Real' instincts are natural necessities, they are 'the free and adaptable response of a living being to the requirements of reality', but instincts that have become egotic will have something violent and obsessive about them and will tend towards determined ends.

It is worth noting that in Künkel's view the primigenial 'we' the *Urwir*, has survived nowhere except in primitive tribes. The relation between a mother and her baby is indeed such an *Urwir*, though partly tainted by the egotic character of the mother. And rudiments of 'usness' do survive in all human beings in the form of a longing for a harmonious community, for a heroic solidarity, etc. When the egotic quality is developed to the maximum, the person's character undergoes a 'crisis', 'breaks' and suffers a catastrophe. This 'crisis' is necessary in order to be cured and to attain 'clarification' (*Klärung*) of the character. The perfect, i.e. the absolutely ripe and clarified 'we', is not of this world; it is the privilege, at best, of a few saints. It is therefore an ideal which we can never attain, but we must aspire to it, though succumbing at times to the egotic part of our nature.

Here again we have one of those psychologies which are concerned with man's conduct within a society and regard his psychological equilibrium as being conditioned by his adaptation to society. Morality invades everything. Ethical admonitions are confused with psychological precepts in a system which offers nothing new, unless it be its terminology which is practically untranslatable.

External and internal 'miseries', Künkel tells us, all help to increase the feeling of inferiority which then takes the form of a vicious circle. The Ego undergoes a veritable 'training' in certain forms of behaviour; either the positive training of encouragement, or the negative training of discouragement. Everyone has an 'arc of tension', of which the span is increased or diminished by a positive or a negative training, and the development of this arc will be arrested if a child is pampered or spoiled. When such a child grows up he will always try to behave like a baby or a child, he will repudiate all responsibility for his conduct. The laws of character, like those of the training of animals, are formed 'automatically, unconsciously and rigidly' in accordance with the old adage that 'the burnt child dreads the fire'. Character traits cannot be altered by reason or conviction; only the 'crisis' will re-establish man's liberty. For the feeling of inferiority, —100 raised to the state of paroxysm, will call forth the 'courage of despair' which comes to the final rescue. Only by returning to the bosom of a primordial community based on the feudal model—loyalty between superiors and inferiors who feel themselves to be members of the same community—will a man be cured of his feelings of inferiority. But the loyalty in question is not that of teacher to pupil, of psychiatrist to patient (or *vice versa*), but of one side of the 'totality' to the other. The trust required must be given to 'the common social group, to the school, to the religious denomination, to the political party, to the state, to the race, to life'.

Thus the ideal set up by Künkel appears to be a character free from inhibitions, but not entirely undisciplined. Such a man will not submit to some imposed 'training', but will let his character grow in response to the tasks which life presents to him. In childhood we are guided by an ideal image: we want to be a hero, a saint, a martyr, a great artist, a successful businessman. Later we try to realise this ideal. Every approach to the ideal causes pleasure, every departure from it a feeling of unhappiness. Every unpleasant experience, mishap, setback or feeling of inferiority, in a word, every lack or *minus*, can be 'levelled up' or compensated for by some special good—a brilliant performance, a revenge, an intensive training, or even an excess of suffering. But every compensation brings with it something rigid and unnatural, something 'false'. It is like a cramp, it is not 'authentic'. To play the violin, not from the love of it, but by way of compensation for a minus, is not to set about it in the right way.

It is just at this point that Künkel proves himself to be a bad disciple, for he drops overboard Adler's fundamental discovery—the idea of compensation—and yet does not succeed in finding a substitute for it in his attempt to re-establish a mysterious community which he labels 'we'. In dealing with special problems he is often brilliant, sometimes

even to the point of genius. But his system is too weakly constructed
to be handed down to posterity as it stands. At the same time he does
not deserve the scorn now evinced by the orthodox Adlerians who,
before his break with Adler, had given him such unstinted admiration.

BIBLIOGRAPHY

Dr. Fritz Künkel's published works are:

Einführung in die Charakterkunde. 7th ed., 1936. Leipzig, S. Hirzel (so far
his best work).
Charakter, Wachstum und Erziehung. 2nd ed., 1934. Leipzig, S. Hirzel.
Charakter, Liebe und Ehe. 2nd ed., 1936. Leipzig, S. Hirzel.
Charakter, Einzelmensch und Gruppe. 1933. Leipzig, S. Hirzel.
Charakter, Leiden und Heilung. 1934. Leipzig, S. Hirzel.
Charakter, Krisis und Weltanschauung. 1935. Leipzig, S. Hirzel.
Grundzüge der Praktischen Seelenheilkunde. Berlin.
Politische Charakterkunde. 1931. Berlin.
Die Arbeit am Charakter. 23rd ed., 1939. Mecklenburg-Schwerin,
Friedrich Bahn.
Jugendcharakterkunde. 11th ed., 1932. Mecklenburg-Schwerin, Friedrich
Bahn.
Krisenbriefe. 3rd ed., 1933. Mecklenburg-Schwerin, Friedrich Bahn.
Das Wir. 4th ed., 1939. Mecklenburg-Schwerin, Friedrich Bahn.
Introduccion a la Caracterologia. (Edited by Oliver Brachfeld) 1945.
Barcelona, Ed. Victoria.
Del Yo al Nosotros (Grundzüge der Praktischen Seelenheilkunde). 1943.
Barcelona.

Several other books by Künkel have recently been issued in the
United States by Lippincott and other publishers.

CHAPTER VII

PAUL HÄBERLIN'S ETHICAL INTERPRETATION

THE term 'feeling of inferiority'—let us admit it—is not a happy one, as will appear from the reading of a book written by the Swiss professor, Paul Häberlin, entitled *Minderwertigkeitsgefühle*. The ordinary translation of this word is 'Feelings of Inferiority'. But the author draws our attention to an interesting distinction. According to him, if we are confronted with something or someone stronger than ourselves we do not experience feelings of minus-value (*Minderwertigkeitsgefühle*) but of inferiority in the strict sense of the word. Feelings of minus-value never reflect a feeling of being weak, small, bereft of strength. To be confronted with something or someone stronger than ourselves will not make us *doubt our own worth*; this doubt is the specific outcome of the feeling of minus-value, and this feeling always arises not from a confrontation between self and not-self, but of an estimative comparison *within* the self. We do not measure ourselves with anything coming from outside, but actually with *ourselves*, or with an ideal which we wish to follow. These 'real feelings of minus-value, arising from our inner communing with ourselves, possess a moral character'. What we are dealing with, then, is a *sense of guilt*.

According to Häberlin, such a feeling could arise only from within. When we ascribe it to an external cause we are grossly misled by appearances. As soon as we examine more closely those feelings of minus-value of apparently external origin we find that in reality we are dealing with 'internal verdicts issued from the point of view of our real self'. Even when we think we are experiencing feelings of minus-value in relation to other people 'it is not the other person's virtue which is exercising this depressing effect upon us, it is the lack of virtue in ourselves'. There must therefore have been already pre-existing in us a 'feeling of inferiority properly so called, born of a critical confrontation with ourselves'.

Following up the idea that no external factor can enter into the formation of genuine and moral feelings of inferiority, the Swiss professor reaches the extreme conclusion that even our *physical* insufficiencies or infirmities, i.e. our organic defects, could never occasion such feelings of minus-value. Our body, he argues, belongs to us in the most intimate manner and yet it differentiates itself appreciably from that other Ego which alone is capable of forming moral judgments and which feels itself to be the author of our actions. 'In this sense', he writes, 'our body belongs to the exterior world, it is the exterior world brought very close', the closest part of the non-ego. We find it difficult to believe, however, that the feeling resulting from a personal infirmity is 'far from having the corroding significance which characterises feelings of moral inferiority'. Thousands of cases give the lie to the Swiss professor's ultra-idealistic and almost theological assertion. Any orthopaedic or plastic surgeon would tell him that the most insignificant defects, such as a leg half an inch too short, a paralysed finger, an outsize nose, can cause the most terrible micromaniacal complexes. Häberlin does grant that the feelings of insufficiency due to an infirmity can 'combine' with the other *genuine* (because moral) feelings of inferiority. But he denies categorically that there is a causal relation between the two. The inferiority, or infirmity, he says, would have first to be considered by the person suffering from it as a punishment inflicted by God. But this, he maintains, would be possible only to one already possessed of the feeling that he deserves this punishment, and this is the very feeling which can be named a *genuine* feeling of inferiority. Alternatively, our physical inferiority might have become the cause of moral inferiority, or a 'lack of emotional control'. But even in such a case, the author claims, the weakness or insufficiency is not the cause, it is only the *place* where the *ethical* insufficiency comes to light. These observations, we may point out, contradict the facts and introduce an *a priori* ethic where only scientific observation is legitimate. In spite of this, M. Häberlin concludes:

'I cannot rid myself of the impression that the theory of the organic origin of inferiority feelings is a trick designed to deceive men of low moral calibre, so that they can abrogate all responsibility and transfer their feelings of guilt from the realm of moral self-criticism to the innocuous realm of the undeserved disadvantages imposed by fate.'

This 'impression' is all the more erroneous as Adler, whose theory M. Häberlin wishes to dispute, denied any *causal* and still more any *proportional* relation between the physical factors and the feelings of inferiority. He too knew very well that there are people with great natural disadvantages who do not suffer from feelings of inferiority as a result of and in proportion to these disadvantages, and that on the other hand, in an enormous number of cases, feelings of inferiority occur without the presence of any physical defect as their basis.

M. Häberlin then tries to establish a classification inside the group of what he calls 'genuine' or 'internal' feelings of inferiority. According to him, we must first distinguish the acute feelings of insufficiency felt by chronic sufferers. All the author is really doing is to reduce the results of the modern psychology concerning the feelings of inferiority to the well-worn categories of morality—a bad conscience, repentance, etc. And when he presents us with ideas such as that of 'an unfavourable congenital ethical constitution', we are frankly unable to follow him, for he is definitely leaving the psychological field of discussion. On the contrary, we assert that feelings of inferiority may be not only *intensified* by suggestions or other influences coming from the outside, but that they may very well be directly *caused* by these. The least practical experience in psychology or pedagogy will be sufficient to convince anyone of this.

'FEELING', 'SENSATION' OR 'COMPLEX'

The discussion of the Adlerian results becomes more complicated when the question (implicit in Häberlin's contentions) is raised as to whether the term *feeling* of inferiority is really a suitable one. Would not *sensation* of inferiority be preferable? It is, incidentally, the expression used by the well-known Chilean authoress, Gabriela Mistral.

I admit that I am at a loss myself as to what term to use. Even if we disregard the popular use of these terms we are no further on, for does not every psychologist use them in a different sense? We need only recall the interminable disputes about these very terms, or the campaign conducted with such vigour by some German psychologists, especially Th. Lipps, against what they contemptuously referred to as 'a psychology which regards itself as a metaphysic' and against what they ironically named the 'Mythology of consciousness' (*Bewusstseinsmythologie*). Cf. Lipps' *Das Selbstbewusstsein: Empfindung und Gefühl*, vol. IX, of *Grenzfragen des Nerven- und Seelenlebens*, Ed. J. E. Bergmann, Wiesbaden, 1901.

The ego or Self is not consciousness, for how would it be possible for one state of consciousness not to remember an earlier one? This means, so Lipps tells us, that it is the *whole individual*, the whole person who no longer remembers. The individual, says Lipps, is the ego, the real Self

PAUL HÄBERLIN'S ETHICAL INTERPRETATION

(*das reale Ich*), i.e. the being which acts through psychic phenomena or which manifests its existence through them. It is what feels, what perceives, what experiences, what wills . . . in a word, it is the *psyche*. Now the Self is the Self of feelings and 'it is the feelings that confer a real and supreme meaning on the word *I*' (p. 39). In theoretical psychology it is important to distinguish clearly between feelings and sensations, though in Lipps' view there is often a danger of their being confused. 'Very often the contents of sensation are called feelings and are confused with feelings proper; people speak of bodily feelings when in reality they mean *the contents of bodily sensations*.' Many authors even consider that there are no feelings without some previous sensations, thus recalling the scholastic adage, *nihil est in intellectu*. . . . In this view, feelings and affects would only arise as the result of external influences, but these external influences would produce the feelings, not as the result of some previous organic sensations, 'but because they conditioned a certain rhythm or mode in the flow of the whole psychic life'. Thus feelings are different from organic sensations. Nor are they to be identified with the famous 'global sensations' (*Gesamtempfindungen*) or synaesthesia.

Lipps maintains very convincingly the 'independence of the feelings from bodily sensations' (*Unabhängigkeit der Gefühle von Körperempfindungen*). There are no feelings, he says, which are not feelings of the Self, of the whole Self. 'The feelings are what constitute the Self.' The self is the totality of the feelings. These do not merely centre around the Self as do the sensations, they merge into it. 'The antagonism existing between the contents of sensation (sensorial data) and the contents of feeling is the most fundamental in psychology. This antagonism is as primary as that between subject and object, between ego and non-ego (p. 16). . . . Both in popular speech and in our own terminology, *feeling* always contains the element of subjectivity. The only difference between popular language and ours resides in the fact that the former assigns a wider field to the term. Which means that it regards as feelings not only those contents of consciousness which serve to designate the Self as such, but also those which belong to it in a special way (*besonders zugehören*), or which appear to be, as it were, bound to it' (p. 22).

We must therefore conclude that the term *feeling* is to be preferred to *sensation*, especially if we accept Janet's definition of the first term. *Feeling*, he says, is *the regulator of conduct*.[1]

---

[1] 'We regard the *feelings* as the regulators of the behaviour which we have called primary. Primary behaviour is that which is determined by stimuli coming

Now daily usage has also consecrated the expression 'inferiority complex', and Adler himself has had to bow to the power of this word, which he had begun by rejecting because of its definitely Freudian ring. The definition of complex given in the *Encyclopédie française* is 'l'action d'une force sur une représentation', a definition which is curiously reminiscent of that of *inhibition* in classical psychology. But clearly it is inapplicable in our case. If we want to judge of the right use of this term in connection with auto-estimative inferiorities, we must first make a rapid survey of the history of the word *complex* in psycho-analytical terminology.

from the external world. The sight of bread is a stimulus to eating, the sight of wine calls for the reaction of drinking, the sight of a path the reaction of walking.' These are 'the fundamental primary behaviours. But later, when actions emanate from inside the person, they become subject to rules and regulations.' (Janet, *La Force et la Faiblesse psychologiques.*)

CHAPTER VIII

WHAT IS A COMPLEX?

THE word 'complex' is in fashion, and is often used as an abbreviation for 'inferiority complex'. This may be a sign that we are making light of the phenomenon, just as the Germans used to speak of a *Mi-Ko*, this being an abbreviation of the inordinately long *Minderwertigkeits-Komplex*.

The term is originally a medical one, e.g. solar complex, etc., but it is also used in the field of commerce. In pedagogy[1] it has a clearly defined meaning, far more so, alas, than in psychology. Thus its meaning varies quite definitely according as it is used by 'classic' psychologists such as G. E. Müller,[2] in the subtle lucubrations of the 'psychologists of thought', or in the Freudian writings. M. Henri de Man is therefore wrong when he states his reasons for preferring 'inferiority complex' to 'inferiority feeling' as follows: 'So that when instead of saying *feeling* I speak of *complex*, it is not from any liking of the uncouth term, but simply because the term "complex" expresses exactly what I mean, whereas "feeling" can mean a whole lot of things . . .' (*Au delà du Marxisme*, by Henri de Man). This can be argued the other way round, for *complex* too can mean a whole lot of things . . . and things much more complicated and diversified than are the different *feelings*.[3]

The term was put into circulation by the Freudian psycho-analysis, though it had not been invented by Freud. It was current already in the

[1] In pedagogy a 'complex' is the method which consists in presenting to the pupils in an encyclopaedic form a large collection of connected problems. An interesting example of this is Mlle. Maria Musis de Nanina's article on the silk worm in *Revista de Pedagogia*, Madrid, June 1935. The exposition begins with the life of the worms and extends to the technological, historical, economic, and moral problems connected with silk.

[2] Cf. G. E. Müller, *Komplextheorie und Gestalttheorie*. Göttingen, 1923, and also F. Krüger, *Komplexqualitäten. Gestalten und Gefühle*. Munich, 1923.

[3] I have in preparation a book in Spanish, in which I try to clarify some of these notions, and in which I reproduce definitions of some 250 'complexes', culled from general literature and the press.

earlier academic psychology, where the idea of a 'complex' was contrasted with that of *psychic elements*, which were regarded as irreducible elements, as it were, of the psychological process. The 'complex' had a certain affiliation with the 'function'. In psycho-analytical literature the term was introduced by C. G. Jung and was immediately adopted by others, for its use was believed to mark 'a very important stage in the relation with ordinary psychology'. (Cf. Ferenczi and Rank, *Entwicklungsziele der Psychoanalyse*, Vienna-Leipzig, 1924, p. 33.)

Jung employed the term 'as a simplification of a highly complicated psychological circumstance, and as pointing to certain tendencies characteristic of the person in question or to a group of interdependent ideas charged with affectivity'. Freud eventually gave it a new meaning and confined it to the unconscious and suppressed parts of these ideas. Certain Freudian psycho-analysts naturally found it inconvenient to assume the existence of these strictly isolated and interdependent 'psychic particles', which could be aroused or displaced only *in toto*. These complexes also appeared (pardon the play of words!) too complex and too complicated not to contain lesser elements which could themselves be separated and analysed. Later, in Freud's own work the notion of complexes figured only as a survival of the first stage of psycho-analysis, and as a notion which really had no proper place in his system of thought after the creation of 'metapsychology'.

Were the complexes then discarded? Far from it, logical though the step would have been. Disciples and master continued to picture the human psyche as a kind of mosaic pattern of such complexes which one tried to 'dissolve analytically' (*herausanalysieren*) one after the other. The personality was regarded as a sum composed of such complexes; the father complex, the mother complex, the brother complex, the sister complex, etc. And since every human being possesses all the complexes it was easy enough to discover them by means of psycho-analysis which assumed their existence *a priori*. After all, everyone in the course of his life enters into relation with the persons and objects around him by forming complexes. The psycho-analysts therefore finally reached the conclusion that the enumeration and analysis of these complexes might be interesting enough for academic and descriptive psychology, but that it had nothing to contribute to the analysis of neurotic patients. It was not even of any interest to the analysis of the *motifs* of ethnographic or literary tradition. *Complexes* and *motifs* could not express the spiritual creations of a people or an author in all their colour and variety; they only reduced them to a dreary and monotonous series of trivial elements. And this poverty was not remedied by giving pre-ference now to one, now to another, of the complexes, nor by the in-vention of new complexes. (Cf. Ferenczi and Rank, *loc. cit.*)

The attempt has also been made to interpret these complexes as one of the four sources of our irrational actions. Thus the philosopher Hans Driesch writes, 'They (the complexes) are not in any way innate—for then they would be "impulses"—but quite definitely acquired, and acquired unconsciously and involuntarily' ('Zum Begriff des Irration-alen', in *Archiv für Philosophie und Soziologie*, 1929. *Hommage à L. Stein*, p. 108). These involuntarily created complexes might thus very well determine a certain number of our irrational actions. And since they remain hidden most of the time, they are unmasked only when they become too powerful and prove to be a nuisance in our lives. But Driesch himself pointed out that even if we assume the existence of these complexes as understood by psycho-analysis they could by no means all, without exception, be regarded as the source of irrational behaviour. Coué, who postulated the existence of complexes favourable to psychic equilibrium, and also Baudouin have shown, moreover, that the general facts known under this name could very well be put to the service of reason itself. The next step would have been to place the complexes at the disposal of pedagogy, of education, indeed of ethics. But this step was never taken, and even in Germany there has never been a pedagogy of complexes, just as psycho-analysis never developed into an analysis of complexes. It is worth noting, however, that Jung's disciples have recently tried to reinstate the term which their master had invented, and since the publication of the tributes to him in 1935 they habitually refer to the totality of his theories by the term *Komplexe Psychologie*. The old formula *Analytische Psychologie* has been abandoned, no doubt because it did not sufficiently emphasise the independence of the Jungian school with regard to Freud. The claim to such independence, it may be added, does not admit of proof; indeed the opposite is the case.

Another definition of the complex has been given by the distin-guished Franco-Russian psychiatrist, Dr. Minkowski.

'In the realm of morbid psychology a complex is a group of memories and ideas bearing a considerable affective charge and cut off from bonds which ought normally to connect it with the unified psychic development of the individual. The complexes do not become integrated in the individual in the course of his life. They remain outside like foreign bodies. But they seek an outlet, and in one way or another break into the patient's life. They manifest themselves in clinical symptoms, amongst others, and determine the latters' psychological content. . . . The complex exercises a patho-plastic influence on the symptoms; it is reflected in them. . . . This does not necessarily imply a relation of cause and effect' (*L'Evolution psychiatrique*, I, 1925). There is a difference between a complex and an emotional shock. The complex does not consist in a violent emotion, a knock-out blow. It is formed by silent griefs, by obscure desires, unfulfilled and sometimes even unadmitted.

Complexes in the nature of 'foreign bodies' which 'do not become integrated in the unified psychic development' of the subject—such an interpretation is incompatible with our way of thinking, which claims that the person is not a *dividuum* but an *individuum*. In the next chapter a brief investigation of the difference between the feeling of inferiority and envy will show that none of the above definitions of the 'complex' will meet our case.[1]

[1] To press the distinction between 'Complex' and 'Feeling' of inferiority too far is pure logomachy. In the United States, moreover, there is a tendency to replace both these terms by the word 'attitude'. We refer the reader to an investigation in which Adler himself took part: *Inferiority Attitudes and their Correlations among Children* by L. Ackerson in the *Journal of Genetic Psychology*, 1943, pp. 62 and 85–96.

CHAPTER IX

ENVY AND THE FEELING OF INFERIORITY.
THE PROBLEM OF AUTHENTICITY

'BEFORE attempting to do something,' said Goethe, 'one must *be* something.' In examining the feelings of inferiority we have been led to the very heart of this problem, which is also the centre towards which gravitates a very powerful tendency in modern philosophy. For it is admitted in philosophy that man *exists* and also that he *is*. But he must also be able to *be himself*. This term has been rendered in French by the word *ipséité*, a happy creation of V. Jankelevitch. The well-known and often quoted words of Nietzsche, *Werde was du bist*, are perhaps the finest expression of this idea, and the phrase which some years ago José Ortega y Gasset flung to the Spanish public, *seamos auténticos* ('let us be authentic'), also bears on the same problem of authenticity, of *Echtheit* which has haunted the minds of the best German psycho-therapists. To give an example: on the boards of a famous music-hall we see a one-legged Negro dancer. The leg which he lost in childhood through an accident has been replaced by a wooden leg. The man performs a number of steps, exhibiting extraordinary skill and courage. And yet, unlike the vulgar crowd, we feel a certain *malaise* in watching him. True, there is no sign of strain or of effort in his dancing (however much there may have been in his training), and yet it does not seem 'natural' to us, the achievement is not 'authentic'. ... Another dancer, going through exactly the same steps, but with the help of both his legs, will, as it were, deliver us from the haunting memory of the Negro's performance, though the latter is by far the more praiseworthy. In the same way a number of noted psychiatrists have tried to discredit the success of Adlerian psychology on the ground that the results of a compensation for some genuine organic inferiority could never equal the achievement which comes of a super-abundance of strength. No matter how brilliant the results achieved through compensation, on the principle that 'genius is an infinite capacity for taking pains', still, it was based on a *minus*, not on a *plus*. The discussion would lead us too far afield into the realm of philosophy.

Our opinion is quite simply that it is impossible to establish a hard and fast distinction between a performance that is authentic and one that is not. The one can merge insensibly into the other, and it may very well be that the factor of compensation comes to be added to a pre-existing and authentic *gift*. Might not the case of Beethoven, who was afflicted from childhood with an organic inferiority of the sense of hearing, be of this nature? Thus Beethoven's genius would be authentic in spite of the compensatory element which went to its formation. On the other hand, when a feeling of national inferiority leads a man like Houston Stewart Chamberlain to renounce his own country and identify himself with a civilisation and a 'Kultur' that are not his own, then, however excellent the resulting intellectual output, there will be something in it that does not ring true. The high intellectual quality of the work, the unchallengeable cleverness of the national and social mimicry will never completely dispel our impression of non-authenticity. According to the school of modern psychiatry represented by Oswald Schwarz and Rudolf Allers, every action can be either a high achievement (German *Leistung*), i.e. something praiseworthy—or a symptom, in the derogatory sense of the term. In order to know which of the two qualifications we are to use in describing a man's actions, we must know him as a whole being and his 'total life situation'.

Take the case of a young and vigorous priest who renounces sex for the sake of a higher spiritual aim, and contrast with it that of a neurotic young priest whose abstinence fits only too easily into his neurosis. In spite of the outward similarity, they are not both chaste in the same sense. It is well known that the Church refuses to admit to the priesthood any man (were it Origen himself) whose virility has been impaired. In this the Church is actuated by the right feeling of the difference which exists between a symptom and an achievement, between false merit and authentic merit. Or take two long-haired young artists in Montparnasse, wearing the same romantic bow ties, frequenting the same haunts, suffering, maybe, from the same neurosis; to the contemporary observer they seem both tarred with the same brush. But future generations will have an objective criterion by which to distinguish between them—their work. The one will have left insipid rubbish, or even nothing at all; the other, if he is 'authentic', will have left works which, whatever their external labels, are immortal masterpieces.

These brief considerations, which should be followed up by a philosopher, will serve as an introduction to the problem before us, viz. what are the relations between two phenomena which one might be tempted to compare if not to identify and thus confuse with one another; envy and the feeling of inferiority? Envy, curiously enough, has been rather neglected by the psychologists; one hardly comes across it except in some disguise, e.g. that of jealousy, etc. And yet, what could one not write by way of subtle commentary on this saying of Goethe's alone, 'When faced with overwhelming envy, the safest thing is to seek refuge in love'?

Envy is the desire produced by the corroding feeling of having been deprived of something which another person possesses. It is therefore the result of a comparison. Now most psychologists who have occupied themselves with the question of the feelings of inferiority have claimed that the latter are always the result of a comparison. But we have shown elsewhere that the presence of feelings of inferiority does not by any means always presuppose a previous comparison. Let us examine the question a little more closely.

As we have seen, the inferiority complex has its origin in the realm of feeling. Now the attempt has been made, and rightly, to establish a distinction between the *feeling that I have* which stands over against the self, which is its *object*, and the *feeling that I am*. Gabriel Marcel, who has concerned himself with the problem of *Être et Avoir*, says very truly that 'at bottom everything rests on the distinction between what one has and what one is. . . . Clearly what one *has* presents a certain exteriority in relation to the self.'[1] Using the author's words we could therefore say that envy represents a 'tension between interior and exterior' and that it consequently belongs to the sphere of having. It is on the plane of having that desire moves; and 'desire is both autocentric and heterocentric'. On the other hand, we would say that the feeling of inferiority belongs to the realm of being; it is a *minus being*. But even the subtle philosopher of *Être et Avoir* is obliged to admit that between the two realms there is a whole series of intervening gradations, 'un dégradé insensible'. Thus envy might very well change from being a feeling of what one has not got into a feeling of something that one is not, though such a transformation need not necessarily take place. Thus envy sometimes produces feelings of inferiority, but not always or necessarily, and still less is it to be identified with them. The distinction between Having and Being is both philosophical and psychological; it will enable us to put an end to the barren discussion which we witnessed above, viz. as to whether the feeling of inferiority

[1] Gabriel Marcel, *Being and Having*, translated by K. Farrer.

presupposes a previous comparison. A number of psychologists have been misled by the term *inferiority*, for to be inferior presupposes the existence of something superior, and logically this implies a comparison. But 'feeling of inferiority' is a conventional expression to designate a state of mind, a kind of self-feeling rather than self-consciousness; it often exists previous to any comparison, and it would be far better to name it 'feeling of imperfection' (Vauvenargues) or 'feeling of impotence'.

So long as envy remains in the realm of Having and leaves the roots of Being untouched it will be a normal and perfectly justifiable feeling of lacking something. But as soon as this lack, this have-not, is transmuted into a being-minus, we find ourselves in the realm of pathology, of inferiority feelings and all their consequences. The authenticity of Being will have been impaired, for envy will have lost its heterocentric character, retaining only the autocentric.

CHAPTER X

FEELING OR CONSCIOUSNESS?

THE modern 'psychology of form' tells us that a man suffering from aphasia is not simply *minus* the function of language, and, as we have seen, anyone suffering from a feeling of inferiority is not *minus* something; like the aphasiac, he has become a *completely different person*. Could not this fundamental change in his state of being which we have called feeling of inferiority be regarded as a kind of knowledge or consciousness? Authors are not lacking who affirm that this is so. One of the best of them is Rudolf Allers, a former disciple of Adler's, at first professor in Vienna and now at the Catholic University of Washington. He writes in a great Encyclopaedia of Pedagogy, 'In what the Adlerian psychology refers to as *feeling of inferiority* (the term *feeling* being once again used in a non-specific sense), we are really dealing with a kind of *knowledge*. It would be more correct to speak of a diminution of personal experience (*Erlebnis*) or of a consciousness of inferiority, though we are bound to admit that this consciousness must not be thought of as something clear and explicit.'

But in that case, if 'consciousness' is no clearer a term than 'feeling', why prefer the former to the latter, especially if its use is in direct contradiction with the facts? Adler has more than once protested against such misinterpretations of his theories, because in his opinion they gave rise to terminological discussions that were devoid of interest. And since the expression 'consciousness of inferiority' shows no signs of disappearing we shall quote here a passage of his addressed to those who continued to make use of it:

'Undoubtedly there is an unconscious knowledge, a knowledge that has taken shape and become mechanised. When a rich man comes into a shop he is probably not thinking at that moment of the figures that express his wealth. And yet he will act, he will behave as though he were so thinking. In the same way . . . one can talk of "unfelt" feelings, i.e. those of which we are in no way conscious but which nevertheless do not cease to influence the movements in which we express ourselves. When, jostled in a crowd, I take care not to tread on my neighbour's foot I am manifesting my community feeling. Yet at the moment when I make the movement so motivated, I experience nothing of the feeling in question. I know and feel myself to be a part of the whole, and especially of the part that must act' (Adler, 'Neurotisches Rollenspiel', *Internat. Zeitschr. f. Ind. Psych.*, 1928).

Thus the feeling of inferiority may very well be conscious, may consist in a form of knowledge, but may equally well remain unconscious. The individual suffering from a feeling of inferiority will be influenced by it in his actions whether he is conscious of its presence or not. We might therefore adapt to our own use Pascal's saying, '*Pour reconnaître si c'est Dieu qui nous fait agir il vaut mieux nous examiner par nos comportements que par nos motifs de dedans.*' ('In order to know if God is activating us we will do better to examine ourselves in our outward behaviour rather than in our inner motives.') Only we would substitute for the first clause, 'In order to know whether our action is authentic and not symptomatic'. Adler himself liked to quote a saying of Luther's which he always put into practice when dealing with a patient: 'Cast thine eye on the hand and not on the mouth'. What counts most for the Freudian analyst is the subject's own introspective material, and in exploring his patient's unconscious he seeks to add to this material, which is sadly restricted by the 'Censor' and the process of 'repression'. The Behaviourist, on the other hand, eliminates all introspective elements and examines only the behaviour of the subject, as though the latter were simply an animal devoid of self-consciousness. The new method inaugurated by Adler combines the introspective and the behaviourist methods and checks the one with the results of the other. Hence its interpretation of *lying*, which is completely different from that of the Freudian school. The latter regards the lies told by a patient as being just as much the expression of his psyche as his true statements. We do not lie as we want to, but in conformity with our psychological configuration. Adler, on the contrary, used to say, 'If a patient tells me all sorts of stories about his personal courage, and if at the same time I notice that he is gripping the arms of his chair like a frightened man, I try not to listen to him any longer and use only my eyes. . . .' Thus the 'unconscious' does not mean the same thing for the Freudian and for the Adlerian, and if both are seeking to probe beyond the sphere of the subject's mere introspection, the depths they are exploring do not lie in the same dimension. In the same way the word 'complex' can never mean the same thing in both systems. Adler never used the term until

1926 when, in the course of his first lecturing tour in the United States, he realised that he had been called the 'father of the inferiority and superiority complex'. After this he began to use the word 'complex' where previously he had spoken only of 'feeling'. It was only towards the end of his life and especially in the last book published in his lifetime, *What Life Should Mean to You (Der Sinn des Lebens)*, that he establishes the exact shade of difference between the two terms.

'I have had to struggle a long time before being able to solve the most important problem in this matter, namely how, from a feeling of inferiority and its physical and mental sequel, due to the impact of the problems of life, there comes to be formed the inferiority complex. In my opinion this problem has never been given priority in the researches made by writers and could therefore never be solved. For my part I have succeeded in solving it in the same way as all other questions of individual psychology; by explaining the part by the whole and the whole by its part. The inferiority complex, i.e. *the abiding consequences of the inferiority feeling and their enforced continuance*,[1] can be explained by a marked lack of the community feeling. . . . We shall always find the proof of an inferiority complex in the subject's life history, in his conduct and attitude to others, in his having been made too much of as a child, as well as in his organic insufficiencies, and in his having felt neglected in childhood. . . . The sexual conduct and individual development of anyone suffering from an inferiority complex will simply be part and parcel of his whole personality as based upon this complex.'

Thus the inferiority complex can be regarded as a chronic affliction caused, as it were, by the residues of inferiority feelings of more evanescent character. But this interpretation, which moreover is in contradiction with the whole spirit of Adler's work, fails to convince, and for two reasons, one theoretical, the other empirical. Theoretically such an interpretation strikes us as over-simplified and too 'energetic', while in practice it is impossible to isolate particular feelings of inferiority from the totality of the complex. We have no means either of measuring or of isolating a state of mind, and the feeling of inferiority is a state of mind. Empirical observation shows us that feelings of guilt, of impotence, of insufficiency, of insecurity, and of inferiority are, with their numerous variants, so like each other that they cannot possibly be isolated and treated separately. However we may label these feelings, they all are connected within the same whole, they all, without excep-

[1] The italics are mine.—O.B.

tion, are a mark of a more or less consciously felt lesion in the auto-appreciative function; in other words, they point to a lowering of the normal level of auto-estimation. It is for this whole group of psychological phenomena that, for want of a better, we have adopted the term *feelings of inferiority*.

Since, however, the word *complex* has been consecrated by use as the synonym of *feeling* of inferiority, we shall continue to use it. The reader will have been sufficiently warned against confusing it with the 'complex' used in the Freudian sense of the term.

There is still one more point to clear up. Does the feeling of inferiority presuppose a previous comparison? Does the word 'inferior', being a comparative term, necessarily imply a comparison? Some critics of the idea of auto-estimation in psychology have objected that the child could not have feelings of inferiority, since he is incapable of comparing, of forming a norm or an ideal to which he felt himself inferior. After all that has been said this argument no longer holds good. In the first place we have shown that the expression 'feeling of inferiority' is only a terminological makeshift, and further, that a child can and really does experience such feelings, probably from the moment of its birth, without any comparison with a superior standard having taken place.

Sometimes a comparison will do away with feelings of inferiority instead of creating them. Here is an example.

A young man, P.B., who works in an office enjoys playing the piano. He is by no means a virtuoso and plays only for his own pleasure. He owns to having very strong feelings of inferiority about his playing because a friend of his, a law student of twenty-two, only an amateur, plays much better than he does. This friend introduces him to the pianist K., a budding artist but very talented. 'Before K.', P.B. tells us, 'I have no feelings of inferiority, although he plays much better than my friend. I feel only admiration for him.' And he himself explains this phenomenon, which is common enough, by saying that K. is—instrumentally speaking—of a superior race to both of them.

It would seem, then, that it is only a slight and not an overwhelming superiority in another person that gives rise in one to a feeling of inferiority. This phenomenon is well known in the psychology of hatred, which in its turn is based on that of auto-estimation. Thus the feeling of inferiority may arise as a result of a previous comparison, but does not necessarily do so. The 'comparison', which in any case should not be completely conscious, is not necessarily an act of reason. It may be made (*a*) between the present self and the selves of others, (*b*) between the present self and a superior self such as might have been manifested in the past or could be manifested in the future, (*c*) between the self and an ideal, a norm or a pattern which the self would like to resemble. This, incidentally, brings us to the threshold of the subject of duty. Finally it is conceivable that strong feelings of inferiority might be felt before the forces of nature; we know that cyclones, tornadoes and avalanches can reduce even the bravest men to a state of paralysis. Man then becomes the feeble 'thinking reed' of Pascal, and his soul will recognise with fearful clarity the utter helplessness of the species to which he belongs. It is this particular kind of weakness, this genuine organic inferiority of the individual from the day of his birth, that we shall examine in the following chapter.

CHAPTER XI

FEELINGS OF INFERIORITY IN THE NEW-BORN, AND PROTO-INFANTILE NEUROSES

IS BIRTH A BIOLOGICAL CATASTROPHE?

FOR nine months the human foetus lies immersed in fluid in the narrow cavity of the uterus. There, in the purpureal cave, as the poet has called it, it spends a purely vegetative existence, indifferent to the changes and chances of the external world, inaccessible to air, light, heat and cold. Throughout its development the embryo is in a parasitical situation. Then, after nine months, it is violently thrust out into the light and exposed to the thermal, auditive, tactile, visual and olfactory impressions coming from its environment. The close symbiosis with the mother has been broken asunder; the vegetative needs can no longer be satisfied automatically and unconsciously as before; henceforth the child must needs receive its food from outside; little by little it will develop a kind of rudimentary consciousness which will not reach its full development until a few years later. How should this expulsion into a hostile and terrifying world not produce in the new-born infant, however devoid it may be of self-consciousness, a vague impression of something extremely painful and really deserving the name given it by Freud of 'biological catastrophe'.[1] In adopting this term from the psycho-analytical vocabulary we must hasten to add that we regard the event as catastrophic only from the *subjective* point of view, that of the infant himself. There is no objective biological catastrophe as the Freudians would have us believe or as might be urged by readers of Calderon, who says in *Life is a Dream*, 'Man's greatest offence is undoubtedly the fact of having been born'.

If the new-born infant could already harbour what are called 'desires', it would probably ask for nothing better than to be removed as soon as possible from this new and terrible situation. The poets have given their own interpretation of our sad awakening from the dream-

---

[1] The finest example of this process which we know is that given by Jules Romains in Volume IX of *Les Hommes de Bonne Volonté, Montée des Périls*.

less sleep within the womb. Baltazar Gracián and many others have told us that 'we are born with tears', and psychologists have taken this as a clue to the interpretation of the myth of paradise which is to be found in Christian and non-Christian religions alike. Writers have spoken, too, of the Birth Trauma and of the Nirvana Complex,[1] i.e. the desire to return to the *néant* whence we arose, and the longing to rest once more in the maternal womb, that place of complete happiness, devoid of all desires and all suffering.

It is therefore senseless to claim, as does the Hungarian psycho-analyst Sándor Feldmann, that the new-born infant experiences in its ego a state of utter happiness and *completeness*. 'The most complete feeling of the self', he tells us,[2] 'occurs in the child at the breast, although even here there may be a certain incompleteness.' (!) The feeling of omnipotence which the child brings with it from its intra-uterine life is continued owing to the fact that at first the infant really receives or thinks it is receiving everything it may need or desire. This, according to Feldmann, is the first stage of the feeling of self. This view is undoubtedly derived from the Freudian assumption that a baby can 'do nothing but desire' and possesses only a 'pleasure Ego', not a 'reality Ego'. But this is not supported by empirical observations and is indeed in flat contradiction with what is said by some of the Freudians themselves.

THE PHYSIOLOGICAL INSUFFICIENCIES OF THE CHILD

Undoubtedly the infant's first impressions are not all of a pleasurable nature. Breathing, we know, begins simultaneously with the extra-uterine life. According to Wallon,[3] it affects the psyche's sensibility in different ways. According to him the 'birth trauma', which the Freudians attribute not only to the 'biological catastrophe' of being ejected into extra-uterine life but also to the first act of inspiration, is a pure myth. But this is by no means to say that the myth lacks any foundation. The truth is that every psychic event of special importance is marked by a change in respiration. Soon the alimentary reflexes make their appearance. (According to Preyer they begin from the moment that the infant's head emerges from the maternal womb.) Here very

[1] The term does not originate with Freud. It was invented by an English-speaking patient of Ferenczi, who subsequently popularised it.

[2] Cf. Sándor Feldmann, *Az ideges félelem*, Budapest, 1925.

[3] Henri Wallon, 'Comment se développe chez l'enfant la notion du corps', *Journal de Psychologie normale et pathologique*, vol. XXXVIII, pp. 9–10.

complex mechanisms come into play : suction, deglutition, the development of buccal activity, the opening and closing of the digestive tube, with all the accompanying connections and mechanisms. The first alimentary reflex is regurgitation. It is only towards the end of the first month that this reaction is transferred to the mouth passage. Sensibility of tongue and lips is highly differentiated and plays a considerable part in what William Stern calls the buccal period. Urinary sensibility also makes its appearance very soon.[1] The sense of equilibrium, however, does not develop as a synergy until about the sixteenth week, while the first attempts at locomotion are made towards the eighth or ninth month. And—taking account of individual differences—the baby will need yet another month before being able to walk upright.

Owing to the enormous differentiation of our species the human child is infinitely more helpless than the young of any other animal. This objective inferiority goes so far that a child of ten weeks, if it is sat up or even has its head raised, is unable to see anything. The eyes will look vague and confused owing to the unaccustomed change of equilibrium. If a child of five or six months is put in the presence of another child, it will make movements towards it as long as the second child remains in a lying position, but as soon as the latter is stood up, the first child will cease to notice its presence. This shows the outstanding importance which the sense of equilibrium possesses for the whole of our psychic life. Nothing, says M. Wallon,[2] interrupts psychic activity so completely as momentary cessation of the sense of equilibrium.

Starting from this important detail we can calculate the extent of the child's disadvantage. It is, so this excellent French author assures us, chiefly to the lack of the sense of equilibrium that we must attribute the child's latent state of anxiety which finds expression in various phobias. Added to the child's real and objective disability is its powerlessness to achieve an exact, regular and continuous adaptation to the objects connected with its activity. This shows in gaps or mistakes in all the efforts it makes, whether motor, sensory or mental. The same thing happens in the normal child's sensory activity, if we rule out the case of the asynergic child. Even in muscular accommodation we meet with irregularities, and the same disturbances exist in the adjustment and expenditure of effort in general. Organic co-ordination, therefore, only

[1] Charlotte Bühler, *Soziologische und psychologische Studien über das erste Lebensjahr*, Jena, 1927.
[2] Henri Wallon, *Psychologie pathologique*, p. 85.

comes with difficulty. Without it there could hardly be any unified stability of action, and still less the *feeling of one's own body*, and with it the *feeling of the self* in general. We are speaking of what specialists have called the *body image*—a notion which until the work of Dr. Lhermitte and his followers seems to have been unknown to all French psychologists, including M. Wallon. The child is still completely incapable of feeling any solidarity between the different parts of its body and the different moments of its activity. The feeling of the self and the sensitivity of the body are still relatively dissociated.

Now all these shortcomings which we have rapidly passed under review are of purely psychological origin in the child. At the same time the life of personal relationships which is simultaneous with them must inevitably be the source of inferiority feelings no less numerous and complex.

PSYCHO-SOCIAL INSUFFICIENCIES IN THE NEW-BORN INFANT

Even if we refuse to regard the event of birth as a trauma in the proper sense of the word, it cannot be denied that the new-born infant finds itself in a state of extreme helplessness. Compared to its pre-natal state, the infant's post-natal state is distinctly a *situation of inferiority*. Some writers have therefore supposed that the child's whole psyche reflects this complex and multilateral shortcoming. Contact with hard and soft bodies would thus produce in the child chiefly sensations of pain but also, in a very small degree, sensations of pleasure. 'It would seem, then, that this sensation of pain is the only thing that can give him consciousness of his own existence', says Martí Ibáñez, in his book *Psicología prenatal*, Higia, 1935, II, 1. There can be no doubt that in the new-born child there is a marked preponderance of painful sensations. And although we have no reason for attributing to the infant a 'consciousness' of its being in the complete sense of the term, these unpleasant sensations will undoubtedly produce in it other kinds of experiences which dimly foreshadow the existence of its ego. Clearly, this ego can be nothing as yet but a bundle of primitive sensations. Thus the 'I think therefore I am' of the philosopher becomes for the baby (and for the psychologist who is observing it) 'I feel helpless, I feel pain throughout my being, I suffer, therefore I am'.

Let us imagine[1] a healthy, well-developed baby of four months lying

[1] The following description is taken from Kurt Seelman's contribution to *Handbuch der Individualpsychologie*, 1926, Vol. I, p. 169.

in its cradle and surrounded with every possible care. In the course of its short existence it has grown familiar with sensations of light and shade, of heat and cold, with the contact of the white linen wrapped around it and with the touch of the persons who look after it. The situation of feeling utterly helpless, utterly at the mercy of what the child vaguely feels to be its non-ego, gradually diminishes. Nevertheless everything around inevitably remains a profound and terrifying mystery. There the little fellow lies, feeble and helpless and trying with his tiny feet to get free of the coverlet which is too warm. Gradually 'convinced', as Kurt Seelman puts it, of the impossibility of his plan he exteriorises his feelings of displeasure and begins to cry. The mother comes to him, looming like a giantess. The little bed shakes as she walks across the room. She speaks to the baby in unintelligible and comforting sounds, removes the coverlet and comes back to him. Her big hands lift him up. Now he feels safe and protected in a completely different world.[1] Everything around the child of a few months old must strike it as pure magic. It knows nothing of this world, even of the part that is very close to it. All it knows is the existence of a magical something which turns it into a suffering object, and of which the source and origin is the whole of the non-ego.

These deficiencies would seem to be quite inevitable. There is not a human being who has not felt helpless and inferior at least during this first phase of his existence. We remember this all too rarely. Otherwise we should have evolved a plan of education that would tend to remove these early feelings of inferiority as rapidly as possible. The task of the educator should therefore be to lead the child through this necessarily slow process as quickly as possible on to the feeling, or—if the reader will excuse the word—to the consciousness of its own worth or *valence* (to borrow a term from chemistry). Unfortunately what happens in reality is exactly the opposite. More or less consciously everything tends to promote rather than to abolish this feeling of weakness and insufficiency in the growing child. Everything tends to inculcate and develop those feelings which we have referred to under the unifying term of *feelings of inferiority*.

Adults like to play with babies as though they were playthings made for their amusement. They often forget that too rapid or sudden a

[1] We part company with the author at this point, for his descriptions lapse into a dangerous *auto-morphism*, attributing to the baby objective observations which it is far from making, e.g. 'The mother can do everything, and can do it so easily'.

movement will seem extremely violent to the child. A single gesture of impatience on the part of the mother, too swift a movement in removing the child from the breast and similar mistakes are often sufficient to throw the tiny creature into a state of distress and to surround it with a completely hostile world. Feelings of this kind due to the behaviour of those around it will be added to those 'normal' feelings of inferiority due to the psychological shortcomings we have outlined above. It possesses as yet only the rudiments of what we call consciousness, and yet, vague though its ego feelings are, it feels marked out, affected, hurt. And if we allow ourselves to endow the infant with an adult vocabulary, we may say that it feels itself to be 'betrayed' by the persons in whom it had placed most trust, the person who till then has surely surrounded it with the utmost sympathy and kindness. At this point, assuming that the birth trauma, of which Rank and Wittels have written, does not take place, something very analogous will happen which may become the starting point of what is nowadays designated as 'proto-infantile neurosis'. If it has not happened before, the expulsion from Paradise will take place at this precise moment. Whenever anyone unconsciously provokes a strong feeling of displeasure in a child at the stage of development of which we are speaking, this may be the point of departure for a desire on its part for a return to the mother as a protection, the enveloping mother of the symbiosis. Consequently, the stronger the feelings of displeasure, the stronger will be the compensating desire to restore (in accordance with rules which we shall examine presently) the original level of auto-impression, or as we shall call it henceforth, of auto-estimation. The child will have 'noted' that as soon as it has given the slightest expression of its displeasure or pain by a scream, by crying or by a gesture, its mother or someone else has come to the side of the cradle to quieten it. It has been picked up, rocked and caressed. Any need it may have felt has been satisfied. Henceforth crying, which at first was only a reflex, will serve to attract the attention of others. A child of six months, which cries when it is left alone, will cease to do so the moment it hears someone come into the room, even if it cannot see him. Of course the baby does not act intentionally and of set design, which would be far beyond its capacity of understanding and volition. In this way a function which at first was purely biological will have been *transfinalised* (i.e. altered in its finality or end) and will be diverted from a purely psycho-biological to a socio-psychological end. From the time that this metamorphosis or rather this duplication of the final 'meaning' of the act of crying takes place, the child will possess a formidable weapon in what was originally simply an expression of physical pain or a means of training the vocal chords.

INFANTILE NEUROSES AND THE PAMPERED CHILD

The number of children is legion who cry not just to train their vocal chords nor from the imperious need to express pain, but owing to the mechanism of 'metamorphosed finality'. It is their way of making adults pay attention to them, pick them up and caress them. In all such cases we may speak of a real infantile neurosis, which presents a difficult problem to the parents and other persons immediately connected with the child. For by yielding immediately to the child's desires and cries one runs the risk of spoiling it. If, on the other hand, one does not give in to it, the still very confused feelings of distress and helplessness will only increase. By taking the latter course we have at least more chance of accustoming the child to endure, to put up with disappointments and bear physical or moral suffering. This constitutes an indisputable advantage. But how much better it would be to avoid causing the evil. The evil was caused, however, on those occasions when we are obliged to produce in the child the sensation of being, not a *subject*, but an *object*, something one picks up or stretches out with a certain roughness or which one callously leaves alone from time to time. At such moments the feelings of inferiority—of helplessness and weakness—are perfectly normal since they correspond to objective reality. Such occasions should be reduced to the minimum. Instead, they are very often artificially multiplied, though in many cases owing to so small a degree of negligence that the person responsible is hardly conscious of it. But such early disappointments imperiously call for a compensation. The greater the humiliation, the greater will be the desire to raise again the lowered level of auto-estimation. To make up for the love which the child 'believes' itself to have lost it will desperately long for caresses from the same person or from another. Very soon it will learn how to 'arrange' ways and means for obtaining satisfactions in compensation for what seems to it to be lost. All these more or less unconscious arrangements and subterfuges will develop on the model or schema we described above as 'metamorphosed finality'. And it is just this craving for the mother's love and caresses which produces the semblance of what Freud and his school have called the *Oedipus complex*. As Adler's brilliant work has shown, this famous complex is nothing but the typical phenomenon of the spoiled child; while psycho-analysis is the study which assumes all human beings, primitive and civilised alike, to be spoiled children!

According to the Freudian theory the Oedipus complex, i.e. the libidinous attraction of the male infant to the mother, is rooted in biology; it is the outcome of our inborn instincts. And yet the same attraction to the mother, the so-called *Electra complex*, exists in the baby girl, where clearly there can be no question of a biological origin. Thus the male form of complex may be as little rooted in the instincts as the female. The truth is that these complexes are not, as the Freudians claim, something primarily biological and instinctive; they appear in response to a deep-seated feeling of fear, of loneliness, of dismay. This sense of weakness (so terrible that some would not hesitate to qualify it as *abysmal*), this basic distress underlying the *infantile neurosis*, finds its compensation in an intense desire for a refuge, a support, a place of safety. And what is love in the child if not a complete surrender of itself to someone stronger than itself, who will defend it against all danger? The greater the number of occasions when a slight violence has been done to the child, the greater will be its longing for love, the more eagerly will it seek the sure haven of the maternal arms and bosom. Lessing did not know how true were the words of his hero in *Nathan der Weise*, 'Ist nicht schon alles, was man Kindern tut, Gewal?' (Is not everything one does to children violence ?)

Thus we reach the conclusion that the famous and wrongly named Oedipus complex, though it undoubtedly exists in the majority of children of our present era, is not something primary, but a phenomenon of a secondary order. It is the compensation for something prior to it, viz. a complex of primary inferiority, based not on psycho-biological factors but on the small and large events of the life of personal relations. It is a socio-psychological phenomenon. It does not represent a regressive desire for an earlier phase, the life within the womb, or it does so only by ricochet; it results automatically from a social factor, viz. the relation between the child and its mother or her substitute, when those relations have taken on a form that is no longer objective or normal. The 'objective' treatment of the child (and this is neither a pun nor a paradox) is to regard it as a *subject* deserving *adequate* treatment. There are two ways of deviating from this normal, salutary and desirable treatment: (*a*) by treating the child as a pure object, e.g. by irritable movements, such as roughly or angrily removing it from the breast, by involuntary pressure, by a blow or any such punishment; (*b*) by spoiling it with an excess of cuddling, kissing, etc.

What happens when the child has been weaned? Unlike the young of so many animal species, the human baby will still be far from attaining the fullness of its powers and a relative autonomy. Even the healthiest child, free from any organic inferiority that might arrest its development, will come up against a hundred obstacles. By means of these very obstacles the child will begin to develop its ego feeling, and, conversely, the ego thus established will realise more acutely, every time the situation arises, its own weakness and the helplessness of its situation. We do not wish to deal at any length with the feelings of inferiority existing in slightly older children, and shall simply pass in rapid review the difficulties which the child will have to face, difficulties which we adults are inclined to forget, though we have all had to go through with them in our time. *Walking upright* is undoubtedly one of the greatest difficulties the child has to overcome. The process of learning is slow and sometimes painful; it is important not only for the physical development of the small child, but also for its mental life, as Karl Bühler has so admirably shown. The many little activities which fill a baby's life, such as learning to control its bodily functions, raise the same problems, although at this later age the child can solve them himself. Not one among these many learning processes but presents the child with considerable difficulty. The presence of illness or of some organic inferiority or defect will only make matters harder. The more developed in the child is the sense of his own impotence, the greater his need to be helped and protected, the longer will be the time required for the process of learning; the feelings of weakness, helplessness and inferiority will only create additional difficulties to be overcome.[1] To pamper the child is no solution; it only brings about the same emotional structure as appears later in passion—a growing desire, best symbolised by an ascending spiral. The pampered child will demand larger and larger quantities of love, tenderness and caresses, for repetition can never produce the satisfaction felt on the first occasion. And as it will be quite

[1] ' "Does every child have inferiority feelings?" is a question we have often been asked. Undoubtedly it does. But, it will be objected, can every child be discouraged? Well, I believe every educator to be capable of such a task with any child, the more so since *humanity as a whole has a tendency to be discouraged*. [The italics are mine.—O.B.] Naturally the energy required to produce discouragement will differ in each case. It may be facilitated by organic defects or arrested by favourable circumstances.' Adler, *Advances in Individual Psychology*, VIIth International Congress of Psychology, 1923; Cambridge Univ. Press, 1924.

impossible either for the mother or for those around him to satisfy this growing desire for love and attention, the child will emerge from the experience with new and more powerful feelings of inferiority.

Take the case of a baby already able to crawl about on all fours and now gradually learning to walk upright. All the objects around him represent something hostile, which could hurt him; the carpet is full of traps that will trip him up, the edge of the table will strike his forehead; in a word all the objects are hard, angular and 'naughty' towards the little fellow who will not fail to show them his displeasure, even his anger. His fear of them will grow in proportion. The more pampered he has been the less self-confidence, and consequently the less courage and agility, he will have, and he will be open to a recrudescence of feelings of weakness and impotence in the face of the objects around him. This will produce a fresh 'inferiority complex' which will reinforce the existing tendencies. It is therefore very hard for the child to get out of the vicious spiral of its inferiority feelings, and in helping him education will have a delicate and a difficult task to accomplish. His genuine and objective debility, due to the differentiation of our species, his lack of bodily strength and agility render the child a *really inferior* being both in comparison to the adults around him and to the lesser or greater tasks he has to undertake. If then his environment creates in him fresh feelings of inadequacy in addition to his existing inferiority, he will be only too ready to succumb to some form or other of infantile neurosis. The child is bound, as we have shown above, to possess a feeling of inferiority which is primal and objective because corresponding to reality; it may be regarded as a 'normal' as opposed to a 'pathological' inferiority complex. It will serve as a point of departure for the vicious spiral of new feelings of inferiority which already are of purely 'nervous' or secondary order. Henceforth there will exist in him a subconscious deposit of feelings of inferiority *in general*, due directly to, if not identical with, the sum of his concrete and particular experiences of inferiority. This substratum (if we may so call it) will predispose the child to all kinds of nervous and neurotic ailments. And if to all this we add, as we must for a huge number of children, an environment of poverty, lack of hygienic conditions, lack of proper medical care, the risks of the child succumbing to further feelings of inferiority will only be increased.

BIRTH OF THE EGO

Owing to the fact that small children have no clear consciousness of their ego, they talk of themselves in the third person, a habit which causes amusement to the grown-ups. It may be assumed, and everything points to this conclusion, that the ego begins to stand out more and more clearly against a background of chaotic sensations from the moment that a certain difference is established in the child's use of the words 'mine' and 'thine'. Most psychologists agree in dating this change halfway through the second year.[1]

From this moment something new enters into the child's relation with the world around it, which now becomes enriched with a new dimension. The growing consciousness of his own self will give the child the possibility of triumphing over difficulties or of enduring failure, of being superior or inferior to others. A *standard of comparison* has come into being. In a word, the whole powerful mechanism of auto-estimation has been released, sometimes with curious results. Henceforth the child will be caught up in the network of human relations. In this new field of action, he will seek to defend his position or to raise himself to a higher degree in the opinion of others and in his own.[2]

[1] Charlotte Bühler, *Kindheit und Jugend*, 1931.

[2] Elsa Köhler describes a very significant case in this connection. The little Anita, after having bitten her younger sister Eva's finger, is punished and apologises to her father. The latter asks her to do likewise to her little sister, victim of the 'aggression'. Then something quite unexpected happens. Anita has a 'brainstorm'. She rolls on the ground screaming 'I'll say I'm sorry to Mummy . . . to Mizi . . . to Oulga (the cook). . . .' She is prepared to apologise to everyone except her little sister (*Die Persönlichkeit des dreijährigen Kindes*, p. 214).

Mme. Charlotte Bühler commenting on this case notes that what arouses such violent protests on the part of this three-year-old child is precisely the humiliation of her ego in relation to the only person whom she can consider inferior to herself, and rightly so—her younger sister.

Without raising the question whether the 'aggression' was not already due to resentment born of jealousy (inferiority) towards the younger sister, we can see that this stupid punishment by the father was bound to do injury to the child's feeling of auto-estimation.

CHAPTER XII

AUTO-ESTIMATION—ITS EQUILIBRIUM AND ITS DISORDERS

AUTO-ESTIMATIVE INSTABILITY AND 'PROTEST'

In studying the young child we were able to assert that the deep feeling of insecurity which he is bound to experience from the mere fact of being a child, i.e. a still very imperfect specimen of the human race, is something perfectly normal. If, however, the feeling of inferiority is too strong, a neurotic *plan of life* will form itself by way of compensation, leading from a real but exaggerated inferiority to a more or less fictitious superiority. The co-existence of these two opposite poles—*inferiority*, regretted with excessive intensity, and *superiority*, desired but fictitious—causes first in the child, then in the adult, a certain instability in auto-estimative experiences.[1]

However, even the child who suffers from no organic inferiority can easily be caught up in the network of inferiority feelings. At times, he will seem the very embodiment of insufficiency and minus-value. This will happen when he is compared to adults who are superior to him both physically and intellectually. The child's wish to be on an equal footing with adults, and even to outstrip them, is, according to Adler, the force which forms his character.[2] The child will therefore find

---

[1] Storch, in the third part of his study 'Zur Psychologie und Pathologie des Selbstwerterlebnis', *Archiv für Psychologie*, Vol. VII, 1918, has tried to describe some of the categories of auto-estimative experience. He contrasts a 'typical mode of auto-estimative security' with another type, that of auto-estimative uncertainty. Weinmann points out very pertinently, however, that auto-estimative instability is a universal human phenomenon, although there may be many gradations of difference within it. Cf. also on the same subject, E. Stern, 'Beiträge zur Psychologie und Pathologie des Selbstwerterlebnisses', *Zeitschr. für Pathopsychologie*, Vol. III, p. 500, 1919.

[2] Cf. a brief study by Dr. J. Marcinowski, "Die erotischen Quellen der Minderwertigkeitsgefühle', *Zeitschrift für Sexual-Wissenschaft*, 1918, Vol. IV, numbers 11 and 12. This author, although not completely Freudian, attributes the feelings of inferiority to erotic sources. In this he is very close to the view taken by orthodox Freudians, for according to them all feeling of inferiority is due to the castration

himself obliged to take up an attitude of protest against the fact of being considered, and of considering himself, inferior. In our present civilisation the expression of 'the weaker sex' implies that formerly the mere fact of being a woman meant being inferior.

If a civilisation automatically condemns one half of humanity to feeling inferior, it is natural that all the representatives of the 'weaker' sex should, at some moment in their life, protest against this attribution of inferiority. 'Only a girl!' These are the words that greet the birth of such a being. And the words are significant, for our way of life is entirely based on man and on the virile principle. Woman's part is still lamentably narrow. Is it surprising, then, that the majority of women should rebel at least in thought and desire against this injustice, and feel 'If only I had been a man'? Now this desire often becomes the starting point of what is called the *masculine protest*, i.e. rejection by a woman of the sexual role assigned to her by nature. Flat-chestedness, the wearing of masculine clothes, a mannish walk, etc.—all these are symptoms of this more or less conscious protest.

Now this masculine protest (mistakenly attributed by M. Piéron to the Freudian school, which completely rejects it in this form) ought, in our opinion, to be completed by a whole series of other protests. By 'protest' we mean the more or less conscious refusal to accept the roles of various kinds which life imposes on us from birth. Every protest against these roles obviously comes from a very intense feeling of inferiority. Thus, there are racial protests, i.e. the rising of the individual against his racial role. The Englishman, Houston Stewart Chamberlain, a follower of Gobineau, disclaimed his English nationality and considered himself a German. Then we have the Jew who imagines himself to be the son of someone else than his father and therefore not a Jew, such as the Nazi-Jew Arnold Bronnen. Or the Jews of the *Action Française*, Pierre David and Robert Herz, fallen for France, etc., who try in this way to be 'on the right side' (see R. Gross, *Enquête sur le problème juif*, pp. 35-8). There is also the linguistic protest against the language of our birth (mistakenly supposed to be a biological constituent of our being). This is true of many bi-lingual 'assimilists', of Catalans in Spain, who refuse to speak anything but Castilian, and of the writer, Joseph Conrad, born a Pole, who learned English late in life

complex, their true 'latent' root. Let us remember in this connection that, according to Freudians, the castration complex exists in both sexes. The same thing holds good, according to Adlerians, concerning the 'masculine protest'; only this protest does not necessarily exist in everyone.

and used it with complete mastery. Finally, let us mention the social protest, i.e. the desire to belong to another class than one's own, such as we find in all social climbers, 'bourgeois gentilshommes', 'nouveaux riches' and parvenus. We must never forget, however, that there are roles that we could, in exceptional cases, reject and replace by others, social or linguistic roles, etc. But nothing can change our race or our sex. Theoretically the list of protests could be indefinitely prolonged, since a child can experience anything as an inferiority, he is always free to protest.

Auto-estimative instability will arise when a normal person is faced with a problem which he feels he cannot solve. Once faced with a task that he regards as difficult, a man's auto-estimation will immediately react and will undergo oscillations of which the degree will be determined by his preparation or lack of preparation for the desired solution. It will also be determined by the degree of difficulty of the task in relation to the forces available to tackle it. The problem which completely defeats the child A may very easily be solved by an older child or by a child B of the same age but better prepared for this kind of test. This explains the law of the ratio of auto-estimation to the degree of maturity attained. The law, says Weinmann, can be formulated as follows: *The oscillations of the auto-estimative feeling before a given problem are in direct ratio to the degree of maturity reached by the subject.*[1]

From the above we may conclude that our auto-estimation tends to remain at the same level. Every time the level is altered by some difficulty, there will be an effort not only to re-establish the old level but to raise it. Very characteristic in this connection is the behaviour of a certain type of mental patient, the schizophrenic. Once they are cured, they laboriously reconstruct their ego-feeling, and in aid of this they suppress every memory of the illness they have suffered (Mayer-Gross).

The level at which the subject wishes to fix his *auto-estimative equilibrium* rises as he grows older. Once maturity is reached the level is fixed, and only inclines gradually with the approach of old age. The problem of suicide is fundamentally only one of auto-estimation. Adler found that the suicide generally acted in response to three different motives: (1) the desire to draw attention to his ego (creation of scandal and sensation, reports in the press); (2) the intention to punish those

---

[1] Cf. also a lecture given by Weinmann at the IXth Congress of Experimental Psychology at Munich, on April 24th, 1925, *Internat. Zeitschr. f. Ind. Psychologie*, 1926, p. 271 *et seq.*

who survive, family and friends, by making them feel remorse; (3) under the guise of heroism, suicide is nothing but a cowardly flight from the difficulties of life.[1]

Recent studies on the *meaning of life* have thrown fresh light on factors which lead people to renounce life. Why are there proportionately more suicides in democratic and liberal countries than in those that groan under a totalitarian government? (T.-G. Masaryk noticed this in 1881.) Why are there more among Catholics than among Protestants, and more among Protestants than among Jews? Those are socio-psychological problems of which we are nearing the solution, and we could not do so without taking the psychology of auto-estimation into account.

The Hungarian psychologist, Margarethe von Andics, devoted her thesis to this problem: What are the reasons which drive people to suicide? At what point does life cease so much to have any meaning for them that they want to give it up?[2]

She examined a hundred persons who had attempted suicide in Vienna and had been prevented and sent to a psychiatric clinic, as was prescribed by the laws then in force. As regards the proportion of sexes, ages and professions of these unfortunates, her results tally with the generally accepted statistics, thus giving them a more universal value. She combines the *Behaviourist* method with that of the *Erlebnis- psychologie*. The hundred would-be suicides explained their decision by two hundred and fifty different reasons. A hard and loveless childhood marked the life of forty-eight of them (orphans and illegitimates). Not one belonged to any kind of group, political or otherwise (and we know what collective security these can give, being mutual insurance societies of auto-estimation). Not one had any friends. Thus loneliness

---

[1] This point of view seems to be very widespread. In a curious work *Der Philo- sophische Arzt*, 1773 to 1778, 3rd edition, by Melchior Adam Weikkard, I found a chapter 'Von dem Selbstmorde', vol. I, p. 185, which says that all suicides die through fear or cowardice, or from a lack of courage. Suicide can be prevented only by encouragement 'through every means, physical and moral'. The French Romantic, Ximenes Doudan, says in *Des Révolutions du Goût* (Bibl. Romantique des Presses françaises, p. xix), 'I do not say that it is cowardly to kill oneself, because that moral antithesis has always made me laugh, but I do say that there is a *desire to create an impression*. Believe me, my friend, I have played with the idea two or three times in my life, and when I look back it does seem to me that the hope of *horrifying the spectators and arousing their pity* at the dénouement of my tragedy played a certain part in my resolution.'

[2] Cf. Margarethe von Andics, *Über Sinn und Sinnlosigkeit des Lebens*. Thesis of Philosophy of Vienna, Gerold ed. 1938.

and the lack of 'community' contributes powerfully towards losing the sense of the meaning of life. The loss of individuality, a widespread malady in these days of standardisation, producing the feeling that one is of no use to others—this is the second great cause of suicide. For the largest proportion of suicides hales from the non-qualified professions. It is the man who practises these who suffers most in his auto-estimation, for can he not easily be replaced? To have a well-defined job, a personal talent or accomplishment, an occupation that creates real values—all this will add to the individual's auto-estimation. The more regular the organisation of his life, the less will he suffer from auto-estimative oscillations. Employees at fixed salaries are the least inclined to suicide; of these, engine drivers appear to be the most firmly rooted, for is their life not regulated in advance with chronometrical exactitude? On the other hand, all casual workers, day-labourers, domestic servants, and all those who earn their living in the so-called liberal professions, with changing incomes and uncertain outlook—all these are exposed to the danger of seeing their auto-estimative level reduced to the minimum. A young woman, a decorative artist, was employed by a large store of fancy articles for which she made the same little object over and over again—a white mouse with a black tail. '*But what I was doing was of no value!*' she declared. In Margarethe von Andics' view modern man is *ein umzingelter Mensch*, a being besieged. Frustrated in his life of personal relations, unable to derive a minimum of satisfaction from his occupation, he feels rising in himself a corroding doubt as to *his own worth*. Duties have thus ceased to be an ethical prescription, they have become the *sine qua non* of auto-estimation and consequently of mental health. Without a minimum of responsibility there can be no auto-estimation. Turned in on itself, its level drops almost to zero.

Nevertheless, the level can never sink below a certain minimal limit, characteristic of each individual; it can never actually reach zero, because, as the brilliant Austrian psycho-analyst Paul Schilder (who became naturalised in America) puts it, 'No human being could live without the feeling of his own worth'. With the loss of the auto-estimative feeling, life itself would lose all value. One could not contradict or refute the suicide's contention in condemning himself. Is he not seizing upon the last way of saving his ego in its perfection? In making his fatal decision, the suicide restores to the self the value which was thought to have been lost (Schilder) and auto-estimation—what bygone ages called *honour*—outlasts the life of the person. 'There can be no possible suicide of our being,' says Maurice Blondel,[1] which, translating ontological language into psychological terminology, we can paraphrase as 'There can be no possible suicide of our auto-estimation'.

This, however, does not exclude the fact that our auto-estimation is often subjected to all kinds of very curious oscillations. This symptom is precisely at the base of a large number of mental illnesses. Many of the fluctuations and changes in our affective tonality are really nothing but the oscillations of our auto-valorative psychic equilibrium. Nervous patients and those of cyclothymic temperament are the most subject to these fluctuations.

Auto-estimative equilibrium is not really very different from what is generally called 'the feeling of self' (*Ich-Gefühl; Sich-Gefühl; sentimiento del yo-mismo*). It may undergo very short, violent and vibratory oscillations, with the result that the individual will (according to Kraepelin) follow two opposite tendencies. He may go downwards, falling into melancholic depression, which is equivalent to saying that the auto-estimative level is reduced to a minimum, at least in appearance; or he may go upwards, rising to a state of exaltation as in cases of maniacal excitation, hypsomania and extravagant boasting, etc.

THE AUTO-ESTIMATIVE IDEAL

The fluctuations of our auto-estimative equilibrium depend to a great extent upon the postulates we lay down for ourselves, in other words, upon our *ideal of auto-estimation*. This ideal is subject to changes and mutations in the course of time, since it is the function, amongst other things, of our maturity. (Weinmann's law of the ratio of auto-estimation stated above.) What an infant can achieve will no longer satisfy an adolescent and *mutatis mutandis* the mature man bases his judgments and actions on a very different scale of values from those held by a young man. An old man, on the contrary, begins to be less exacting with himself and no longer suffers on this point, unless it be on account of his *gerontomania*, i.e. the mental disorder which sometimes resembles persecution mania and culminates in the sentiments: 'I no longer count' (in my family, in my office, etc.). '*They* never tell me anything.' '*They* no longer take me seriously', etc., etc. This is why

---

[1] Cf. this author's masterly work *L'Être*, p. 46. We find in it a confirmation of the psychological theories on the theme we are now concerned with—suicide and auto-estimation. The most unworthy being cannot but 'will himself' and persist in spite of himself.

many pensioned Civil Servants or retired business men try to keep up an external show of their former habits; they behave as though everything was as before, as though they still held their post or exercised their profession. Inferiority feelings of this kind are very common in the aged of both sexes, and we may therefore note that every age has its own specific group of inferiority feelings.

To sum up, we have found that *there is a close correlation between the ideal and the auto-estimative equilibrium; while on the other hand the said ideal depends to a great extent on age and individual maturity.*

CLASSIFICATION OF THE AUTO-ESTIMATIVE OSCILLATIONS

Our auto-estimation fluctuates as a result of widely differing causes. The oscillations may be due (*a*) to factors of a purely physiological order, such as fatigue, hunger, exhaustion, or to psychological causes, such as fear, terror, anguish, pleasant or unpleasant surprise, discouragement, or returning courage. It is precisely in experiences of this kind that one finds the proof of the great elasticity of our auto-estimative feelings. Psychology as well as psychiatry contains innumerable descriptions of typical reactions due to the lowering of the auto-estimative level, from the tears of the infant to the brainstorms of the adult. Mention should also be made of the outbursts of anger, the acts of vengeance by which human beings try to compensate for feelings of inferiority due to the lowering of their auto-estimative level.

There are, too, all the different kinds of escape—illness, first and foremost; excessive and, in such cases, useless or merely simulated activity—toxicomania, travelling, reading and even the acquisition of useless knowledge.

We need hardly point out that (*b*) certain social and political circumstances play an important part in causing disturbances of normal auto-estimation. Poverty, the feeling of being exploited, of depending upon a boss or a clique, a sense of injustice due to such factors as unemployment, economic depression, etc.—all these are so many causes of our 'inferiorisation'. The tendency to re-establish the level of self-esteem will then (so long as we are dealing only with individual reactions) take the form of crime, neurosis and all kinds of asocial activities. Psychoses also find the soil prepared for them in such conditions. If we turn to forms of collective compensation, we find the compensatory tendency asserting itself in such things as public scandals, social unrest, street fighting, lynching and local wars. All this goes to show that one cannot with impunity offend the auto-estimative sense. And this is true not only of the individual but still more of the group, such as a school class, a social class, a minority or any other kind of human collectivity.

In the social *milieu*, we have (*c*) the third group of causes acting upon our auto-estimation and often putting it to very hard tests. Any change of surroundings, whether physical or social, confronts us with problems which are not without importance for our auto-estimation. Without a minimum of security in this connection it would be quite impossible for us to face new human relations and new situations. In this group of factors we find all the phenomena that Adler in his time described with such acumen in his works relating to the *problem of distance* and that of *aggression*. (It should be recalled that he regarded melancholia as a direct aggression against the patient's *milieu*. A variant of this type of aggression is the behaviour which consists in our making a great effort, ostensibly to do someone a service, but taking very good care, though unconsciously, that the person in question never reaps the fruit of our sacrifice.)

Whenever a person arrives in a *milieu* to which he is not accustomed, such as the fiancée's family, a new academic community, a new job, a holiday resort, etc., he will have to fight, as it were, to obtain the place that is destined to him but which is not yet clearly defined in the unconscious hierarchy of inter-personal relations. The inferiority feelings are thus Janus-faced; the individual may enter his new surroundings with great apprehension and many mental inhibitions; on the other hand, the situation may stimulate him to get the better of himself and appear to be more than he is, or at any rate more than he is held to be in his habitual or professional surroundings. It may also be that earlier social valuations, of which he had previously been the object, were of no concern to him at the time and caused him no feelings of inferiority, but that now, *a posteriori*, as it were, he is troubled by the memory of them. This may be what happens in the case of a lazy and badly behaved schoolboy who is moved to another school. Once in his new setting a complete change comes about. The boy is encouraged by a better master, by more mature companions or by the inferiority of his new school-mates. At any rate, his conduct is completely changed: instead of being lazy he is industrious and he has abandoned his violent ways. He happens to meet some of his former companions and they address him by a nickname which was habitual to them. The boy is extraordinarily vexed and turns his back on them. The nickname, which he heard with delight in the past, has become as distasteful to him as a discarded garment. The same thing can happen to anyone who rises in the social hierarchy. In such cases we can talk of genuine feelings of inferiority caused *retrospectively*.

Finally (*d*) we must take into account the individual's sexual life, which is a veritable forcing-ground of auto-estimative experiences, both positive and negative. For it is chiefly in the domain of sex that our auto-estimative ideal will make its appearance, and this is particularly the case in southern countries. But although in our opinion sex, while far from constituting an autonomous system, represents only one facet of the life of relations in general, the study of the auto-estimative oscillations connected with it is so complex that it deserves a chapter to itself.

CHAPTER XIII

INFERIORITY FEELINGS AND THE
FAMILY PATTERN

ANYTHING in life can become the source of inferiority feelings, just as there is nothing which is unfitted to give rise to feelings of superiority. The best example of this is the beggar who wears his tattered rags with the dignity of the monarch. The facts are nothing; everything depends upon the opinion which the individual consciously or unconsciously connects with them. The facts are there only to act as a framework which limits the necessarily subjective feelings. But these are subject to infinite gradations according to different individuals, and even according to the changes of age, social situation, etc., of the same individual. The man who in his youth hears the opera from a seat in the gallery will, in later life, forgo the same musical pleasure unless he can enjoy it in his dinner-jacket from the stalls. A woman who scorned to wear jewellery in her youth will feel it to be indispensable once she has passed the dangerous age. The village youngster who ran about barefoot and hated to wear shoes, when he comes to live in a town would die rather than cross the road unshod. One could multiply such examples indefinitely.

In children, feelings of inferiority arise mostly as the result of sudden changes in the routine of everyday life. A completely new situation always acts as a kind of test for the child, and he will react to it either positively or negatively. He will be either encouraged or discouraged by what has happened, whether it be the birth of a little brother or sister, the death of one of the household, the arrival of a new nurse or the departure of an old one, the first day at school, an innovation in the school or class, a new teacher, his first contact with playmates of the other sex, etc., etc. The child's response to every new problem will be determined by his previous experience and by the more or less conscious estimate which he can make of his own strength. This dialectical play between constantly occurring new situations and the child's autonomous and unpredictable response to them is what will determine the ever-fluctuating equilibrium of his auto-estimative feelings. This is the very thing which Adler called the *style of life*.

Now, although conditions vary in individual cases, there are in life a certain number of situations which are more or less common to all human beings. The scale of 'responses' is theoretically infinite, yet Adler himself must have realised that if a child occupies a certain place in the family constellation he will adopt a *style of life* in its main lines closely analogous to that of the immense majority of children placed in a similar constellation. To every child the fact of being the eldest or the youngest is of the greatest importance. The directing lines of his life will develop in virtue of this situation and as a response to it. The eldest child—and we now know why—will naturally be of a bossy disposition. In life he will tend to fill places of responsibility and authority. He will be ambitious, and this ambition will be the result of his intense, though unconscious, desire to reconquer his former privileged situation of only or favourite child, the happy condition from which he was as rudely expelled as Adam was cast out of Paradise. Very often he will be a Conservative in politics, as witness the cases of General Francisco Franco and Charles Maurras. The younger child is more likely to become a rebel or revolutionary, witness Victor Hugo and Ramon Franco, the brother of the Spanish general we have just mentioned. Nevertheless, there are cases where the first-born will feel himself to be at such a disadvantage that he will deviate from the normal directing line towards crime and rebellion. Cain and Esau are biblical examples of this, while Isaac and Jacob are the typical 'good boys' of the family. Equally characteristic in this connection is the case of Karl Moor in Schiller's play *The Robbers*. In a word, the fact of being eldest or youngest born exercises a very profound influence upon the formation of the individual's style of life, and consequently upon his character.

We shall now give a number of examples from our own observation which will illustrate these principles in greater detail. It must be borne in mind from the first that the words 'eldest' and 'youngest' are to be taken in a relative and not in an absolute sense. Here is a family of five children: Robert (13), Pauline (10), George (7), Sylvain (4) and Yves (1). In the ordinary sense there is only one eldest and one youngest, but in the psychological sense of the family constellation things are quite different. The two youngest children form a separate group, in which the one plays the part of eldest and the other that of youngest. The birth of these two children has had no effect on the child immediately above them (George), because at that time the latter's style of life was already more or less fixed. He was then the youngest and had been so, in the psychological sense, for three years; his style of life will therefore be fixed accordingly. Pauline, the only sister, has developed a style of life typical of the 'second child', which we shall discuss in a moment. But what determines her place in the constellation is the fact of belonging to the opposite sex. She too has been the youngest for three years, but this was not enough to establish her style of life quite definitely. Pauline's situation was perhaps the most difficult of all, and she must have had very acute inferiority feelings owing to being 'only a girl', and to being smaller and weaker than her elder brother. After the birth of the third child, Sylvain, she even found herself, as it were, between two fires. Not only did the elder brother outstrip her in all his superiority, but she must also have felt herself threatened in her position within the family by the presence of the younger children. She must therefore have developed a kind of double 'family complex' formed partly by the fact of being the 'younger' child, and then by that of playing, up to a point, the role of 'elder' child. According to Adler's principles the general rule that we can formulate from the psychological point of view is that if the difference between children's ages exceeds four years, the style of life of the older child, being already established when the younger one arrives on the scene, will not be altered by any subsequent addition to the family. It is obvious that if the children are brought up with others of the same age, such as cousins or friends, the position of eldest, second and youngest will not be determined by blood-relationship, but by the psychological relations between the children living under the same roof. Generally speaking, the least favourable position is that which befalls the second child where there are three in the family, or in a wider way, the child who occupies the middle position. The case of Pauline among the four boys in the family we have just been examining will supply the explanation. This situation of being attacked on both sides is the least favourable because it means that one's energies have to be deployed in a struggle on two fronts—against the child immediately above one and against the child immediately below one in the age sequence. And indeed it is mostly among children occupying this middle place that we find cases of complete discouragement resulting from a two-way inferiority complex. They are generally the least brilliant, the least intelligent in the family.

We must now give our attention, as briefly as possible, to the *variability* of the situations that occur within the framework of the family constellation. Let us take the case of four brothers—Louis, Othon, Willy and Rudolphe. Louis dies at the age of ten. Othon, who is only a year and a half younger, is not slow to take his place, pleased enough to pass to the position of eldest in the family. He feels himself his brothers' 'protector' in the bad sense of the term, and he takes full advantage of the unexpected circumstance that he is now the biggest and strongest. During his elder brother's long illness he seemed, as it were, to be serving an apprenticeship for this new position, but he was diffident in the role and felt himself to be something of a usurper. As soon as his brother Louis was dead, however, these inhibitions disappeared and Othon's newly acquired power went to his head, to such an extent, indeed, that his father saw fit to intervene. And yet the child was over six years old when his brother died, and already possessed a well established style of life. We are therefore in the presence of a *change of role* within the constellation of brothers, a change which, on this occasion—but not necessarily always—entails a change in the style of life.

Henceforth, Othon adopts the style of life of eldest brother; Willy, that of the second brother who finds himself fighting on two fronts, while Rudolphe continues his role of younger brother. The respective ages of the three brothers are eight, six and five. Othon is the most ambitious, but Rudolphe is the most intelligent, whilst of Willy his parents say that he is the best behaved. He is also the quietest and mentally the slowest of the three. Obviously, Willy can hold his own against such powerful rivals only by using a weapon which they have both neglected, that of 'being good'. By this attitude he hopes, despite the lack of such qualities as intelligence and industry, to win the sympathy of his parents and of the rest of the household. To-day, ten years later, the most interesting case psychologically is still that of Othon. He wants to be a business man, somebody very straightforward and decided. Rudolphe, the Tom Thumb of the family, will probably go to the university, while Willy can only catch up little by little, and at the late age of sixteen embarks upon a musical career.

If there are children of both sexes in the family, the situation changes and there will be even more occasion for an exchange of roles between first and second children, between youngest and eldest. For, as everyone knows, the rhythm of evolution is different in girls, slower at the start and lagging behind that of boys till the first stage of puberty; after that they catch up and even outstrip the boys, and very often between the ages of fourteen and twenty-one they are definitely superior, both as regards intelligence, industry and maturity of character.

Another family we had occasion to study consisted of three girls—

Flora, Irene and Hermine. Flora has the role of the 'brilliant eldest child'. She is both the prettiest and the cleverest, and is admired by everyone. She is ambitious too, equally at home in the kitchen and at the piano, playing Beethoven's sonatas with a skill that has been compared with that of professionals. Irene finds herself fighting on two fronts between this brilliant elder sister, three years older than herself, and Hermine who is a year and a half younger. The latter is very brave, as often happens with the youngest in the family; it is one of their most powerful weapons, adopted not from ethical motives but in order to make their worth felt. Hermine is industrious in every field of activity and leads one to believe that when she reaches Flora's age she will outstrip her. All that is left for poor little Irene is the mediocre role we saw adopted by Willy in the last example. For she must seek an outlet in another field of activity if she does not want to be completely eclipsed by her two sisters who have the advantageous positions of eldest and youngest. So she turns to purely manual and practical occupations. She can't play the piano like Flora, nor muddle her way through Latin or English or German like Hermine. But she can cut out a doll's dress, she can make a hat with a little material and wire, and thus develops a practical sense which is totally lacking in her more intellectual sisters. Later, when all three are married and have families of their own, it is to Irene that the other two will turn when they have practical problems to solve, such as the dismissal of a servant, the purchase of a house, etc. It is interesting, too, to compare their handwriting. Flora's is that of a fashionable young lady who has been to one of the best convent schools; Hermine's is childish and has remained so since she has grown up; being the youngest, she will always remain the 'baby' of the family. But Irene's is original—rather heavy, and less 'brainy' than the other two; hers is the handwriting that shows most independence. Here, once again, we see the middle child taking a completely different line from that followed by her two sisters, with whom she cannot compete on their own ground.

But when Hermine is five, Roger, the son and heir, is born, and the grandmother remarks to the mother, 'Now you will no longer be so devoted to that ugly, dark-haired little girl.' Hermine's whole life may have been affected by this, whether she actually hears it or not. Such things should never be thought, let alone said before the child in question, nor before its brothers or sisters, who will be only too ready to repeat them. To do so is a real sin from the pedagogical point of view. These actual words may never have been pronounced. What matters is the fact of having felt and *behaved* as if they were. From the day of her brother's birth, Hermine must have felt that she had lost her mother's affection. Henceforth she will carry on a terrible fight against the heir, Roger, although the weapons she uses will be those of filial and fraternal love carried to excess. Roger has become the centre around which gravitates the whole life of the family, and this inevitably affects Hermine's style of life. From being the good little girl, full of promise, she becomes the 'neglected child'. Later on, one could see very clearly these two separate psychological strata formed by two different attitudes—that of the youngest child and that of the child who is at a disadvantage.

An exchange of roles in the family constellation may on rare occasions lead to a complete reversal of the situation. Here is the case of two brothers, Frederic and Victor. They are no longer children, as their ages are twenty-five and twenty-one respectively. Frederic has violent feelings of inferiority, is unable to cope with the minor problems of everyday life, and is obliged to consult a psychologist. The latter soon discovers the cause of the young man's neurosis. It lies in the most complete reversal he has ever seen between the roles of eldest and youngest. Like Esau, the eldest seems literally to have sold his birthright. The reversal of the roles was due to a long illness suffered by Frederic, whom most of his friends now believe to be the younger of the two. Victor made the most of the advantage he gained over his brother during the latter's illness, and to this day he still exaggerates his triumph. One day someone reproached him with allowing his brother to vegetate in a very modest situation when he himself was earning big money and had many influential friends. 'What', he exclaimed, 'a better job for Fritz? That one suits him perfectly and he shouldn't aim any higher.' What Victor really wants is to be and to have more than his brother. One might accuse him of heartlessness. In a general way the accusation would be unfair, but in his attitude towards his brother he is under the sway of his old inferiority complex. A friend of the family who, though not a psychologist, has a certain knowledge of human nature, once said to us, 'It will end badly, you'll see. One day Fritz will kill his brother, or at any rate he will bash his face in!'

This case reveals one of the most frequent causes of an exchange of roles between brothers, the younger taking on the attitude and style of life of the elder, and *vice versa*. Anyone treating these two brothers will think from Victor's balanced and serious attitude that he is the elder, while the fundamental uncertainty of Frederic's character will make everyone think that he is the younger of the two. Such cases are fairly often to be found where the eldest child has suffered from a long illness or has lived for a time in a *milieu* that was unfavourable to his physical and moral development. Illness, infirmity, retarded development, the fact of having grown up in less favourable circumstances than the younger brother, or of having been outstripped by a younger sister or girl cousin—such are the most frequent causes of this reversal of roles in the hierarchy of brothers. Needless to say that parallel phenomena take place in girls.

We should add that *mutual* feelings of inferiority exist between children of both sexes in the same family. It is a very delicate question and one that is often fraught with consequences for the children's style of life in their most formative years and therefore for their whole future.

Let us return to the case of the three sisters, Flora, Irene and Hermine, who are suddenly presented with a little brother, Roger. The little boy finds himself surrounded exclusively by girls who are all bigger than he is. Roger will therefore very soon form an 'opinion' on the female sex, of which he knows only representatives who are stronger than he is—his mother, grandmother, aunts, servants, sisters, including their friends, all of them strong and overpowering. Inevitably he will experience acute inferiority feelings in the presence of the other sex. At puberty he will adopt a number of 'flight' attitudes towards young girls, and will eventually marry and be dominated by a woman much stronger and more energetic than himself. He suffers from marked *gynaecophobia*, due to the fact of having been surrounded in his earliest years by women who were older than he, women who spoiled him and coddled him but also dominated him. Let the pedagogues draw the moral of the story.

CHAPTER XIV

THE PROBLEM OF COMPENSATION

THE idea of compensation plays, as we have seen, a very important part in all the theories dealing with organic deficiency and with various feelings of inferiority. The idea is not a new one and has long been familiar to biologists.

'Compensation', says M. Claparède, 'is a means or a stratagem used by nature to guard against an organic deficiency and re-establish as best it may the faulty equilibrium. Where too short a leg causes the body to lean to one side, the spine will form itself into a "compensating" curve. The heart that has a lesion will become hypertrophied so as to compensate, as it were, for quality by quantity. Where the brain has been injured, supplementing cells will be formed in aid of the functions that have been impaired.'

From the earliest times doctors have known this wonderful 'reply' of the organism, and have made use of the latter's plasticity. Plutarch in his *Life of Demosthenes* gives the following curious tale of compensation:

'They tell that Laomenes of Orchomene, in order to cure himself of an illness in the diaphragm and in obedience to his doctors, went in for the training for long-distance running. Once hardened by these exercises, he began to take part in the games for the crown (the Olympic Games) and in the end became one of the best athletes on the stretch of the two stadia.'[1]

We have here a remarkable anticipation of some of the most modern medical results.

[1] Cases are not rare of an organic inferiority leading a young man to athletic training and hence to the compensation, even the over-compensation, for his physical defect. Hungary's best all-round swimmer is the one-legged Oliver Halassy, who is also an excellent player of water polo.

Even more remarkable is the case of Glenn Cunningham. As a schoolboy he lost the big toe of his left foot and the doctors declared that he would never be able to walk without crutches. But he tried to do without them and concentrated his attention upon forms of movement. Having discarded his crutches he became interested in walking races and in 1934 established the world record for the mile race.

143

Goethe, owing to his marvellous intuition, was their precursor in a completely different field. In his philosophical poem which he named *The Metamorphosis of the Animals* we find the following verses:

Siehst du also einem Geschöpf besonderen Vorzug
Irgend gegönnt, so frage nur gleich, wo leidet es etwa
Mangel anderswo, und suche mit forschendem Geiste,
Finden wirst du sogleich zu aller Bildung den Schlüssel.

('If thou seest a creature endowed with some special advantage, enquire forthwith what it lacks in some other way, and seek with an enquiring mind. Quickly then wilt thou find the key to all culture.')

Before examining the question of compensation in greater detail, however, we must turn our attention to that of *organic minus-values*, to their classification and to the specific compensations they evoke.

ORGANIC MINUS-VALUES AND THEIR CLASSIFICATION

The notion of organic inferiorities or *minus-values* is based on a comparative or differential evaluation in relation to a norm. The organs submitted to comparison have suffered a certain diminution, a lack, a minus. These minus-values can be divided into four groups: (*a*) the morphological, (*b*) the functional, (*c*) the relative, and (*d*) the transitory.

The *morphological* minus-values appear in the defective formation of an organ, or of some of its parts, and can even extend over a whole set of organs. The *functional* minus-values appear in the work done by organs or organic systems that are not carrying out the task assigned to them. A subdivision of these is formed by the *relative* minus-values which occur whenever an organ has a specific task to carry out and is unequal to it. The *transitory* minus-values are a subdivision of the relative. Thus in the violent changes undergone by the female organism at puberty, in pregnancy, and the menopause there is undoubtedly such an increase of function for a number of organs that for the time being these appear to be defective. We are therefore entitled in this connection to speak of transitory minus-values. One could probably discover parallel phenomena in the male organism, but observations on this point are still awaiting verification.

The above classification covers only the minus-values of the body. From a higher point of view, i.e. starting from Adler's integral conception of man as an individuum (lit. 'undivided'), the arbitrary separation of body and soul is one that cannot be made. We are therefore left with two big categories: A, the objective minus-value, and B, the subjective. Each of these admits of two subdivisions. Beginning with A (objective) we have:

1. Objective minus-values of a somatic order, such as weakness or deficiency of the sensory organs, bodily malformations, arrested growth or mental infantilism, that can be noticed in the whole bodily constitution, having become localised in particular organs. This would include all paralysis and weakness due to anterior causes, chronic illness or secondary pains, loss of an organ through accident or injury or surgical operation, loss of sight or hearing owing to latent hereditary disease, etc. Speaking generally, two further subdivisions could be established here: (a) *hereditary* minus-values, and (b) organic defects *acquired* as a result of some serious illness suffered in childhood.

2. Objective minus-values of a psychological order, or those appertaining to character, are of infinitely greater importance. Under this heading would come all psychopathic cases, as well as those of 'inferior characters' (*minderwertige Charaktere*). Their study would, however, take us beyond the limits of this work.

Turning our attention to Group B, i.e. the subjective minus-values, we find that these are the actual subject of our research, viz. the feelings of inferiority proper. These admit of the following subdivisions:

FEELINGS OF INFERIORITY

They may be: 1. The projection of the organic minus-values of category A on to the conduct of the individual. An organic minus-value, although existing objectively, might remain unnoticed, provided it was not projected on to the psychic screen. This would be the case of a population consisting entirely of blind or deaf persons. An external observer of such a community would say that its members were very imperfect specimens of humanity. But since all the individual members of this imaginary nation (which exists only in a story by the German writer, J. Chr. Gellert) are equal in their inferiority, no one of them can become aware of the common defect, which comes under the category A (a) (Objective somatic minus-value not projected on to the psychic screen). But suppose that representatives of normal and complete humanity one day arrived in this country. Confronted with these superior human beings, the blind people would inevitably experience an acute sense of inferiority. The landing of the Spaniards in America had a very similar effect upon the natives, and we shall have occasion later to speak of the inferiority feelings of the Indians in Latin America.

In our example the possibility of *comparing* two different states is essential. This has led to the supposition that *all* feeling of inferiority or minus-value is due to a previous comparison with a norm or value taken as a standard to which one feels oneself to be inferior. But as we have shown in earlier chapters, this is not necessarily so, and the feeling of inferiority or insufficiency can be a direct and concrete experience.

2. In addition to the subjective feelings of inferiority caused by objective minus-values, there are analogous feelings due to minus-values which we may call *conventional*. Under this group we would place the variants below the human norm, where the minus-value is not an objective one. We have in mind a phenomenon which has received more attention than most minus-values and has been the object of special study by the Viennese woman doctor, Alice Friedmann. We are speaking of left-handedness. It would seem that forty per cent of the human race are born left-handed and that the preponderant use of the right hand is conventional rather than congenital. It is society that changes the situation. Left-handed children are always being told 'Do it with the right hand', 'Don't take it with the wrong hand', and they soon become accustomed to the preponderant use of the right hand. Training and practice make up for the lack of congenital inclination. All the same, many children remain left-handed, and teachers know what ravages are caused by the inferiority feelings which result.

Analogous with this is the case of persons who suffer from an acute sense of inferiority on account of their hair. It is not only the bald, the albinos and the red-headed who are victims. Many whose hair is quite normal will envy the blond hair of others, as frequently happened in Hitlerian Germany, where the Nordic type was in favour.

3. A third category might be formed by those inferiority feelings that are due to a diminution or repression of the individual in his life of personal relations. Such would be the case of a coloured man living among whites, or *vice versa*; also that of the self-made man, the *nouveau riche*, and even of the poor man (though the latter can adapt himself more easily to his situation by seeking refuge in religious convictions, etc.).

THE PARADOX OF ORGANIC MINUS-VALUES

Feelings of inferiority arising solely from *situation* will be treated in greater detail in a later chapter. For the moment let us turn from this rough classification of minus-values to the curious phenomenon of *compensation*. It has been considered by some as a fundamental property of life. And, indeed, every living being shows a marked tendency towards a form more perfect than that which it possesses. According to Monakow every normal and healthy being possesses the germs of perfectibility in a given material. Anatomically speaking, he calls this phenomenon 'the displacement of the function towards the skull' (Cf. von Monakow, *Arbeiten aus dem Hirnanatomischen Institut*, Zurich, t. X, 1916).

Compensation is undoubtedly a phenomenon inseparably connected with life. It is at the same time an admirable means by which imperfect individuals of all the animal species, including our own, may seek and find improvement. For are we not all, without exception, in one way or another, imperfect beings? Are we not all aware of having *points of lower resistance*? We shall confine ourselves to a few well-known examples. The man who loses an arm and is obliged to make the remaining arm work extra hard will inevitably and involuntarily develop it to athletic proportions. The heart that owing to excessive activity in sport or otherwise is obliged to work harder than normally will grow larger, become hypertrophied in order to perform its increased functions. The phenomena of compensation are even more obvious in the case of more acute minus-values, such as that of the blind with highly developed sense of hearing and touch; the man suffering from otosclerosis who, from being indifferent to music, becomes an enthusiastic devotee; the short-sighted person who takes up drawing, etc. There seems, therefore, to be a curious correlation, not only between the deficiency of one organ and the relative perfection of another, but also between the initial deficiency and the eventual perfection of one and the same organ, and this to such a degree that the process has been called *over-compensation*. In many cases, the process of compensation takes place automatically and on the organic plane itself. In many others, on the contrary, powerful psychic factors are at work. A careful analysis will show that, consciously or unconsciously, the feelings of organic minus-value gradually become a spur and a stimulus to the individual, constantly urging him towards the development of his 'psychic organ' of compensation. Physiologically the result is seen in a strengthening of the nervous tracts, both in quality and in quantity. The mental aspect of this compensation and over-compensation could only be explained by means of psychological analyses. In the animal hierarchy, man is a very incomplete being. The brain itself is only a

147

general psycho-physical organ which is there to compensate for the weakness of our species. The child who is burdened with an organic deficiency has a negative estimation of his own body and, through it, of his ego, for however young a human being may be, he always has a confused estimation of himself. The insecurity which he feels in the face of a powerful and hostile world is increased owing to the struggle to which his inferiority condemns him from his tenderest years. This struggle becomes an actual training, conscious or unconscious, and the term borrowed from the world of sport is not out of place. The point of least resistance is surrounded with all kinds of 'securities' and 'arrangements' so that the child's auto-estimative feeling should not suffer any diminution. Two sharply opposed reactions are possible, as the following examples will show.

Case No. 1. A child of seven, born left-handed. He carefully avoids using his right hand on all occasions and confines himself to the use of his left hand and arm. Neither coaxing nor punishment can induce him to use the 'right' hand. It is probable that he will retain the defect all his life. We have known several adults who, from lack of self-confidence and lack of training (the latter being only the natural result of the former), gave up once and for all the compensatory struggle (under-compensation).

Case No. 2. A child had been operated on the eye shortly after birth, thus incurring the danger of blindness. Great care was taken of his eyesight, which, nevertheless, remained weak. In spite of this his attention was always attracted to visual objects, and these aroused more interest in him than the solicitations from the external world reaching him through any of his other senses, and this by reason of the very difficulty he had in perceiving through this organ (of sight). Thus the point of least resistance is always covered up with a network of concentrated attention and special efforts. Psychologically speaking, we are in the presence of the same phenomenon which, on the purely physiological plane, builds up a greater quantity of cells than is strictly necessary to repair the damage.

The process of training in this case becomes almost an obsession, and sure enough, it is not long in bearing fruit; the eyesight becomes more and more perfect and can soon detect the smallest details. The excessive attention given by the child to everything visual, the unstinting effort he makes to receive all the optical impressions coming from the world around him (efforts far greater than those ever made by children whose eyesight has given them no trouble) result in the abnormal eyesight very soon becoming normal, and even more practised than the average vision of children of his age. We are in the presence of an *over-compensation*.

Here is a classification with illustrative diagrams of some inferiority feelings and their compensations.

1. The loss of a kidney as a result of a surgical operation determines the development of the remaining kidney which now does the work of both. The loss of an arm incurred in hunting or at war results in abnormal development of the other arm enabling the subject to make it more or less serve all purposes (as e.g. the famous pianist, Zichy, who gave recitals, playing with one hand only). This is a direct and purely *somatic compensation*.

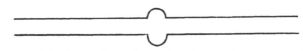

2. A wound heals up through an abundant and even superabundant production of cells by the skin. This is *physiological* or even, if you prefer, *somatic* over-compensation.

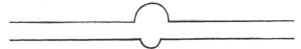

3. Complete loss of sight cannot be compensated for directly in the same organ. But compensation apart from the affected organ is possible, as e.g. by the development of 'internal vision'. It is not by chance that in mythology the Fates, justice, and human seers are represented as blind. In other cases the loss of sight may initiate a marked development of another sensory organ, such as touch or an ear for music. We have known cases of blind sculptors. This, then, is *sensory compensation*, but shifted from one sense to another.

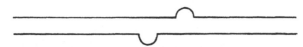

In such cases, however, it is extremely difficult to distinguish (*a*) between pure compensation and over-compensation, and (*b*) between physiological and psychic compensation. What matters most is the *degree* of the feeling of personal minus-value, for this is what determines the degree of over-compensation. At bottom, the organic inferiority or weakness does not compensate itself automatically but by working through a psychic superstructure.

4. Let us suppose a case similar to the last one described, as e.g. complete loss of sight by progressive atrophy of the optic nerve. This loss will cause considerable psychic depression and will be a serious blow to the subject. At first he will do everything to hide his condition, if not from his immediate *entourage*, at any rate from acquaintances and strangers. He is never completely successful in this attempt.[1] In such a case the development will be very similar to the case described in 3. 'Inner vision' will become more intense, but at the same time another function will develop which was not present in the former case. There will, e.g., be a powerful curiosity and lively desire for special kinds of knowledge.

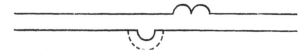

5. Let us now take a case where the defect or minus-value is really negligible, such as having red hair, being left-handed, etc. These 'inferiorities' are so only because of the subject's over-estimation of differently coloured hair, of the right hand, etc. Trivial as these things are, the subject attributes enormous importance to them. These inferiorities depend entirely on social valuation and are therefore purely *situative*. A left-handed person can undergo a training, first of the left hand then of the right, which may lead to great manual dexterity. He may even learn to draw with both hands simultaneously, which is an over-compensation. (In Spain, the case of Dr. Adolfo Azoy, the Barcelona physician, is well known. The famous Rastelli jugglers, father and son, were also left-handed.)

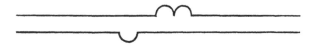

5(*a*). Let us now imagine the case of a child whose faulty education has left room for no favourable compensation of the kind just described. There will be no development of manual dexterity. Compensation will, however, take place, but only in the psychic sphere. It will take the

---

[1] A Hungarian patient (an Adlerian) once came to see me in Paris. She was leaning on her companion's arm and I took her to be ill or even suffering from a kind of agoraphobia. It was only later that I learned, to my astonishment, that she was completely blind. I have known many similar cases and they often deceive strangers who happen to speak to them.

form of great intellectual versatility; thus a kind of *over-compensation* will be realised, but indirectly and in a different sector of the personality.

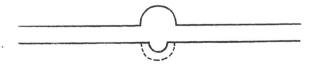

There are many cases of compensation among famous musicians and artists. These will be mentioned in the chapter on Psychogenesis of Art.

The above analysis raises a whole series of purely theoretical problems. The question arises whether a compensated sensory organ, i.e. one which began by being inferior and owes its superiority only to the systematic, if sometimes unconscious, training of compensation—whether such an organ is 'as good as' another organ whose superiority is inborn and natural. There may very possibly be qualitative differences between the two. But it is none the less true that compensation (or over-compensation) has succeeded in turning a minus-value into a plus-value. It is a process that has enabled an infinite number of persons to overcome their congenital handicaps as well as the inferiority complexes to which these give rise.

Certain famous cases of over-compensation are known to everyone, such as the stutterer Demosthenes who became the greatest orator of his time. Beethoven and Clara Schumann, both struck down with deafness, the result of a congenital inferiority of the ear which had formed the starting-point of their compensation. We shall quote more examples in a later chapter, which will deal with the Psychogenesis of Art.

We must point out at this juncture that organic variants above the norm can also call forth inferiority feelings, and the resulting compensations. (This has been disputed, but unsuccessfully, by the author Oberndorf.) Too large a male organ is functionally as inferior as one that is insufficiently developed, as it may often make sexual intercourse difficult. The same thing can be said of the hypertrophy of the clitoris in a woman, or insufficient development of the vulva. Subjects often complain of having 'too small' a male organ, although the doctor can tell at a glance that their genital organ is perfectly well developed. The dimensions of the organ vary considerably during erection, and one that is relatively small in its normal state can achieve larger dimensions than one that normally seems bigger. Subjects who attach great importance to the problem of their virility are usually unaware of this.

In general, it is never the real and objective deficiency that is in question, but always the subject's evaluation of the matter. There have been cases of twins each complaining that the other was more developed sexually when, in fact, there was no difference between them in this respect.

UNDER-COMPENSATION AND OVER-COMPENSATION

The subject's reaction to an organic deficiency (as on the psychological plane to a problem that induces feelings of inferiority) can be of two different kinds. He may 'give up the game' in discouragement, i.e. there may be an under-compensation; or the reaction may be positive, leading to results that go beyond the normal, the process we have called *over-compensation*. M. Claparède speaks in more popular terms of a *dissimulatory* or *protective* compensation on the one hand, and of a *triumphant* or *heroic* compensation on the other. The latter 'attacks the obstacle directly and overcomes it; the other is content to circumvent it'. He adds yet a third type, the *consolatory* compensation, which finds an escape in *fiction*, as in Robert de Traz's story *L'Ecorché*, a 'fine type of inferiority' who used to enjoy thinking about 'the favourite dream of his childhood . . . the dream of becoming invisible'.[1] Claparède also mentions cases of *derivatory* compensation, such as that of the unintelligent schoolboy 'who puts up a good show in class by learning his lesson by heart (i.e. substituting memory for reflexion) and by behaving with perfect discipline'. This nomenclature of different types of compensation does not seem to us very happy, and we claim to be nearer the truth in distinguishing only two categories—the positive and the negative. How, for instance, would M. Claparède classify a left-handed subject who, unable to overcome his defect in childhood, has continued to eat and write with his left hand but has (and such cases are frequent) become a first-class swordsman?

These two possible types of compensation were known to the Ancients. Ulysses, the most wily of the Greeks, is described by Homer as a man of weak physique. He has made up for his bodily weakness by an increased development of his mental faculties. His is the useful and social type of compensation, whereas that of another Homeric figure, Thersites, is useless and asocial. Finding himself unable to achieve the ideal of the καλὸς κἀγαθός, Thersites makes up for his physical in-

---

[1] Cf. the same idea in a curious little story by Henri Gallis, *Mon visage fait horreur*. Ed. Les Étincelles, Paris, 1930.

feriority by indulging his slanderous tongue, by what Janet would have called the *péjoration* of other people.

Certain cases of compensation (anagogic or catagogic, or both) are too well-known to be discussed here. Emil Ludwig has given us a searching study of the Emperor William II; Claparède (*loc. cit.*) also analyses his case; while Wilson Lee Dodd states that the deformed arm of the ex-Emperor was 'the most dangerous deformity that European civilisation has ever known'.[1]

THE PSYCHOLOGY OF THE DEFORMED

The case of William II has brought us to a special chapter of psychopathology which we can only touch upon here—the psychology of the deformed. It is a subject that leads to very interesting results, for even if the bourgeois precept of *mens sana in corpore sano* is absurd there can be no doubt that physical deformities nearly always entail certain curious mental twists.

The psycho-pathology of the cripple confirms the Adlerian ideas on every point. In his important work *Das Seelenleben des Krüppels* (Leipzig, 1921) Hans Würtz reaches the conclusion that the cripple, owing to feelings of inferiority which he is bound to experience, suffers from a very serious complaint—the inclination to think too much. Unless those appointed to the task can snatch him in time from his meditations on his infirmity, he will be plunged into the darkest pessimism. Comparing himself with the healthy and normal people around him, his attention will be directed to what is favourable for others and unfavourable to himself. He will try to escape from these depressing feelings by some of the various forms of compensation, but at the same time he will be either proud and hypersensitive, to the point of arrogance, or lapse into a state of apathy and melancholia.

Ugliness may certainly be considered as a kind of infirmity. A nose that is too big can produce all sorts of psychological complications. It is said that the Comtesse de Noailles was accustomed to show the front of her face only, as her profile was spoiled by her nose. Many blind and deaf persons try to conceal their infirmity, and they are sometimes remarkably successful. Deformity or ugliness often leads to a kind of ambivalent compensation, made up of de-compensation and over-

[1] Cf. W. L. Dodd, *The Golden Complex. A Defense of Inferiority* (New York, John Day Co., 1927). The author regards the inferiority complex as something to be defended, and cites Byron as its supreme example.

compensation, of which we have a brilliant characterisation in Rostand's *Cyrano de Bergerac*. In spite of its exaggerations and its pompous verse, this play contains an understanding of character which might partly be envied by many professional psychiatrists.

Cyrano is ugly. His 'pauvre grand diable de nez' ruins his chances of being loved. He has only to see the shadow of his profile to be reminded of it. On the one hand, no one must make the slightest allusion to his nose, for that is his 'point of least resistance' and the slightest remark will make him draw his sword. But on the other hand, he himself can say anything he likes about this highly prosaic organ. The tirade on his nose in the first Act is a masterpiece; in Adlerian language we would say it was an expression of over-compensation. Only the feeling of inferiority can explain Cyrano's ambivalence on this point. He will allow no one to mention this nose of his, as though he wanted to forget its existence, but at the same time he boasts of it ironically. As Richard III accepts being a miscreant, he accepts his misfortune. He feels incomplete and says to the handsome but commonplace Christian:

> 'Veux-tu me compléter et que je te complète?
> . . . Je serai ton esprit, tu seras ma beauté.'

Cyrano de Bergerac gives us a caricature of the deformed neurotic in general. The mechanism of compensation (whether fictitious or real) led Würtz to speak of a veritable daemonia on the part of the invalid. No one has embodied this daemonia more completely than Byron, whose work, shot through as it is with the psychology of compensation, exercised so great an influence on the literature of his epoch. Only a cripple could have become the founder of the romantic Titanism of the Romantics.

THE CASE OF BYRON

The character of *Lara* is a kind of self-portrait of Byron himself, a man who is fundamentally asocial owing to his club-foot. 'He was surrounded by a kind of magic circle which kept everyone at a distance and obliged him to lead a solitary life.' To use, for once, a mechanistic form of speech, we would say that the impossibility of discharging the 'affects' in the isolation of solitude led to an emotional accumulation in the psyche and the many conflicts which this entails. After all that the Adlerian school has told us about the genesis of sexual perversion, we shall not be surprised to learn that Byron's love-life was very definitely marked by perversity. 'I wish that all women had but one mouth that I could kiss', exclaims that Don Juan whose eroticism has been so ably analysed by André Maurois. Byron's admiration for power and energy can be explained only by his feelings of inferiority. He professes the utmost hatred for Napoleon's tyranny, but at the same time he admires Napoleon for his energy and will-power. (The same thing happened to many weak-souled men towards Hitler and Mussolini.) Throughout his life, Byron tried to escape from his feelings of inferiority. He liked being in Venice because by travelling about in a gondola he avoided exposing his limping gait to the public. He excelled in swimming (a favourite sport with the lame) and revived the antique exploit described in 'Hero and Leander' of swimming across the Bosphorus. Finally, he fought and met with a hero's death in Greece.

In the souls of such tortured beings there occur what Würtz calls 'spasmodic knots of the will and the emotion'. These lead straight to 'mystical inferiority' and the 'romanticism of horror' (cf. Würtz, loc. cit.). The deformed subject finds himself in open conflict with society, bound as he is to feel inferior to its more fortunate members and to hate them unconsciously. It is this hatred that explains the demoniacal character of the deformed 'who recognize their own image in the devil'. Very often intriguers are deformed in some way. Benjamin Constant says of Talleyrand, who was lame, 'Talleyrand's feet were the decisive element in his character'. During the last Civil War in Spain, the chief of one of the Anarchist *tchekas* in Barcelona was a lame hunchback, who was wont to remain invisible (problem of 'distance').

The intimate relation between ugliness or deformity and horror has found symbolic expression in the figure of the 'club-foot devil' and of the gargoyle, one instance of the many fiendish and terrifying masks that appear in so many religions. According to Würtz, the demoniacal character can be explained by a secret despair, for which diabolism is one of the forms of compensation; hence the abundance of demoniacal characters in Byron's works. Thus in the English poet the psychic accumulation found a more or less satisfactory canalisation in literary creation. We are dealing in the last resort with phenomena which, although they come to be woven into the tissue of somatic symptoms, do not necessarily spread beyond the psychic sphere. The mechanism of compensation is sufficient to explain them. We find ourselves almost entirely in agreement with Würtz when he says, at the conclusion of his analysis of Byron, 'It may therefore be stated that deformity gives rise to volitional obstinacy which in its turn hardens into diabolism; diabolism then becomes the subject's conception of the world, which conception is finally metamorphosed into the fundamental affective tone of the subject's life; the task thus constituted must be one of mental repression or of artistic creation' (Würtz, *loc. cit.*, p. 61).

In *Individual psychologie u. Religion*, written in collaboration with Adler by a Protestant theologian, Jahn, who had previously accepted his theories only with certain reservations, a close parallelism is established between the results obtained by Würtz and the Adlerian ideas. And indeed the results do tally, and the authors' ideas supplement each other. Each, independently of the other, has invoked the lame gods of mythology, both Greek and German, Hephaistos and Weland (or Wieland). 'Hephaistos manufactures for Zeus the lightning that flashes forth from thunder. Weland invents wings which carry him freely through the air' (Jahn, *Minderwertigkeitsgefühle*, p. 130).

SOCIOPATHS AND COENOPATHS

Although they were reached in complete ignorance of Adler's theories, Würtz's results certainly confirm these. The cripple, 'deep down, never feels quite sure of himself when deciding upon a course of action. He begins to doubt again of his own worth and finds himself obliged to repress with all the force at his command the lack of self-confidence which fills him. This repression, however, does not have very agreeable results. Self-distrust produces in deformed persons a desire for greatness which can reach fantastic proportions' (Würtz, *loc. cit.*, p. 3). From the examination of these phenomena, Würtz draws conclusions that apply to sociology in general and to the sociability of cripples in particular. 'Before normal persons the cripple is in a state of inner tension. . . . He does not want to come out of his shell. The ease and spontaneity of the community man, the good mixer (*Gemeinschaftsmensch*) are often unbearable to him.'

Würtz then makes use of a terminological distinction introduced by the sociologist Tönnies, and applies it to those cases of *diseased sociability* which he has observed in cripples as a result of their violent feelings of inferiority. Tönnies divides human collectivities into two fundamentally different categories—those that have a deep emotional foundation, and those that are organised on a basis of reason and convention. The first he calls 'communities' (*Gemeinschaft*), the second he designates as 'societies' (*Gesellschaft*).[1] Thus according to Würtz a difference should be made between 'mental' patients, i.e. those whose suffering is chiefly due to psychological causes, the psychopaths, and those whose trouble is due to a physical defect or deformation. Thus the psychopaths suffer in their relation to 'society' in the sense that Tönnies gives to the word, while the mental anomalies of the deformed arise from their inability to become integrated into a human 'community' of an affective order. Thus we would have to say that the psychopaths were asocial, but we would be at pains to find a term that adequately described the suffering due to a faulty integration in the 'community'. We should have to create the word 'coenopath' (from the Greek, κοίνος=common).

It is surprising that no attempt has been made to draw from Tönnies' two fundamental notions—*Gesellschaft* and *Gemeinschaft*—consequences that would be useful to the psychology of neuroses and to psychiatry in general. For obviously there are people perfectly adapted to a superficial and rationalised *society* who are quite incapable of achieving any intimate contact with another person. And there are others who can only live in relationships of an intimate and emotional type and are incapable of adapting themselves to the social life of the *Gesellschaft* type. The French style of life is more of the societary type, while the German style of life approximates to the communitary. Even ethno-psychology could apply the Tönniesian dichotomy with profit.

In any case, and quite independently of this possibly hair-splitting distinction, there can be no doubt that the psychology of the deformed constitutes one of the most interesting chapters in the strange study of the inferiorities experienced by the human race. For if from one point of view inferiority feelings are an infringement upon the patient's will-power, his energy and his stability, what we have seen above shows that from another angle they can be regarded as a disease of our 'community feeling'.

[1] Schmalenbach, it will be remembered, added a third type of human association—the 'league' (*Bund*). Durkheim, reviewing Tönnies' chief work, *Gesellschaft und Gemeinschaft* (first ed. 1888) in *L'Année sociologique*, pointed out that these terms, including *Bund*, are frankly untranslatable into French (or any other language).

CHAPTER XV

THE INFERIORISING EFFECTS OF INDUSTRIAL STANDARDISATION

THE increasing standardisation of modern life and consequent levelling out of individual differences has, by compensation, only exacerbated the desire for individualism. Workers coming out of a factory all look the same height, wear the same clothes, tilt their caps at the same angle, and show the same expression on their faces. Thus the factory produces its own standard type of man. In his excellent thesis *La Technocratie*, Paris, 1934, M. Joseph le Breton de la Perrière mentions an illustration in the book, *Men and Machines*, by Stuart Chase.

'The picture', he writes, 'shows a row of machines all exactly like each other, in front of which stands a row of men all exactly similar. Their right hands are raised, for they are all making the same movement, and each right wrist is imprisoned in a large ring attached to a heavy chain. We are reminded somewhat of a street in Pompeii at the time of Ancient Rome, when the house slaves were chained to their loggia. These men are workmen. When they arrive at the factory they voluntarily hold out their wrists to the foreman, who locks them on to the chain and puts the key in his pocket. The reason for this is that the machine, which punches a small piece of material they hold under it, goes so fast that there is not always time to withdraw the hand, which might therefore be crushed. So the machine gives the chain a sudden pull and the lazy hand is removed from danger. This seemingly barbarous measure is therefore dictated by humane feeling. Of course, the pace at which the machine works might be reduced, but that would mean a diminished output.'[1]

[1] The extent to which such a contraption humiliates the American workman has been shown very clearly in *Social Problems in Labor Relations*, by Pigors, McKenney and Armstrong, New York, 1939. These three psychologists worked for two years observing the personal relations between men, foreman, and chief in big factories. They found that the men are obstinately opposed to safety devices that hinder the liberty of their movements when working on dangerous machines; hence the increasing number of accidents. The workman's auto-estimation will make him accept the risk of danger rather than the feeling of being inferiorised.

Industrial civilisation is becoming inhuman, for it is outstripping the measure of man. What must these men feel subjectively, who are chained to their job, as slaves were once chained to the galleys? No one cares, the *output* is what matters, let the output be assured, *pereat mundus!*

Standardisation also entails the disruption of family life, thus increasing the general sense of instability.

'The rapid increase of large buildings divided into small lodgings is reducing more and more the importance of what used to be considered the characteristics of family life. Every five years 78 per cent of the population changes its address. This constant migration takes place even in centres where 84 per cent of the population are owners of the dwellings they inhabit' (Dr. J. S. Plant, 'Social Factors in Integration', *American Journal of Psychiatry*).

This state of things is bound to react on the economic structure of which it is the outcome. Such 'statistics of instability', as they have been called, explain many of the idiosyncrasies of the home market of the United States. 'A people suffering from so marked a lowering of its social worth and the part it plays in society will naturally tend to spend its money on the satisfaction of its personal needs and pleasures rather than on the requirements of its social life' (Elton Mayo, Professor of Industrial Research at the University of Harvard, in 'La Stabilité Économique et le "standard of living"', in *Le Travail humain*, vol. 1). We are in the presence of a vicious circle. Whereas formerly life, both in intensity and variety, was regulated down to its smallest details in accordance with the existing economic stability, to-day cyclic depressions, unemployment, and war are constant causes of instability. This factor has been duly studied by the psychologists of American labour conditions, and notably by Rexford B. Hersey, and they have found that although the fear of losing his job incites the workman to work with a better will, his output both in quality and quantity is none the less reduced. The flagrant drop not only in the social value but in the auto-estimative level of these vast working-class groups creates a problem of which, as yet, no solution is in sight. The learned professor concludes on a disillusioned note. 'Our cyclic depressions are only a reflection of our profound ignorance of the conditions that control economic consumption.' This discouragement and a sense of impotence extend from the university professor to the humble working-class masses. But the psychologists are content to go on with a great wealth of statistics, laboriously examining the problem at the surface. '1000 situations of nervousness in 120 individuals'! The result is lamentable in its poverty.

Is it surprising after all that men who were systematically inferiorised by the world war and by the subsequent shocks of economic depression should have shown in the ensuing period the reactions of primitive races reduced to the service of civilised masters? The psycho-pathological phenomena that occur in Java and have been described by Kraepelin and Van Loon are now part of the European picture. The phenomenon of *panic* can take two forms which are more or less complementary to each other. They are the *running amok*, already familiar in Europe, and the *latah*. Both are of interest to us as instances of an exaggerated drop in auto-estimation. The wild behaviour of the *amok* often takes place after serious illness, such as marsh-fever, pneumonia, etc. It generally arises in states of hallucinatory confusion, the fear of dying, or in a situation of danger. The individual then reproduces the phenomena which in Europe we have so far witnessed only in crowds under the influence of panic. *Running amok* is a kind of individual panic, an extreme response of the 'diminished' individual, in whom the feeling of impotence is expressed by violent affective changes.[1]

And yet there is also a 'gay' form of this extreme diminution of the auto-estimative feeling. According to Van Loon (*Zeitschr. f. Völkerpsychologie und Soziologie*, 1931), instances of it are to be found in 'good' society in Malay-European circles. Thus a native servant who has been frightened by her European mistress will, as a result of the affective disturbance, fall into a state of hyper-imitation. She will repeat every word she hears and imitate every gesture made before her. In a word, she lapses into a state of complete submission, which once again reminds us of a reaction which in Europe is known only in its collective form when people are gathered in masses.[2] We need only recall Hitler's speeches. He seemed to be running *amok*, and the hypnotised crowd

[1] It would seem that the *amok* belongs to a primitive stage in the evolution of the nervous system, the protopathic stage, which has been studied by Head, Rivers and Riddoch. The acute pain which we feel at the cutting of a nerve is due to these protopathic sensations (*Gefühlsempfindung*). Certain parts of our body, such as the skin of the penis under the prepuce, still retain the memory of these early stages of nervous evolution.

[2] Involuntary imitative coughing in a crowded room, which the psychoanalyst S. Szalay has called a 'collective parapraxis', is considered by Van Loon as just such a manifestation of *latah*.

seemed to be identifying itself with him in a complete state of *latah*. This mass reflex was a lamentable regression on the part of the European crowds towards a primitive form of affective life, based, we may assume, on a protopathic stage of our nervous system. That was the state to which the systematic inferiorisation of the masses had reduced humanity before the last war.

Is it surprising, then, that under the weight of the gigantic problems created by industrial standardisation man should still appear inadequately adapted to his new conditions of life? This inadequacy appears even more clearly in what we might call the labour complex, which will be the subject of our next chapter.

CHAPTER XVI

THE LABOUR COMPLEX, OR FEELINGS OF INFERIORITY DUE TO THE CIRCUMSTANCES OF ECONOMIC LIFE

THE PROBLEM OF WORK IN CONNECTION WITH PSYCHO-TECHNICS AND THE KNOWLEDGE OF MAN

BEYOND the family constellation and before reaching sexual maturity (Oswald Schwarz dates this at the age of 40!) the majority of human beings have to face a problem of paramount importance—that of work. School, which anticipates, as it were, both industrial and social tasks, is only an imperfect preparation for them. Thus the subject's relation to his 'neighbour', his relation to the opposite sex, and his relation to time[1] constitute the three major problems of human life. According to the Adlerian psychology, the degree of precision with which a man succeeds in solving those three problems is a measure of his psychological normality. The problem of the self in relation to time, the problem of work and of daily occupations (for even the millionaire must 'kill' time) is no small task for the neurotic, whom an accumulation of inferiority feelings have predisposed to 'escapes' and 'protests'. It follows that the relation of time to a man's profession becomes, in virtue of the law of the 'vicious spiral', a fresh source of inferiority feelings and compensations.

It may be noted in passing that if the current Existentialist philosophy plays havoc with the notion of time, it was a German contemporary of Goethe's, the German Romantic philosopher, Franz von Baader, who gave a very interesting account of 'the sufferings of temporised man' (*Die Leiden des verzeitlichten Menschen*). Like Proust, he believed that time has a 'corrosive effect' upon us, like 'the water of mineral springs

---

[1] 'Time is the neurotic's worst enemy', Adler was wont to say. Paul Valéry also detected this modern illness. 'J'ai mal à mon temps' is a remark made by a speaker Monsieur Teste in one of his luminous dialogues. In Marcel Proust, too, time is the great enemy that must be overcome, or suspended by music, by dreaming, by love, or by memory. Cf. our study on Proust, *Revue de l'Université de Debrecen*, 1930.

on the objects immersed in it'. A curious modern Spanish thinker (cf. my article 'Diego Ruiz, Philosophe de la Révolution espagnole', *Revue Mondiale*, 1932), writing at the beginning of the century, laid down as an axiom of his philosophical system: *Tempus est Dolor*.[1]

Unfortunately a 'science of labour' worthy of the name is still only in its infancy. Apart from the excellent work of Laugier, the late J.-M. Lahy, Schreider, and Mlle. Weinberg, who have brought about a revival of the subject in *Travail humain*[2] (a review published by *L'École des Arts et Métiers de Paris*), this new 'science' is very often nothing but a weapon wielded in the class war by psycho-technicians in the pay of vested interests. Thus Arnold Dünkmann and Horneffer, directors of the psychological department of a big technical institute in Düsseldorf, openly declared that they used industrial psychology or psycho-technics to oppose the demands made by the workers. At the same time, turning to political uses some of the propositions of the late Giese, they fostered differences between all categories of workers and employees 'so that the proletariat should be unable to organise itself' (Cf. *Thesen der Fachgruppen der Berliner Gesellschaft für Individual Psychologie*, Berlin, 1932).

Fortunately this tendency in Industrial Psychology is on the decrease. It is akin to F. W. Taylor's brutal postulate 'to simplify work to such a point that it can be done by a tame gorilla'. We need hardly say that from the scientific as from every other point of view the use of the psycho-technics as a political weapon should be vigorously opposed.

The psychology of work, like all modern psychology,[3] must entail two types of enquiry, (1) *Qua* psycho-technics, it must examine all processes of work under the multiple aspects of rationalisation, (2) It must regard the working-man as a total human being, starting from the integral conception of man as both subject and object in the ergographic process. This second part of its work is connected with anthropology, in the modern sense of the word, which means the science or knowledge of man. It is chiefly from this point of view that the

---

[1] Cf. my study in Spanish on 'Chronophobia as a nervous symptom', in the *Revista Medica de Barcelona*, Nov. 1932, and the *Revista Balear de Medicina*, 1933.

[2] See also special numbers of *Esprit* edited by Em. Mounier and Touchard and devoted to this subject, as also of *Les Nouveaux Cahiers* (N.R.F.) and the Documents of the Centre Polytechnicien d'Études Économiques.

[3] Cf. the interesting *Introduction à la Psychologie* by Paul Schiller de Harka (in Hungarian: *Pszichotechnika és Emberismeret*, Budapest, 1934). See also *Die Aufgabe der Psychologie*, Springer, Vienna, 1947, by the same author.

psychology of the feelings of inferiority can make a very valuable contribution to the scientific study of human labour.

THE FEELING OF SOCIAL INFERIORITY

The man who no longer possesses the tools which he uses for his work but simply hires out his time and his energy to an employer, has lost first and foremost the *joy of work*. It is for this reason that Henri de Man,[1] the well-known expert on the Belgian working-class movement, has stated that 'Any psychology of the working-class movement must start from an examination of the affective state of the isolated worker considered as a type, and of the normal influences of his life and work'. This author, whose starting-point is excellent though many of his conclusions can be accepted only with reservations, shows very clearly that what brings down the auto-estimation of the working-man is not so much his lowered wages as his curtailed social independence and his lack of joy in his work. In addition to this, his material security is constantly being threatened by recurring economic depressions and by the effects of standardisation. 'This process is still going on and is creating in the working-classes a social resentment characterised by feelings of exploitation, oppression, social injustice, working-class solidarity; also by religious belief in a better future life.' This would explain why 'resentment is felt against the bourgeoisie less because of its riches than because of its power'. This state of things is due to the fact that European capitalism, unlike the American brand, has been built up on pauperism. In the United States, according to our author, there are no inferiority feelings, because all its citizens are equal before the law. We may note in passing that the studies carried out by American specialists on the psychology of the workers in their country, e.g. the work of Hersey mentioned in an earlier chapter, do not lead to such an optimistic conclusion. In a word, what de Man reproaches capitalism with is not the surplus value exposed by Marxism, but an infinitely more complex phenomenon, and one far more deeply rooted in the affective life of the worker—'what modern psychology has called a social inferiority complex'. Now it is a curious fact that in the whole of modern psychology prior to de Man's study there is not a single detailed

[1] Cf. Henri de Man, *Au delà du Marxisme*, Paris, Alcan. The work has been translated into German, *Psychologie des Marxismus*. Another interesting work of de Man's is *Der Kampf um die Arbeitsfreude*. See also, for a summary of de Man's theories, the thesis of Marie-Laetitia Roux, *Le Socialisme d'Henri de Man*, Paris, 1938.

study of this complex in a sense remotely resembling that given to it by de Man. We therefore have only his own statements to go by. Actually, de Man, who is quite familiar with Adler's work,[1] would seem to be the first to have tackled the theory of this so-called social inferiority complex, and he therefore deserves that we should pause to examine his interpretation of this widespread social ill.

De Man admits the existence of an 'instinct of auto-estimation' which he claims to be identical with the English 'self-assertion' and the German *Geltungsstreben* (actually the term was used exclusively by Adler, *Selbstwertgefühl* being more in use with other German psychologists). The nearest French term would be *amour-propre*, but our author rightly considers it as not giving exactly the same meaning as the words in the other languages. This instinct of auto-estimation which, he asserts, colours all the animal instincts in man, could be defined as 'the disposition which causes men to seek those affective states that are accompanied by a heightened sense of their personal worth, and to avoid states of the opposite nature'. Pursuing his idea with more consistency than does Adler, he hastens to add:

'This is essentially the social instinct . . . We must beware of confusing it with pride (*amour-propre*) in the popular and negative sense of the term which identifies it with vanity. It can be the mainspring of the most sublime as of the basest actions, for it is morally neutral, as are all the instincts. . . . Thus it is by means of the instinct of auto-estimation that our conscience exercises its activity, i.e. that we make judgments of value, or give effect to our innate or habitual estimates of right or wrong. . . . In civilised man the instinct of auto-estimation absorbs all the others into itself, as it were, or at least it does so in so far as it

[1] Cf. Henri de Man, *loc. cit.*, p. 137: 'This orientation, that namely of the American instinctive school, is very similar to that of the so-called Individual Psychology. Adler's fundamental idea is that most nervous disturbances can be explained by a discouraged communal feeling and by the compensating wish for reassurance through artificially exacerbated auto-estimation. There is no difficulty in making this the basis of a social conception, in which the point of view of mental health will coincide with that of social ethics: to be well one must cultivate altruism. The psychology of Alfred Adler certainly seems the boldest attempt that has yet been made to justify a thesis of social morality from the standpoint of the advanced biological sciences. The attempts at systematisation that have been made on this basis are, however, too imperfect to enable us to conclude that this ambitious plan can be carried out successfully. The causal synthesis that Adler looks for, in other words, the justification of ethics by mental hygiene without the help of a metaphysical scale of moral values, is a thesis that still remains to be proved.'

proceeds from emotional reactions capable of being excited by ideas associated with the notion of the self.'

This instinct arouses a complete transfinalisation or transmutation (in the Darwinian sense) of the activities emanating from more primitive instincts.

'Our industrial civilisation, imbued as it is with the spirit of individualism which makes an idol of the thinking ego, and of competition the supreme law of preservation, has brought about a widespread release of this instinct of auto-estimation. The great majority of neuroses and psychoses in this epoch of nerves and neurasthenia is due to the repression of this instinct.'

Any repression of the instinct in question inevitably leads to the birth of an inferiority complex, and this complex is equivalent to a diminution in self-appreciation.

'This does not necessarily mean that one forms an unfavourable judgment of oneself; one need only feel it in the form of an emotive appreciation. The inferiority complex engenders resentment of the real or imputed causes of this disagreeable appreciation. It tends to bring about the performance of actions which will eliminate the causes of this unpleasant state and thus deliver the subject from his depressed feeling of self.'

It is gratifying to see that the language adopted by M. de Man is free from the pseudo-rationalism which falsifies the writing of most French psychologists. At the same time he sees very clearly that the resentment is not, as the late Max Scheler supposed, the same thing as the feeling of inferiority, but that the latter is the psychological root of the former. This is what Roffenstein (too soon lost to science) meant when he said that 'resentment had its origin in an unadmitted inferiority or insufficiency, whether imaginary or real, whether personal or objective'.

Unfortunately, in trying to explain how 'the inferiority complex . . . tends to compensate for a diminution of auto-estimation', de Man seems to be saying that a complex compensates itself (see above his definition of a complex, quoted from p. 24 of his book). Nor can one see why the compensatory representation of a complex is always a 'representation of the will', for there are also illusory compensations, such as day-dreaming, turning to useless and asocial activities or to neurosis. The Freudian idea of repression seems to be in unhappy partnership with the inferiority complex here, in spite of the fact that the two ideas come from two different and even opposed ways of thinking.

Nor does one see exactly how de Man manages to bridge the gap between the individual inferiority complexes examined in the auto-biographies of a certain number of workmen, and the same social inferiority complex which he assigns to the whole of the working-class. This is what proved the stumbling block of the Adlerian school, and de Man does not seem to have been more successful in dealing with it, despite his valuable contribution to working-class psychology.

The fact remains, however, that the working-class, as such, is inferiorised because, according to our author, it feels itself to be so. Its inferiority complex 'arises from the fact that the conditions under which the men live and work interfere with the satisfaction of a whole set of instinctive and habitual needs, and thus bring about a chronic repression of auto-estimation'.

Thus the whole of the working-class movement is nothing but a form of compensation for the vast inferiority complex which besets the toiling masses of Europe. Another form of compensation is the fanatical interest in sport, which is nothing but a quest for the imaginary exaltation of the ego by means of the psychological tension inherent in struggle and adventure. The less initiative is required of a man in his work and the more he is inferiorised, the more in consequence he will tend to become a sport 'fan'. Where work is most unskilled, as among dock labourers and factory hands, the cinema constitutes another form of collective compensation. In view of all these facts, de Man believes that the chronic discontent of the working-classes has causes that go far deeper than the question of wages or the unequal distribution of wealth. The cure for the social inferiority complex 'is something more than an economic question'; it is related to the question of auto-estimation rather than to that of self-interest.

The inferiority feeling arising from the situation of the modern working-man is 'identical neither with the idea of political inequality nor with that of economic exploitation. . . . The state and the work-shop are not the whole of society. From the start, the workman feels himself inferiorised by something more than his lack of political rights and the unfair distribution of surplus value.'

The man of independent income who voluntarily enters the ranks of labour in order to study its conditions will never 'in spite of his horny hands and soiled garments feel the moral humiliation of social inferiority'. De Man made the experiment himself, and the few days when he was obliged to work, not as a dilettante, but actually for his bare subsistence, taught him more about the working-man's mentality than he would have learned in ten years of the most arduous amateur work (European and American 'Jacques Valdours' should take note of our author's judicious observation). 'The insecurity of his existence, the uncertainty of getting work, and the resulting state of chronic anguish—these are the essential marks of the social inferiority of the working-man.'

Omnia ex opinione suspensa sunt (Seneca). M. de Man repeats *ad nauseam* the theme of the Stoics which Adler recalled in connection with the inferiority feelings of the individual. He claims that if the working-class ceased to believe in its inferiority the result would be a real inferiority, but *without* the accompaniment of a disagreeable complex, *without* resentment, a condition we find in the 'Untouchables' of the Indian caste system. Since the publication of de Man's book other more practical politicians have tried to apply his ideas on a vast scale. Nazi-ism, by placing the Jew or the 'negroid' Frenchman, or other 'inferior' people occupying German *Lebensraum*, below any Aryan member of the *Volksgemeinschaft*, succeeded in considerably reducing the inferiority complex of the German working-classes. The question will always remain as to how long this provisional and fictitious solution of the class struggle would have lasted.[1]

'The feeling of social inferiority of the working-class', continues M. de Man, 'rests on three assumptions. First that the working-class must regard itself as constituting a class in a permanent manner; secondly that it must look upon the situation of the non-working classes as an enviable one, thus establishing a hierarchy of inferior and superior classes; thirdly that this hierarchy must be regarded as not immutable, thus allowing the lower classes to hope for a general social levelling' (p. 65).

A different belief, our author pursues, would create a different social situation and thus transform the working-man's social inferiority complex into a feeling of superiority. It seems that such a transformation may have taken place in Russia (*vide* Stakhanovism), but it remains to be seen whether such a feeling of superiority is not, just as in the mental life of the individual, merely a compensation for what was originally a feeling of inferiority. The sane opposite of, and real cure for the feeling of inferiority is, as we have already said, a 'sense of being' (*sentiment de l'être*).

[1] Written in 1939.

For was not the feeling of superiority of the German crowds, due to their identification with the Führer-God, built on sand? Such a feeling of superiority will save no one from suddenly falling into the most acute inferiority complex; on the contrary it predisposes him for such a lapse. According to M. de Man's own testimony,

'Millions of people in Germany passed abruptly, and without a transitional stage, from the feudal subjection of the peasant to the neo-feudal subjection of the workman to Big Business. They felt themselves to be Proletarians, and as such, members of a class needing protection, before they could feel themselves men, citizens or individuals. *Their inferiority complex was from the first a class complex.* . . . With them the individual vindication was derived from the class vindication, whereas with their Western neighbours the class vindication was only the integration of individual vindications.'

In giving the resumé of Henri de Man's ideas on the importance of auto-estimation and its effects on the working-man and in the labour movement in general, we shall not repeat all the criticisms that they aroused on the part of the Adlerian school, and still less those that came from his political opponents. With him unquestionably rests the honour of having first attacked the vast problem of modern working-class conditions from the point of view of the psychology of auto-estimation. It was by a cruel irony that his ideas, those of a moderate socialist, should have been first applied by a totalitarian regime, which under-took on a vast scale to alter the workers' mental superstructure, though it was unwilling and unable to ameliorate the existing substructure of their lives.

INFERIORISATION OF THE UNEMPLOYED

In the decade that preceded the last war interesting evidence of the 'inferiorisation complex' was supplied from within the working-class concerning that section of it which had lost even the provisional security of work and pay—I mean the vast army of the unemployed. De Man has pointed out the dangerous part which unemployment plays in the inferiorisation of the workman; other studies supply us with an instructive account of the mental state to which the unem-ployed are reduced during periods of prolonged economic depression.[1]

[1] Mme. M. Jahoda and H. Zeisl, *Die Arbeitslosen von Marienthal*, Leipzig, 1933. G. Jacquemyns, "Les Conséquences psychologiques du chômage", *Revue de*

A profound resignation, a kind of *taedium vitae*, takes possession of the unemployed worker. It is not confined to his private life; his political interest drops to zero, social groups disintegrate, and instead of feeling the urge to take part in political activity the individual turns to the cheap compensations of gambling and drink. One by one his links with society are severed (a process which incidentally has no analogy with the neurotic who is the victim of complexes). From being a member of society he has become an atom devoid of individuality, for he no longer has a place in the social hierarchy. The unemployed man turns in on himself and his moral backbone is broken. Economic impotence is more distressing than any other. All the securities with which he had thought himself protected have proved useless. He is obsessed with the feeling that the individual is nothing, the state everything. Henceforth he is ripe to become the supporter of any kind of totalitarian regime, though with its vast bureaucratic organisation it is the opposite of a genuine human association. All the psychology in the world is powerless to help. The man is 'prepared'; he is only too willing to enter a labour camp or any other pseudo-military organisation.

In speaking of unemployment we must not forget the 'odd job' men or casual workers who may be regarded always as potentially unemployed. It is a case with them of a profound sense of impotence rather than of an inferiority complex. They, far more than workers who have a regular and continuous job, are exposed to *assécurose*, to the neurosis of accident, and to all kinds of escapes because of the extreme instability of their instinct, or rather their *sense*, of auto-estimation.

SHOULD INFERIORITY FEELINGS BE ELIMINATED?

We may well ask ourselves what sort of a world it would be in which everyone was 'assured' and free from all feeling of insecurity. At the 1947 Health Education Conference of the American Academy of Medicine, Dr. W. W. Bauer, director of the Bureau of Health Education of the American Medical Association, aptly pointed out that 'in recent years the trend has been to try to get away from fear as the basic motivation', and he goes on to ask what kind of a world we should have if safety really came first.[1]

l'Institut de Sociologie, Brussels, 1934. It should be noted that unemployment is due not so much to technical progress as to lack of skilled qualifications among a large section of the workers.

[1] W. W. Bauer, *Motivation in Health Education*, New York, Columbia Univ. Press, 1948.

In Spain no workman can be dismissed unless he has been guilty of a serious offence. The result is deplorable and the output has fallen excessively. This law was due to the fact that wages were very low—below the cost of living. But psychologically the worker (pompously named *producer*, just as formerly the Hungarian peasant was euphemistically called 'small agrarian'), who is thus assured of not losing his job, shows no ambition or initiative. The provision of a minimum security, inspired by a sense of social justice but resting on a mistaken psychology, is therefore completely negative in its results. And to think that a Spanish so-called sociologist recently asked the State to go a step further and to convert all the workers into state employees! A world of absolute security, both social and economic, even if it could be realised, does not seem desirable either from the social or from the psycho-hygienic viewpoint.

AFFECTIVE CONDITIONS THAT ACCOMPANY WORK

It will perhaps be instructive at this point to reproduce a schematic table drawn up by the German specialist in psychological problems of labour, Dr. W. Eliasberg. In it he seeks to correlate the affective states produced by non-autonomous work with endogenous psycho-pathological affective states.

PRIMITIVE AFFECTIVE STATES OF DEPRESSIVE MANIACS	AFFECTIVE STATES OF THE PAID WORKER
Religious experience, ideas of guilt, ecstatic experiences.	Abstract feeling of duty; feeling of insufficiency.
Primitive sexual affects.	Tendency to assert oneself; vanity.
Fear; depression without motive or object.	Feeling of being exploited, oppressed, and made dependent.
Depression with attacks of rage.	Bitterness, envy, desire for possession.
General type: Affects devoid of object. Appearance of unmotivated feelings which spread to the whole psycho-physical person. This explains why the feelings can be expressed without any inhibition, thus leading to the popular opinion that the insane are closer to the primitive and ancestral sources of life.	*General type:* Existence of feelings of which the causes have real existence: hatred of the exploiter. Inhibition of any exteriorisation of the feelings, which explains why the *whole* person is not affected: the individual can still control himself. The affects are violently repressed.

(Cf. Eliasberg, *Grundriss der Arbeitspsychologie*, Leipzig, 1924, p. 24.)
Yet in examining the question of work from the standpoint of the

171

psychology of auto-estimation we should be wrong to think that only the working-classes suffer from feelings of inadequacy, impotence, and inferiority. Those who occupy posts of authority are, in principle, no more exempt from such afflictions than is the humblest of their workmen. Such a personal crisis will, however, take a different form in a captain of industry from what it does in a manual worker.

M. de Man, the late Célestin Bouglé and others have shown very clearly that the love of risk, the will to power, the desire for authority act as very powerful factors in the mentality of business men and in particular of those at the head of big private concerns. For such a man's work will naturally give him ample opportunity to satisfy the needs that arise from the categorical imperative of auto-estimation—a satisfaction that is denied to the great majority of industrial workers. But if the workman is dependent on his superior, both are dependent upon the state of the market and all the complicated processes of our economic system, the interconnections of which are often no clearer to the mind of the chief than they are to that of the workman. The more a man owns, the greater his fear of losing it, and psychiatrists long ago pointed out how easily industrial chiefs, who have to bear such heavy responsibilities, are inclined to neurasthenia (Hellpach, 1924), whereas the wage-earner is more inclined to hysteria. These terms have nowadays lost much of their meaning, but the fact remains (let the reader remember the French strikes and lock-outs of June 1936, and the ensuing panic) that masters and men, owing to the mutual inferiorisations inherent in their relation to each other, work up between them a kind of collective neurosis à deux. It is not without cause that 'industrial relations' have become the subject of such careful observation in the United States, where psychologists have invaded the workshops to carry out long-term investigations. Three of these—Pigors, McKenney and Armstrong—have given an excellent report of their observations. Refraining from all argument or polemics, they have confined themselves to stating the facts. Is not modern enterprise, they ask, a field in which tendencies of an extra-economic nature manifest themselves, in which purely personal desires and ambitions have play? The situation our industrial chiefs have to face when confronting their workers, so these authors claim, is as dangerous as that of 'an air pilot flying blind'. The non-solution of this problem 'might well lead to a collapse of the whole system'.

Thus the all-powerful bosses, the big capitalists, the captains of industry are also—I am not saying this to enlist the capitalist sympathy—

exposed to the shock of attacks on their auto-estimation. Eliasberg attaches a certain importance to the fact that such men, especially the 'self-made', suffer from a sense of inferiority towards intellectuals, who regard them as 'Philistines'. Such a naïve view might have been held before 1914, but not to-day.

Nevertheless, the fierce hatred that surrounds them, inspired by the envy of the dispossessed, even if it hardens these men, cannot fail to break down their auto-estimation up to a point. All this will probably arouse in them a 'superiority complex', but we know how easily this complex can assume a negative form. Nor must we forget the fierce competition, both national and international, which still obtains in the business world in spite of the rapid growth of trusts and syndicates.

At the dawn of the capitalist era, according to the remarkable studies of Max Weber, the industrial chiefs still had the support of religion, since it was on the soil prepared by religion that capitalism took root. But to-day this support is failing, and the captains of industry are involved in an inexorable competitive struggle. The result is a state of tension which may lead to nervous breakdown of greater or lesser magnitude according to the subject's predisposition (the result of infantile inferiority feelings) and to his capacity for resisting inferiorising events.

Nothing could be further from my mind, however, than the attempt to establish a parallel of any kind between the vulnerability of the employer and that of the worker in the matter of auto-estimation. The rich are infinitely less vulnerable than the poor, the commanders than the commanded. The advantages are all on the side of the 'haves' as against the 'have-nots', and cannot the *Beati possidentes* always add to the many safeguards that protect their auto-estimation the final luxury of culture?

Nor must it be thought that work carried out in a state of complete dependence, such as that of industrial workers, need necessarily lead them to neurotic conditions. True, it is hard for them to escape from their inferiority complexes, because the class struggle, so Eliasberg[1] categorically asserts, cannot be *discharged* as the Freudian complexes are said to be released (*Abreaktion, abreagieren*). The working-class, therefore, has recourse to all kinds of compensations, suitable and unsuitable, real and fictitious. We shall add a few to those already mentioned in connection with the ideas of M. de Man.

[1] Cf. W. Eliasberg, 'Der Arzt und das Wirtschaftsleben' in *Psychologie und Medizin*, III, 1928, Stuttgart.

Hatred of the bourgeoisie is one of the most characteristic of these compensations. Its function is to act as a prop to security. The class struggle, like neurosis, and even like many purely physical illnesses, is in a sense its own cure. This struggle and the successive gains of the working-class in the matter of social reform have considerably reduced the psychological gap that until fairly recently still stood between bourgeois and proletarian. Are not workmen on holiday with pay visiting the same seaside resorts as their masters more likely to recover their auto-estimative equilibrium than those who never get any holidays at all?

Among other institutions that help to repair the harm done by the 'work complex' we may mention trade unions, insurance societies, unemployment clubs, co-operative and sports clubs. A political party has also been called a collective safeguard against feelings of inferiority, and Eliasberg stresses the compensatory value of speech and gesture in Latin peoples. In districts where the economic system is still that of early capitalism—small business concerns with a limited number of workers (as in Spanish Catalonia)—emancipation by culture was until recently still the fashion. The compensation was an easy one, because in the absence of an established middle class and of any secondary education worthy of the name, the workers, who were generally very gifted and spoke a language common to both upper and lower classes of society (such is the wonderful democracy of the Catalan and Spanish tongues), could easily equal and even surpass the cultural level of their petty bourgeois masters.

Before closing this chapter we must mention the interesting experiment made by the Czech industrialist Bata, who began life as a shoemaker. In his factory he contrived a skilful combination of workshop and technical school, of work and education or amusement. He did this by a system in which the workers shared in the profits, and thus created a certain spirit of competition between the different workshops of the factory. By trying to interest his workmen in every phase of production, by teaching them the meaning of each operation, without any previous commercial instruction, Bata[1] hoped to transform the mentality of wage-earner into that of an employer. It was his merit to have understood that by eliminating any irritation of what M. de Man calls the instinct of auto-estimation and by combining a team spirit of close

[1] For further information cf. M. Vitèzslav Rec's legal thesis, *Essai de Rationalisation industrielle—La Maison Bat'a*, Toulouse, 1930, and *L'Expérience Bat'a*, by M. H. Dubreuil, Grasset, 1937.

collaboration with a clear understanding of every process of manufacture (from the purchase of raw materials to the sale of the finished product, including even a knowledge of the state of the market) he had found the way not only to social peace but to a successful conduct of his business. In the technical schools housed in the factory itself young workers, while earning their living, were trained from the age of fourteen in a spirit of austere self-government. 'In order to ensure the success of his enterprise he took psychological factors into account.'

In conclusion, the problem of the work complex which we have only outlined here is still very far from finding its exact formulation, still less its correct solution. If, in his *Psycho-therapy of Accident Neurosis*, Eliasberg advises psychiatrists to see to it that the workmen 'express themselves' in singing, in debating societies, in amateur theatricals, etc., in order to avoid the harmful effects of inferiorisation, it is obvious that this is only a treatment of the symptoms. The remedy is still lacking that would attack the trouble at its roots. There is a regrettable lack of interest on the part of working-class movements in the problem of inferiority feelings, individual and collective, though the question is being taken up by psychologists and sociologists on both sides of the Atlantic. In conclusion we may say, in the words of one of Adler's disciples, 'We do not begin to realise what a barrier the feeling of inferiority is, and how it arrests the onward march of the proletariat'. The feeling of inferiority is discharged (*abreagiert*) in the wrong way. The proletariat indulges in illusory over-estimation and in the 'bourgeois protest', which means that the workers accept and over-estimate the bourgeois scale of values. They adopt the external ways of bourgeois life, and unconsciously make bourgeois aims and ideals their own. On this point Adlerian psychology is awaiting more material before it can give fruitful results.[1]

[1] Cf. Dr. Paul Krische, 'Die psychologische Erweiterung des Marxismus', *Intern. Zeitschr. f. Ind. Psych.*

CHAPTER XVII

THE COMPENSATORY FUNCTIONS
OF CIVILISATION

I N this distracted world, with its crumbling foundations and growing insecurity, modern man has nevertheless at his disposal a choice of compensations far richer than that available to his forebears. For a small sum of money the doors of the modern 'dream factory' will open wide to him and there he can identify himself with Tyrone Power or any other film star who, in spite of every obstacle, always ends by winning the most beautiful girl in the world; or with any of the characters who live in houses more sumptuous than the kings' palaces of yore; or with the G-men who always end by killing or capturing the gangsters. At home he can turn on the radio and enjoy the music from the Savoy Hotel, from a music hall, or from the classical concert hall.

But perhaps the most powerful of these modern compensations is one which exercises both a physical and a mental effect—the cult of speed. Adler always told his pupils that modern man, in his cult of speed, was seeking to identify himself with God (*Gottähnlichkeitstendenz*). This explanation is perhaps a psychologist's rationalisation, for the effect of speed is really pre-psychological.

Those who are in a position to investigate the cause of street accidents know very well that the great majority are due to fast driving that is nearly always unnecessary and lacks motivation. Does this mean that all these are cases of 'accident neurosis', which is well known to psychiatrists and to which we have already made allusion in our study 'Psicoanálisis del automovilismo' (*Europa*, No. 5, 1935, Barcelona)? By no means. And if 'the tendency to resemble God' were what stimulated those who cause all these accidents, no doubt they would prefer the aeroplane to the motor-car or motor-cycle. And yet the aeroplane, which enables us to soar above vast regions and to develop a very high speed, intoxicates us far less than the vehicles that cover the ground and give us strong feelings of *subjective* speed. Sail-boats, speed-boats, skijöring, and other 'harnessed' sports, such as surf-riding, produce a great sense of speed, and this is obviously sought after for other reasons than from the wish to resemble the Deity. The favourites in this respect are the motor-cycle on the road and the speed-boat on water. It is on them that one can best appreciate speed, and what is even better—*acceleration*. For, as a connoisseur on the subject asserts, 'it is *extra* speed rather than speed itself that acts on our senses' (Marcel Stani Ducaut, 'La Vitesse', in *L'Aérophile*, Nov., 1939). And he adds, 'The impression of speed can be enjoyed much better after a good meal, which, by nourishing the organism, enriches its experience'. It may be added that a large number of road accidents can be laid to the charge not only of too succulent a repast but to too great an indulgence in alcoholic drink.

There can be no doubt that we have here a purely gratuitous compensation for inferiority feelings. 'The driver attributes to himself', says the author, 'the power and the merits of his machine. This illusion is fairly universal, for in this way the strong keep their habit of domination and the weak find an artificial means of satisfying their desire for superiority.'

Indeed, if we have the shillings to pay for it, a ride in a taxi can supply us with a cheap dose of superiority. Those small doses are sought after by far more people than one would think. We all know the man who somehow (no doubt unconsciously) 'arranges' to start too late and thus finds himself obliged to take a taxi and arrives at the last moment. These arrivals at the last moment are a very easy form of compensation.

Another of these gratuitous compensations—although it costs a good deal of money nowadays—is *tobacco-smoking*. A painstaking study carried out by the Hungarian professors Schiller de Harka and J. Varga on the motives and habits of tobacco smokers in Budapest throws some interesting light on the subject. Apart from its pleasant physiological effects, smoking is determined by a number of psychological motives. The two Hungarian specialists, one a psychologist, the other an economist, point out the enormous part played by our feelings of inferiority in the establishment of our habits. Smoking is pleasant, they tell us, chiefly because of the agreeable forgetfulness it brings with it; although this is in the main a physiological effect. 'Habit is another important reason. There can be no doubt that for those who have contracted the habit, not for pleasure but under influences of a social nature, the fact of smoking possesses a value due less to its actual effect than to the personal tradition that binds the individual to an inveterate habit. Every act resulting from an old habit has a certain familiar character which makes a man feel that in the midst of all the uncertainties of life he can find a certain stability within himself.' The use of tobacco, moreover, with its complicated ritual, is peculiarly fitted to establish all kinds of habitual movements. Those persons will therefore take to it more easily who are inclined to mannerisms and stereotyped gestures and who like to express their personalities by purely external traits.

Questioned as to the motives which urged them to contract the habit, a large proportion of smokers of both sexes alleged reasons which the authors collected under the inclusive name of 'infantilisms'. The answers they gave were, 'to seem grown up; from childish cunning; from vanity; to boast; to impress women; because it is elegant; because it struck me as virile; from thoughtlessness, etc., etc.' These results lead one to consider smoking as a substitute 'inadequate' action which takes the place of other 'adequate' actions. Now in those cases where the smokers themselves allege an 'infantile' reason it is not so much a case of performing a substitute adequate action as of showing a *tendency to opposition*, arising from a lack of adequate actions. 'In childhood pranks, in the tendency to impress other people, etc., we see the signs of a certain revolt against authority which expresses the opposition of the person suffering from inferiority feelings. Thus when an adolescent smokes "as a lark" or when a man of humble status does so in order to impress a woman, we are in the presence of an inadequate act which apparently confers a greater superiority on the smoker than he would have normally if he were in fact virile, rich, adult, etc.' After a passing reference to Ortega y Gasset, our authors proceed to remind us of the series of habits—inexpensive but showy—which modern technical invention puts within reach of the masses. In our terminology we would call them 'gratuitous compensations' for feelings of inferiority. It should be noted, moreover, that the motives which led young men to smoke in the past no longer obtain to-day. Far fewer men than women owned to smoking for 'infantile' reasons, the explanation being apparently that 'men possess a much stronger inadequate desire for power than women'. Here, too, it would seem that women will soon catch up with men, for their participation in this gratuitous compensation is on the increase.

It is highly probable that our civilisation will seek to add to the number of these gratuitous compensations in so far as the international situation will allow.

We mentioned in an earlier chapter several of the typical forms of compensation for the feeling of impotence recently elaborated by Dr. Fromm. To these we may now add his curious statement that 'one cannot exaggerate the frequency with which ideas of grandeur appear among members of the middle classes and among bourgeois intellectuals'. This seems to us rather an over-statement, but the fact remains that our epoch is marked by a dual tendency: on the one hand the individual is submerged in the crowd, on the other he stands out and is valued as in no previous period in history. Mass photographic reproduction[1] has conferred upon everyone a new privilege: anyone of us, even the most insignificant, can be interviewed as the 'man in the street', his name and his photograph may appear in the papers; in the same way anyone may be filmed. The individual name is triumphantly coming into its own again, by a kind of 'augmentation of function'. Such is the conclusion of a very witty article by Leo Löwenthal.[2] Actually we are in the presence of a temptation, a gratuitous compensation. Man has never been so 'de-particularised' as he is to-day, has never deserved so little the attention of other people. And when (till recently) people used to greet each other with the name of a dictator, all they did was 'to show their own importance'. In a period when the 'crushing authority of facts' leads to the standardisation of everything, down to the last shred of thought, down to the last pulse of emotion, people learn an enormous number of names in record time, and then forget them all the quicker for it.

Many other no less gratuitous compensations come to be thrown on the screen of collectivity. In the first place, sport—not as it is practised but as supplying a spectacle for onlookers and experts. Another no less important compensation, for it embraces an enormous public, is art. The public that enjoys music, the theatre, and especially the radio and cinema, includes practically everybody. Everything in the way of 'light entertainment' is intended in the last resort to fill the void, the feeling of emptiness and passivity created by the sense of impotence. The man who reads a detective story and identifies himself, now with the criminal, now with the clever detective, enjoys imaginary triumphs; the spectator in the cinema, the listener who turns on his radio and hardly attends to the music that fills his home, however humble— all these are only actors in the more gratuitous compensations that are taking place on a world scale. To complain of this, as does M. Georges Duhamel, is old-fashioned. We must accept the inevitable with our

1 Walter Benjamin deals with their social importance in his brilliant study 'L'oeuvre d'art à l'époque de sa reproduction mécanique' (in French), *Zeitsch. f. Sozialforschung*, t.v. 1936.

2 Leo Löwenthal, 'International Who's Who 1937', *Zeitsch. f. Sozialforschung*, C.V. 1939.

eyes open; and it may be that by becoming conscious of the compensatory character of those entertainments that entertain us so little, we shall eventually give them meaning by completely removing their gratuitousness.

Art of to-day is thus only a form of compensation for the feeling of helplessness and impotence that has invaded the mind of twentieth-century man. 'The soul that is chained but wants to expand seeks and finds its satisfaction in the quick succession of images in the film. The story is felt by the spectator as being enacted in his own soul and thus becomes the realisation of situations which life has refused him. This illusory experience (*Erlebnis*) almost succeeds in canalising the bitterness that has accumulated under the inexorable constraint of life and society.' So says Hönigsheim, the excellent German sociologist. Art, then, is nothing but an escape from the feelings of inferiority and impotence which torment us all. The élite may seek in it a higher form of experience; for the masses it is nothing but a compensation.

But did the part played by art in past epochs differ fundamentally from that which sociologists attribute to it to-day? It would seem not, for what the cinema does to-day was represented in former times by the epic. The epic was something more than a factory of dreams; it was a collective means of compensating for a collective evil. That at least is the conclusion reached by a young Spanish thinker, Angel Sanchez Rivero, who died prematurely in 1930. In some interesting notes in his *Posthumous Papers* (*Papeles Postumos, Revista de Occidente*, 1931, published under the title *Los Héroes*) he develops a new theory of epic poetry and of the social functions of the hero.

'The *Chanson de Roland* might very well have originated as follows. After a long series of conquests Charlemagne enters upon a less glorious period—the expedition into Spain and the failure to capture Saragossa. Then retreat and finally the disaster inflicted by the mountaineers of the Pyrenees on his rearguard in the Pass of Roncesvalles. The imagination which created these legends selected this weak point in the Emperor's career from amongst all others so as to give an explanation compatible with the glory of the hero. *It is a work of compensation.*[1] As though one were to isolate from the life of Napoleon his only genuine defeat—Waterloo. . . . The Iliad is undoubtedly a similar work. A moment of disaster for the Greeks when they were on the point of being driven back into the sea had to be purified, and the imagination created the

---

[1] The italics are mine—O.B.

myth of the wrath of Achilles. Here just as in the case of the *Chanson de Roland* the legend emerges to prove that the disaster was due not to the enemy's real superiority but to a situation in which allies had been brought to grief by their own fault. In the Iliad through the wrath of Achilles, in the *Chanson* by the treachery of Ganelon.'

At the time when Sanchez Rivero was jotting down these ideas Freudian theories were beginning to influence literary circles in Madrid. As Adler's theories of compensation were unknown to him, Sanchez Rivero tried to link up his discovery with the general body of Freud's ideas. That is why, having discovered the idea of collective compensation, he adds, 'What happens here is something Freudian in which the imagination tries to sublimate under an ingenious fiction a (historical) moment full of shame'.

The diagnosis is correct; only the terms used are wrong. According to Freud, sublimation is the transformation of certain instincts or impulses, but it is obvious that we are here in the presence not of instincts or impulses but solely of a feeling of inferiority, provoked by large scale national disaster. This feeling must have extended to the whole community and therefore imperiously called for a levelling-up compensation. Sanchez Rivero, fully conscious of the value of his discovery, uses the same theory to explain the birth of the Spanish national epic, the *Poema del Mio Cid*.

'There can be no doubt that this process by which moments of national shame are sublimated (we should say *compensated*, O.B.) is of great importance in the explanation of legends and myths. This means that the imagination is employed not so much to extol positive moments as to save those that are negative. The first would be superfluous, the second indispensable, from a vital point of view. For in reality, is not all spiritual creation the fruit of a sense of *détresse*? This is a rude blow to optimism, for if epic poems are themselves the children of anguish . . .'

THE COMPENSATORY FUNCTION OF CIVILISATION

Sanchez Rivero's ideas give support to the attempts made by some of Adler's disciples to interpret all civilisation and culture as the direct result of those feelings of distress which have fallen to the lot of humanity from all time. Primitive man paints on the walls of his cave the bison against which he must measure his strength on the morrow. And in fixing this magic figure on the wall he is, as it were, giving himself up to a kind of training in sport. The training is directed against the instinctive feeling of inferiority which comes over him in the presence of the dreaded animal. He wants to familiarise himself with this presence so as not to lose his courage when brought face to face with it. In this way the art of painting is born. According to the well-known sociologist and dramatic critic, Julius Bab, drama obeys the same motives and is the compensation for man's terrific feelings of inferiority. In this way the art of ancient tragedy was born. Egon Friedel (the luckless historian who committed suicide when the Nazis entered Vienna) in his three-volumed *Kulturgeschichte* likewise attributes to feelings of inferiority and their compensation a major part in the genesis of human civilisation.

Thus quite a number of authors seem to have hit upon the same idea independently of each other. To return to Sanchez Rivero and his reflections on the genesis of national epics, we find him drawing fresh consequences from his discovery. In expressing them he sounds that note of awe which accompanies any disclosure of profound truth.

'Thus it would seem that the will to power is the great creative force; but not directly, as Nietzsche thought, but by a Freudian *détour* [i.e. he should have said *Adlerian*, O.B.]. . . . The terrible thing is that this means that the sublimation of *détresse*, this one and only spiritual mainspring, is transformed both into Marxism and Fascism.'

Sanchez Rivero did not live to develop the political consequences of his theories. In any case, what mattered to him most was the explanation of national epic poetry. He saw very clearly that modern epics written by well-known poets did not show the same compensatory traits. And the final conclusion to which he comes is not without interest for the study of inferiority feelings.

'What we mean is that the epic poem is not written in praise of history but in a Freudian [i.e. Adlerian, O.B.] defence of certain historic depressions. Imagination works in all its intensity only when it is a question of curing a *détresse*. . . . The poem emerges not to exalt history but to veil it. Caesar, Alexander and Napoleon are not really epic heroes, just because they are important persons. This is what shows the profound difference between the spontaneous and the learned epic. Erudite poets thought that the important personages of history were those most suited to become epic figures. Virgil chose the founder of

Mother-city Rome, Lucan chose Caesar, and Voltaire chose Henri IV. But it was not Achilles who built Troy. Legend takes good care to stress his final ineffectualness. . . . The ineffectualness of Achilles' life is expressed by Homer with tragic clairvoyance.'

The author was aware, moreover, that 'the subject swarmed with problems which could be solved only by prolonged and detailed study'. Nevertheless he saw in a flash the vast scope of the problem of inferiority feelings and their compensation on a collective plane, and his hastily written notes supplement in an interesting way the work which is being done to-day on the compensatory function of art in the period of its mechanical reproduction and diffusion on a wide scale.

CHAPTER XVIII

THE DIAGNOSIS OF INFERIORITY FEELINGS

W E have seen that the feeling of inferiority is a state of mind that does not admit of objective measurement. But just as the height of a pyramid can be measured by its shadow, without climbing to its summit, so we can up to a point calculate the level of auto-estimation of our subjects. Psychology, in spite of its elaborate methods of tests for the measurement of our aptitudes, has been little concerned so far with a genuinely objective measurement of the feelings we are concerned with in this book.

The Americans use vast questionnaires—from fifty to a hundred and fifty questions to be answered either by yes or no or by an evaluation in points which are afterwards added up to yield a 'degree' of auto-estimation similar to a degree of temperature on a thermometer. But this sort of thing is fit only for readers of the popular press or of women's magazines. To ask someone if he has feelings of inferiority simply doesn't make sense.[1] Auto-estimation is a complete phenomenon, of which only a small portion emerges above the level of consciousness, like the summit of an iceberg above water. With the best will in the world the subject himself cannot tell us much about it. The tests elaborated by Adlerian psychologists—Mme. Marthe Holub has published some in the *Internat. Zeitschrift f. Ind. Psych.*—are also quite inadequate to serve as a starting-point.

We must therefore fall back upon indirect signs—the tilt of the head, the movements of the body, gestures and mime, the subject's walk and even his position during sleep. *Ego-fugal* movements and gestures point to our having a high feeling of our own being, whereas *ego-petal* movements are a sign of discouragement, of a drop in the auto-estimative

[1] A typical example of such an enquiry is that of E. S. Dexter, 'Personality traits related to Conservatism and Radicalism', in *Character and Personality*, VII, 1939, pp. 230–7. Out of 267 students divided into two groups according to their 'Right' or 'Left' political opinions 73 per cent. of the 'Lefts' and only 30 per cent. of the 'Rights' answered in the affirmative to the question 'Do you experience feelings of inferiority'. And yet, says Dexter, those of the 'Left' were far the more brilliant, especially intellectually!

level. This broad principle, perhaps too general to fit all cases, has given rise to the elaboration of a system of graphology, that of M. Nöck Sylvus, for handwriting can supply valuable indications not only concerning the intellectual level and artistic sense of the writer but also concerning his auto-estimation. But even the subtle methods of graphology are not altogether adequate and can be trusted only in extreme cases. The indices of handwriting are polyvalent. A feeling of inferiority can find expression in an excessively small handwriting (where this is not simply the result of short-sightedness) or owing to the mechanism of compensation in its exact opposite—an excessively big handwriting.

Some people suffering from an inferiority complex show in their whole bearing the nature of their complaint. They often look as if they were carrying an invisible burden. Their movements seem weary, their shoulders are hunched and they drag their feet as they walk. Others greet us with a strained smile on their lips, they stretch out a hand timidly as though they were afraid we would refuse to take it, and then squeeze ours too eagerly as though they were afraid we would withdraw it at the last moment. The victim of an inferiority complex lies down to rest in a hunched-up position which recalls the 'passive defence' of the boxer and even of certain animals; if some circumstance obliges him to lie in a different position he will have difficulty in going to sleep. If, as in a case mentioned above, a child called Charles has learned without difficulty to shape all the letters of the alphabet, capitals and others, but sticks over the capital C, the initial of his own name, we may be pretty sure that he 'feels inferior'. It is not outside the realm of possibility that a child with arrested development in spite of a perfectly normal infancy may be suffering from an inhibited functioning of certain glands under the weight of his inferiority complex. This, however, is only a hypothesis, based on the fact that the disappearance of the complex following upon a change of surroundings often brings about an accelerated physical growth as though an obstacle had suddenly been removed.

But all these indices are extremely unreliable; they would have to be correlated and compared and their results checked by each other before we could use them with scientific accuracy.

A second group of facts which will allow us to conclude the existence of inferiority feelings in a subject are what we may call *inadequate reactions*. Giving an exaggerated importance to the least little setback, beating a retreat before the most insignificant obstacle, reacting as though a catastrophe had occurred (the *Katastrophenreaktion* of German psychiatry)—all this serves to point to an auto-estimative disequilibrium. Such is the case of the young schoolmaster who, on being unexpectedly asked a question in class to which he cannot immediately give the answer, rushes out of the room and never returns to the school or perhaps even the town; or of the schoolboy, who knows his lesson perfectly, has repeated it to his mother without a mistake, but when questioned at school cannot remember a word of it. One could easily multiply these examples; our feelings of inferiority, our *esprit d'escalier*, often play us very mean tricks.

Among these inadequate reactions, i.e. out of proportion to the real difficulty to be mastered, we could also mention the behaviour of the subject who goes about as if he were in enemy country. The looks, the laughter, the smiles of everyone are directed at him. He is eternally on the *qui vive*. Unconsciously (though showing no signs of genuine agoraphobia) he will avoid going through a hall by the central gangway, will always sit in a corner or against a wall in a restaurant and in the back row at a lecture or concert as though seeking protection from behind. There is no end to the variety of such symptoms.

And yet the Adlerian psychology has put at our disposal far surer methods of discovering the existence of inferiority feelings, their specific nature and even their intensity. *Everything* can be a symptom. We have already surveyed a whole series of signs in external behaviour. But we can also analyse the subject's dreams. It is not a question of 'attributing meaning to that which has none', of splitting hairs in an attempt to explain the minutest detail, but of bringing out the 'style' of the dream. Nightmares, dreams of falling, of being killed, of missing a train, of arguing with a superior, etc., may express in symbolic form mental states of inferiority; on the other hand, flying, overcoming of difficulties, getting to the top of a mountain are all, in the language of dreams, manifestations of courage.

The interpretation of the earliest memories of childhood is another fertile source of indications. Thus a young man of nineteen, questioned on the subject of his earliest memory, tells us, 'I see myself sitting on the floor; in front of me is my mother, very big, sitting in a very high armchair. Her feet are on a footstool. She is feeding my little brother at the breast. So I must be—since my brother is two years younger than I am —about two or three years old.'

His brother, who is seventeen at the time we question him, gives us the following earliest memory. 'I see myself in the corner of our nursery where a portion of the wall is used for making marks showing our height and bearing the initials of our Christian names. I see myself standing against the wall to see if I have reached the mark of my elder brother.'

We could in the case of these two brothers speak of complementary or parallel inferiority complexes. The elder feels 'inferior' to his brother who is placed 'so high' in his mother's love, while the younger one suffers from the same feeling because his brother is 'bigger' than he is. It is the 'Cain complex' in the one case, the 'Jacob complex' in the other. (Cf. Edmond Schlesinger, 'Jacob, second *enfant*' in *Courage*, July 1938.)

The *style of life* of these two young men is perfectly clear to the psychologist once he knows of these two 'complementary' memories. The elder brother will always be very liable to inferiority feelings in all situations where he may believe himself to be slighted; the younger, on the contrary, will always suffer from not being assigned the 'first place', everywhere and in all matters.

All these methods, which we have briefly passed in review, make it a very difficult matter to run to earth the concrete and specific inferiority feelings in any specific case. With children it is a relatively easy job, even on a collective scale. For instance, one can set a whole class little essays on such subjects as 'What do you remember about the time when you were quite little?' or 'If you were a magician . . .' or even make them tell stories or fairy stories on their own initiative. But the day may not be far distant when we shall have at our disposal methods sufficiently reliable to make more headway in our study of auto-appreciation in our subjects. This will form the subject-matter of our next chapter.

CHAPTER XIX

UNCONSCIOUS AUTO-ESTIMATION

INFERIORITY feelings, then, are so complex in their nature and so equivocal and vague in their external manifestations that it would seem impossible to create a method of discovering their existence and deciding upon their nature. If, however, we could obtain from the subjects themselves, *unbeknown to them*, evaluations of their own ego, would this not bring us nearer our aim?

Every human being possesses an 'opinion' about himself, mostly of an affective nature, and nearly always unconscious. How then can we capture this opinion on our subjects and describe it?

With primitive man it is relatively easy. When Dr. Moskowski was exploring in Central and Southern Africa he took photographs of the Hottentots and the Kaïs, who do not know the use of mirrors and have never seen their faces reflected except on the surface of water. When he showed them the photographs each native recognised his companions' faces quite clearly, but was unable to identify his own. One Kaï who was shown a photo of himself even exclaimed, 'Why don't you kill that disgusting beast?'

This violent affective reaction to one's own image is all the more interesting because experiments made in our own civilised surroundings do not belie it. We all react to pictures of our own ego, *when we do not recognise them*, in a very special way. Let us take as an example the recognition of one's own voice.[1]

We take records of a few ordinary sentences spoken by twenty different persons in succession. Some time later we turn on the record for each of these persons to listen to. They will recognise the voices of their friends and acquaintances, but *they do not recognise their own voices*.[2]

[1] The experiments we describe were devised by the ex-German psychologist Werner Wolff, and carried out at the Psycho-technical Institute of Barcelona.

[2] There are a few rare exceptions, such as professional reciters and radio announcers, etc. André Malraux has an interesting bit of dialogue on the subject in *La Condition Humaine.* 'One very rarely recognises one's own voice, you know, when one hears it for the first time—You think the gramophone record distorts it?—No, it's not that, because one can easily recognise other people's voices, but

The subjects are then asked to describe or *characterise* one by one the different persons whose voices they have heard. Roughly speaking, the recorded voices are characterised in much the same way by all the listening subjects. There is only one voice on which the descriptions differ—*the voice of the listening subject himself, which he had been unable to identify earlier in the experiment.*

Thus we react to our own voice, *unrecognised as such,* as though we had recognised it. This shows that we have recognised it unconsciously, and our way of characterising it will come from the depths of our unconscious. Let us now compare the individual subject's judgment of his character by his own unrecognised voice with the inter-agreeing judgments of it given by a certain number of the other subjects. We reach the following conclusions. (1) The judgment formed unconsciously of one's own character is never neutral but will always be coloured affectively, either too favourably or too unfavourably. (2) The tendency to judge oneself unconsciously in too favourable a way is always more definite and more frequent than the opposite tendency. It was easy to control these results. Each subject was handed ten sheets of paper with ten characterisations of his own voice, and he was asked to arrange them on a descending scale going from the most favourable to the most unfavourable. The subjects were not influenced in any way. The psychologist in charge of the experiment left the room. *The judgment made by the subject on himself was always either at the head or at the bottom of the list.*

After comparing the judgment given by the subject himself with those, more or less the same, given by the other subjects, it was found that the former was generally 'deeper', much nearer the truth than the judgments given by the others, which were necessarily rather superficial. For example, the other subjects hardly ever guessed the profession followed by the owner of the recorded voice, whereas the unconscious owner of the voice nearly always guessed right on this point.

The next step in the experiment suggested itself automatically—a comparison between the subject's unconscious appraisal of his own character through his recorded voice, and his *conscious* auto-appreciation. So several months after the first experiment the subjects were

you see one is not accustomed to hearing oneself . . .' And a little further on Malraux gives the explanation. 'It's probably a case of how we hear. We hear other people's voices with our ears—And our own?—With the throat. Stop up your ears and you'll hear your voice. Interesting.' We may add that we also hear our own voice in the cranial cavity.

given five sheets of paper each with five characterisations, one of which was their own unconscious and already forgotten estimate of themselves. Each was then asked to arrange the characterisations in order of the degree to which he thought they applied to him *personally*. It was then found that the unconscious auto-appreciation was either at the top of the list, or at the bottom, or occupied an intermediate position on the scale. Needless to say, the subjects' conscious estimates of themselves were far from being objective; they corresponded, not to their unconscious auto-appreciation, but to an ideal which they consciously wished to resemble.

We shall not give the statistical tables showing the relations of the favourable to the unfavourable judgments given by the subjects of their own unrecognised voices. Such tables, much to the taste of American psychologists, would prove nothing, for the experiments carried out were not sufficiently numerous for statistical treatment to give strictly conclusive results. The normal subjects (who were in the majority) were very kind to themselves. They also gave their judgments unhesitatingly, whereas those who gave adverse appreciations did so after a great deal of hesitation. Both groups were inclined to talk at greater length about their own voices than about those of the other subjects. But those who gave unfavourable judgments clearly *would have liked to be different from what they were*. They criticised themselves immoderately, but with much hesitation, because it is not very easy to disapprove of oneself, even if one does so unconsciously. These were clearly recognisable cases of persons suffering from feelings of inferiority.

These experiments were not confined to the unconscious characterisation of the subjects' own unrecognised voices. Photographs were taken of their faces, their profiles, their hands, etc., and their movements were 'filmed' without their knowing it. The results, which we need not give in detail, were always the same. In every case the unconscious appreciation made by the subject of himself yielded a much more real and plastic picture than did the judgments of the others. Moreover, the image which each subject unconsciously held of himself seemed to be guided by a rather exacting ideal picture of the ego. The only slightly unusual case was that of the walk. The subjects found it easy to recognise their own walk although they had never seen it, except in this specially taken 'film' in which, moreover, by a photographic trick the subject appeared swathed in a long cloak, and everything about him was thus unrecognisable except his walk. Even so, the subjects took up an obviously defensive attitude against their ego as it appeared on the screen. *One clearly felt the pull between what they were and what they would like to be.* Any judgment about ourselves is bound to be coloured with affectivity; this is something that our conscious mind can do nothing about. Thus the affective participation in these 'characterisations' can be affirmative or negative—favourable or un-favourable. We never describe our character as it is, but as we wish it to be, or as we fear it may be. When the gap between the real self and the wished-for self is too great, an internal affective separation or dis-junction takes place in the subject which is analogous to the separation that takes place in dreams. This separation, now accessible to experi-mental discovery, is what subjects endowed with a faculty for self-observation describe as the essential feature of their 'inferiority complex'.[1]

To translate this into the language of psycho-analysis, let us recall that Freud recognised three forms of 'resistance' in our psychic system. There is resistance against the *ego*, resistance against the *super-ego*, and a third kind of resistance against the *id*. The super-ego is a sort of ideal that contains everything in the way of divinity, authority and 'con-science'; it is formed by the rudiments of the *imago* which the child has formed of his parents and of all the persons commanding his admira-tion. Thus it would seem that the gap between the ego and the super-ego is the source of most of our feelings of inferiority. It is also the reason why the super-ego stands in the way of a favourable self-appreciation. For when man judges his own character, *he never starts from what he is, but from what he would like to be.*

This conflict is already present in primitive man and in the child. It explains the birth of magic as a consequence of the gap existing be-tween the world of reality and the fictitious world of desires and dreams, where the subject tends to be omnipotent, like God. This mirror or double of the self (*alter ego, Sosias, Doppelgänger*) explains the

---

[1] One part of the mental flux becomes detached from and even opposed to the rest. No one has described this state of mind provoked by the feeling of inferiority better than André Gide in *Les Faux Monnayeurs*. 'Whatever I may say or do, there is always a part of me which stands back and watches the other part com-promising itself, which observes it, which cheers or hisses or doesn't care a damn. When one is divided like that, how can you expect one to be sincere?' (p. 469).

This is really at the root of what Janet calls the feeling of self-shame, the feeling of incompleteness, in a word, of inferiority. 'This self-contempt, this disgust with oneself that can lead the most undecided to the most extreme decisions': *Les Faux Monnayeurs*, p. 235. This is the secret cause of everything we regard as neurotic. (The page references are to the original French publication.—Tr.)

great part played by all ideas of magic. And this conflict is closely related to the psychology of compensation, which has been regarded as the fundamental feature of modern neurotic man. The inability to reconcile reality and dream produces a sort of moral shock which gives rise to a burning sense of inferiority, of inadequacy, and of insecurity. Hence the longing for *security*, for *superiority*, however skin-deep, and for *power*, however fictitious.

Thus in addition to the *research methods* practised chiefly in America, we are beginning to have at our disposal in Europe *the method of unconscious auto-appreciation*. Once it has been developed and perfected, this method will undoubtedly supply us with a relatively reliable method for detecting the existence of feelings of inferiority in our subjects.

CHAPTER XX

THE WISH-IMAGE AND THE NEGATIVE IDEAL
IN RELATION TO INFERIORITY FEELINGS

T HE experiments described in the last chapter showed the possibility of applying the method of *tests* for the exploration of the unconscious. They led their author, Werner Wolff, to formulate the theory of *wish-image* (*Wunschbild-Theorie*), and to carry out further experiments which we shall now describe.

(*a*) He presented his subjects with a series of graphological specimens which had been photographed in a mirror so that the writer could not be identified. Each subject was then made to 'characterise' his own unrecognised handwriting by a method similar to that which had elicited the unconscious auto-appreciations described in the last chapter.

(*b*) He read short narratives to his subjects—generally fables or popular tales—and asked each of them in turn to repeat the story. The recapitulation was taken down by a stenographer. Later on, these recapitulations were submitted to the subjects, who were asked to characterise the narrator or recapitulator in each case (cases where the subject recognised his own version were discounted).

(*c*) He obtained full-face photographs of his subjects, took *reversed* copies of these (by turning over the film), so that what was normally the right side of the face appeared as the left. He then bisected these portraits longitudinally and stuck the 'left' half of the reversed photo to the left half of the original photo, and the 'right' half to the corresponding right half. He thus obtained, in addition to the normal left-right portrait, others—a left-left and a right-right. He then carried out his previously described experiments in auto-appreciation. All this led him to the formulation of a theory described in a very long volume which has not yet been published. It makes stiff reading and is not always very clear. At the risk of not doing it full justice we shall deal only with that part of Wolff's theory which has a special bearing on our subject. According to him, there are within each personality two fundamentally different systems which are active in different proportions—his *character* and his *wish-image*. In the case of *optimistic* subjects the wish-image predominates very definitely; the subjects seem, as it were, to draw their life sustenance from it. With *pessimistic* subjects on the other hand, i.e. those suffering from an inferiority complex, the wish-image is dissociated from real life; it is not derived from the 'id', but from the 'super-ego'. To such persons real life falls short of the wish-image, and the whole of their mental life is dominated by the dynamic of this fundamental divergence. To know their characters it will not be sufficient to study their behaviour and bearing it will also be necessary to explore their wish-image with the method of unconscious auto-appreciation. Now the wish-image can help to mould the actual face of a subject and even bring about organic changes. Thus the desire to have a child may, in a hysterical woman, bring about the symptoms of a miscarriage, imitating those of a real confinement.

But our author goes further and reaches the following somewhat startling conclusions. The wish-image, he says, which is the yard-stick for all characterisation, is not merely a personal and individual ideal representation; it has a collective character. When the wish-ego I and the real I are intimately fused there will be profound harmony between the 'individual form' and the 'collective form'. But where the individual is burdened with feelings of inferiority, the individual form is 'confronted' with the collective form and slinks away condemned from the ordeal. The subject then judges his own character as inferior and inadequate to the demands of collectivity. The wish-image contains not only the polarity : conscious-unconscious, but also the polarity : individual-collective. In primitive man or in the savage tribes of to-day this divergence between the individual and the collective forms is not present; both exist in organic communion. Their dissociation and even complete separation has thus taken place only since modern man became isolated from the collectivity. In children the separation is less complete, and since, as a general rule, the right side of the body corresponds to the individual while the left side expresses the collective aspect, it is found that bodily symmetry is more pronounced in children than in adults. But modern society wants to 'activate' everything that is individual so that the individual can be held responsible for his actions, and it therefore severely represses our call upon the magical forces that are latent in the collectivity. And since the left side represents what is collective, this side is considered 'inferior'. (For example, society regards left-handedness as an inferiority from earliest childhood.) Now in persons whose vital *tonus* is poor, any preponderance of collective features will bring about an inferiority of individual functions. Those, on the other hand, who enjoy a rich and vital *tonus* are able to call the collective forces into action in *support* of their individual energies. Thus the division between reality and wish-image is to be explained by the 'organic division' between the collective function and the individual function, which are localised (in accordance with the law of diametrically opposed localisation) in the right and the left cerebral hemispheres respectively. Every time an individual function is inhibited, this function, localised in the left hemisphere of the brain, brings about the reactivation of a part of the right hemisphere which is generally completely inactive. Thus forces of a collective origin come to the rescue of the failing individual forces. And this, adds our author, explains, incidentally, the curious fact which has been experimentally established, that rats, which generally use their right paw to take food out of a hole, use their left paw as soon as they are deprived of Vitamin B. (!)

We have expounded this curious theory here in order to remind the reader that the cerebral localisation of feelings of inferiority is by no means outside the realm of possibility. Has not Professor Piéron, basing himself on Pagano's experiments, postulated the existence of a 'centre of fear'? There might very well be a special centre of the emotions in the encephalum at the level of the caudate knot, where the feelings of inferiority would find their organic localisation.

THE COUNTER-IDEAL—THE WORK OF PROFESSOR L. SZONDI

Some ten years ago we tried to develop a theory of the *negative ideal*. We had noticed in a number of subjects the existence not only of an ideal which they seemed to follow and imitate, but also that of a *counter-ideal*, which they either hated and shunned or, on the contrary, pursued with pathological ardour. Subjects suffering from inferiority feelings due to 'confrontations' with others were especially inclined to practise symmetrically opposite confrontations so as to shield their complex. Here are some examples.

An old lady tells us: 'When I was young I was unhappy because I was not as rich, or as beautiful, or as sought after by young men as the beautifully dressed young Countess I saw driving past our home every day in a magnificent carriage. But one day I said to myself, "What a fool you are. Why do you always compare yourself to the Countess? Compare yourself to the *concierge's* daughter." And true enough, I found that I was richer, more beautiful and more sought after than this other girl, and immediately I felt a weight had been taken off my shoulders.'

A young German Jew with very dark hair is profoundly envious of blond Aryan young men. He seeks their friendship and in all his attitudes towards them his inferiority feelings are clearly discernible. Whenever he sees a young Jew or an Aryan with hair darker than his own he has a feeling of joy which expresses itself in 'incomprehensible' laughter which makes him look rather an 'idiot'. The psychologist has no difficulty in discovering the origin of the young man's secret satisfaction; it could be stated as follows: 'It's dreadful for me not to be fair and have blue eyes.[1] But what luck, all the same, not to be as dark (i.e. as definitely a Jewish type) as X or Y.'

In a boys' school the pupils A., V. and P. were the least proficient in physical exercises. Now each one had a marked inclination to talk about the other two to the rest of the class, and seemed to take a special pleasure in it. Again, their attitude could be formulated as follows: 'What luck all the same not to be as inferior as V. or P. (A. and V., A. and P., respectively).' For each one the other two represented the negative-ideal or counter-ideal, and this counter-ideal helped to restore their auto-estimative equilibrium.

The theory of the counter-ideal has found a brilliant confirmation in the work of Professor Lipot Szondi of Budapest. This psychologist has devised a remarkable affective test which consists in presenting the subject with six series of eight photographs each; in every series eight different types of mentally abnormal persons are represented. The subject is asked to pick out the two faces which he finds most sympathetic and the two which he finds least so. The choice must be repeated ten times. The photos are numbered and have been selected in such a way that they can be regarded as representing so many abnormal affective types. By dint of careful combinations it is possible to obtain interesting character sketches even from normal subjects. The test is easy to carry out and enables one to penetrate without difficulty to the deeper layers of the subject's character. It is based on the ideal and counter-ideal, both factors which exercise a paramount influence on anyone's auto-estimative level. We have here a method which, once it was perfected, would bring us appreciably nearer the goal of an absolutely

[1] John Löwenthal in his study of Walter Rathenau, and alluding to Thomas Mann's well-known novel, has called this type of inferiority feeling the 'Tonio Kröger complex'.

objective and scientific way of diagnosing feelings of inferiority, both in children and adults, both in the normal and the abnormal.[1]

I underwent this test in 1939 under Dr. Szondi's first assistant, Dr. Ferenc Mérei. In 1947 the test was made public and is now available for commercial purposes. (In German by Hans Huber, publishers in Bern, Switzerland; in English by Messrs. Grune and Stratton, New York.) Szondi claims that the subject's choice is based on an 'affinity of genes' (*Genverwandschaft*) existing in his reproductive cells and in those of the owner of the face to be judged. I would hesitate to support this view.

In contrast to Szondi's *theories*, the test itself seems well adapted to practical use, even if one does not share the author's belief in the possibility of 'diagnosing the instincts'. In any case, it is a very good test of character. I have used it on several hundred subjects of all ages with varying results—some excellent, others mediocre, others nil. One very feminine little girl placed twenty-three women among the antipathetic faces and only one man, who, as it happened, might have been taken for a woman. Among the sympathetic faces she placed twenty-two men and only two women, of whom one might have passed as a man. Some *feminine protest* certainly came into play here! A subject of twenty-eight, who had a strong father-fixation, chose as sympathetic all the bearded faces. Such facts cannot be explained simply by the operation of the genes. The personal equation is involved, and not least the feelings of inferiority.

This is the place to mention the latest test that has been devised for the study of wish-images. The Spanish psychiatrist Dr. J. M. Pigem-Serra asks his patients: What would you like to be if you were not a human being? He then asks the subject to name two other wish-images of the same kind. The subject must answer by naming two things, an inanimate object and an animal. (Typical answers are: lion, eagle, statue, tree, fresh spring; but also church monstrance, dove, pig, etc.) Finally the subject is asked what he would not like to be if he were not a human being. (Again he must give three answers.) In most cases the answers enable one to unearth inferiority feelings in the subject.

[1] This chapter was already written when I came across Carl Schmeing's book, *Ideal und Gegenideal*, Leipzig, 1936. The author emphasises the importance of the *counter-ideal* in education, on the basis of an enquiry carried out on a large number of children of different ages.

EGO-IMAGES

It would seem, in conclusion, that we have three kinds of images of our ego which determine our auto-estimative level, so that it changes when they change. They are the *image of our own body* (the *Körper-schema* of the German psychologists), of which Professor Lhermitte has made a remarkable study; the *wish-image* expounded by Werner Wolff; and the *counter-ideal* expounded by myself and Szondi. Our *auto-estimative image* would thus result from the interference of all three. A minute examination of these three factors would therefore be equivalent to an exact diagnosis (in so far as anything can be exact in psychology) of the feelings of inferiority experienced by our subjects.

CHAPTER XXI

MAJOR FORMS OF THE INFERIORITY COMPLEX: NEUROSIS, PSYCHOSIS AND CRIME

> We deny the existence of any organic predisposition to neurosis, but at the same time we believe we have shown more clearly than most writers the way in which organic inferiority tends to create certain mental attitudes, and the mechanism by which bodily weakness gives rise to the feeling of inferiority.
> Adler, *The Neurotic Constitution*. Preface.

WHEN the burden of inferiority feelings becomes too heavy for the shaken equilibrium of auto-estimation to be restored by useful activity, the forces of the psyche are inevitably side-tracked in the direction of aims of fictitious superiority. The child who has been scolded by his father will go off somewhere where no one can see him or hear him, and will heap abuse upon his parent; in psycho-analytical language he is abreacting. In reality, the child is trying to experience a very small and fictitious superiority over the person who has just shown his own unquestioned superior strength. Another child, having suffered some humiliation in class, will buy sweets and compensate for the attack upon his auto-estimation by the pleasure of sucking them. Our own life is full of such tiny and sometimes grotesque compensations, determined in each case by the subject's personal equation. Thus a young man, if he has met with some setback, however trivial, during the day, cannot sleep at night except by lying flat on his face—the position of 'virile' superiority. Another, younger one, in a similar case, can perhaps only get to sleep after masturbating. These forms of compensation are not serious; they will become so only when they have taken on an obsessional character. Once they have become the rule, instead of relieving the injured auto-estimation they only complicate matters by producing fresh feelings of inferiority.

In such cases a vicious circle is formed. One day the child whom we saw sucking sweets has no money to buy any; and yet, the need to compensate his inferiority-feeling having become acute, he feels he *must* have those sweets, with the result that he 'pinches' them or steals the money to buy them. This act will not fail to arouse, if he is 'well brought up', a fresh oscillation in his inner sense of auto-estimation. He will be torn between the feeling of superiority at having overcome the obstacle to his desire, at having committed a forbidden act without being found out, and the feeling of inferiority at having done wrong. If the first feeling—that of superiority—disappears and the second one prevails, he will do the same thing again on the next occasion.

This dialectic, or shall we say this mechanism, is present in all the major forms of compensation—neurosis, psychosis, delinquency, drug-addiction and sexual perversion.

PSYCHO-NEUROSES

Neuroses are considered the least dangerous of the major forms of compensation of inferiority feelings. For this very reason we should be all the more on our guard against them.

A young student at law in his first year spends all his time in the Library of the Faculty, turning over the leaves of books on jurisprudence. He shows all kinds of nervous symptoms. He is irritable, has no appetite, sleeps badly. The doctor comes to see him. He prescribes sedatives and suggests a rest cure, but thoroughly approves of the young man's assiduous reading (which is not reading at all) on the ground that the knowledge thus acquired will be helpful to him later on. The situation shows no change and the symptoms persist. An Adlerian psychologist is then called in, and is not slow in discovering that the so-called reading in the library is nothing of the kind, but merely a way of killing time. He tries to find the obstacle, the inner conflict which has caused the young man to be side-tracked into this pseudo-activity. The obstacle is not far to seek; it is the examination at the end of the school year which is terrifying the student without his being quite aware of it. The treatment consists entirely in encouraging him, in showing him that his fears are without foundation. The 'invalid' eventually passes his examination and all his nervous symptoms disappear. The daily 'reading' which the doctor, unversed in Adlerian psychology, failed to unmask as a little neurotic 'arrangement', no longer being required, had been replaced by rational study.

This, of course, is not a serious case, though if left unattended the situation would certainly have deteriorated. Inferiority feelings are, according to Adler, 'up to a point our common lot, since we are all bound at one time or another to find ourselves in a difficult situation or faced with an obstacle that we have to overcome'.

These feelings will arise where the individual, in the face of problems for which he is inadequately adapted or equipped, expresses the conviction that he cannot solve them. Of course one can express this conviction with words, with complaints, but one does so primarily by one's bearing and attitude, by the 'language of the organs', etc. Every difficulty creates a tension resulting in a 'delimitation of the field of action'—hesitation, retreat or rest. At the same time, not all persons suffering from an inferiority complex behave outwardly in the same way; they are not all of them passive, humble, submissive and inoffensive. 'Inferiority feelings can be expressed in a thousand ways.'

There is no neurosis which expresses so clearly what Adler meant as the example he gives himself as the most typical—agoraphobia. The subject is oppressed with the invincible feeling that he cannot get out of the room, the house, etc. In such cases, the field of action is physically reduced to its minimum. The 'arc of tension', as Künkel called it, is visibly reduced.

And yet it would seem that all the other forms of neurosis followed the same pattern. We have described elsewhere cases of *chronophobia*, i.e. the fear of 'traversing periods of free time'.

All neuroses, whether hysteria or neurotic obsessions, have fundamentally the same structure. The *accident-neurosis*, which Professor Laignel-Levastine had rediscovered under the name *assécuroses*, is the most typical, since in the last analysis it contains the schema that appears in all the others—flight into a false security, the *buen retira* of the insurance premium. What is not easy to foresee is the form of neurosis which the discouraged individual will choose. Readers of Adler's works will find in them a large number of detailed analyses. What we want particularly to stress in the understanding of a neurosis is the paramount importance of detecting the specific discouragement which is at its root. Adler tells an amusing anecdote to illustrate this point. Three children are visiting the Zoo with their mother. At the lions' cage they all have inferiority feelings, but this discouragement shows itself differently, according to each one's *style of life*. 'I want to go home!' exclaims the first; 'I'm not a bit frightened,' asserts the second; 'Would you like me to spit in his face?' asks the third.

DELINQUENCY AND CRIME

These are, at bottom, only specific forms of discouragement. The opinion that the criminal is nothing but a neurotic is gaining more support every day.[1] The causes of crime are economic depression, poverty, misery. But this does not give a complete explanation, since offences, both trivial and serious, occur in the social classes that have a secure economic background. This points to the existence of *subjective* causes for crime, which are nothing but the expression of profound social discouragement. The criminal, like the neurotic, suffers from an intensified sense of inferiority; both, therefore, will try to 'cheat', and will become sidetracked into a makeshift behaviour which is easier than activity in the 'useful' domains of social life. Both the neurotic and the criminal put their own interests before those of the community. But they retain some vestiges of the community sense, and the criminal has therefore to root these out before committing his crime. Dostoyevsky's wonderful analysis of Raskolnikov in *Crime and Punishment* is a striking example of this slow process. He shows how, intellectually and emotionally, the hero of the story gradually overcomes what remains in him of community feeling. Before killing the old money-lender, he stays in bed for two months and tries to imagine all the good he could do with her money. Even so, he is not yet 'ripe' for the crime at the end of the two months, and he asks himself the spurious question: 'Am I Napoleon or am I a flea?' Henceforth, his decision is made. The image of superiority, 'Napoleon', carries the day, and Raskolnikov kills the old woman. Genuine criminals seem to make use of similar false dilemmas to screw themselves up to action. The famous American murderer who had forgotten his spectacles had said to himself, 'What does this fellow matter? We have millions like him.' Another murderer, before killing his brother, had thought 'One or the other—him or me!' In the same way, the employee who steals his boss's money will say, 'Why, the man's got plenty of money in the bank. What will it matter to him if I help myself to what he has left in this drawer?' These 'auxiliary constructions' of thought are merely so many aggressive 'arrangements', so many mis-stated problems. It should be noted that these

---

[1] Cf. Eugène Schmidt's *Das Verbrechen als Ausdruckform sozialer Entmutigung*, Munich, 1931. The movement in France, *Pour l'enfance 'coupable,'* 12, Rue Guy-de-la-Brosse, Paris, Vᵉ, was animated by the same spirit and had the collaboration of such excellent specialists as Mme. Magdeleine Bonnefoy-Madras, M Van Etten and others.

dilemmas always presuppose a comparison, and come from the subject's feeling that he is 'worth' less than other people. That is why we find among criminals so many deformed or ill-favoured persons, such as cripples, hunchbacks, etc., in a word human beings who are already physically or morally 'inferiorised'. Not only children who have been neglected, but also pampered children who have had too much attention, are particularly drawn to criminal activity when they grow up. In adult life they will try to 'pamper' themselves. The exclamation of Richard III, which we have quoted above, gives the quintessence of the delinquent's state of mind.

Criminals differ from neurotics, however, in certain important respects. The delinquent is aware of the anti-social nature of his conduct; the neurotic has no idea of it. The criminal fights against the feeling of his own responsibility, whereas the neurotic pleads unfavourable circumstances and thrusts the responsibility of what he does or fails to do on to those around him, on to the times he lives in, or on to the world. The criminal will blame only his own stupidity for letting himself be caught, while the fact that he can escape the hand of justice will cause him agreeable feelings of 'superiority'. The criminal, moreover, has a greater disposition to activity than the neurotic, who generally takes refuge in a camouflaged pseudo-activity, and he also has a stronger community feeling—witness the well-known 'honour among thieves', and the Robin Hood legend of the kindly bandit who only robs the rich and helps the poor. The neurotic, on the other hand, if he does help a fellow creature is being kind in order to raise his own sinking level of auto-estimation. It is a case of the psycho-pathology of kindness. Neurotics repress their impulses and inclinations; criminals openly defy society. The neurotic adopts no less aggressive an attitude to those around him than does the criminal, but in his case the aggressive attitude remains veiled or disguised, it takes on furtive and insinuating forms, he is always anxious to 'save face', to keep up appearances. To sum up, we may say that the criminal represents a special type of neurotic, and that if we value human beings by the extent to which their aggressiveness leads to action, the criminal will have more good marks than the neurotic proper.

Before leaving the subject mention should be made of the attempts that have been made for some twelve years at the Stateville Penitentiary by Dr. John F. Pick, one of America's leading plastic surgeons, to 'cure' criminality by plastic operations. It seems that this 'Operating on Inferiority', as it is called in the United States, has met with some success.[1] The assumption is that the true cause of crime is a sensation of inferiority. Only the future can tell us the value of this method—rhinoplasty is the name given to it—as an adjunct to psycho-therapy.[2]

PSYCHOSES

If we except cases of psychotic syndromes due to cerebral lesions, we may say that psychosis differs from neurosis through the acuteness of the experiences of inferiorisation, discouragement, guilt, pessimism, etc. Whereas in a neurosis the trouble is only partial, in psychosis it pervades the whole being. In the first, the goal of superiority is fictitious, in the second, it is rigid and dogmatic. What the neurotic feels as a future menace, a more or less distant possibility, becomes in the psychotic the anticipation of terrible events, such as the end of the world or similar catastrophic events. Psychotics are completely without any understanding of their own illness. What to a neurotic are only obstacles and difficulties become veritable disasters for the psychotic. Fear, an affective expression of inferiority feelings, sets its mark on the neurotic; but in the psychotic it grows out of all proportion, and the patient's life unfolds with terrific intensity. Constitutional psychosis is an anomaly of the whole affective set-up, and could therefore be regarded as an organic inferiority in the Adlerian sense of the term. Here the emotion of fear takes the form of a vicious spiral, such as the 'fear of being afraid', whereas for the neurotic it still plays the part of an 'insurance' against danger. The psychotic patient, finding himself defenceless against the affective mechanisms, succumbs, in obedience to the law of the vicious spiral, at an increasing speed to a state of general demoralisation. In other forms of psychosis the patient becomes apathetic and endeavours to exclude all affective experiences from his life, as may be seen in some cases of schizophrenia; this leads inevitably to a severance of all personal relationships. This total withdrawal from reality springs fundamentally from the desire to eliminate all possibility of conflict. This is the one and only solution by which the patient feels he can consider himself in 'security'. Leonhard Seif regards this absolute suppression of all conflict (*absolute Konfliktlosigkeit*) as the supreme goal of the psychotic. The self-deification which can be observed in neurotics and

[1] Cf. David Anderson and Robert Cromie, 'New Faces—New Lives', in *This Week Magazine*, New York, May 1949.

[2] Louis Linn, M.D., and Irving Goldman, M.D., 'Psychiatric Observations Concerning Rhinoplasty' in *Psycho-somatic Medicine*, XI, 5, 1949.

psychotics alike is, in the last analysis, the outcome of this tendency, which we may describe as an attempt on the part of fear to come to terms with reality. 'The psychotic's fear is fear of catastrophe' (Seif).

Our study of neurosis and psychosis shows us, therefore, that fear (the affective equivalent of conflicts arising from a sense of inferiority) depends in each case upon psychic energy, a factor which varies with the individual. Each has his *own* neurosis, just as one day he will die his *own* death. These individual differences determine the different forms of the flight from the demands made by life. It is in virtue of them that the inferiorised individual becomes a psychotic, a neurotic, a drunkard, a criminal, or a sexual pervert.

CHAPTER XXII

INFERIORITY FEELINGS AND SEX

'. . . *comme la sous-vitalité donne soif autant que la sur-vitalité . . .*'
H. Montherlant.

SOCIETY AND SEX

ONE of the most frequent errors committed in treating of sex or even of human psychology in general is to consider the individual in isolation, apart from the collectivity. And yet, as Adler said, sex is not just a private matter. Moreover, there is a tendency to regard sex as a 'little being' within the human being, relatively independent of him, and often even opposed to his desires and inclinations. 'I can't cope with it' (*C'est plus fort que moi*) we often say when speaking of our sexual instinct, and in this way endow it with a kind of separate existence which does not belong to it by right. The biological instinct is then alone held responsible for our love-life, the *libido* becomes our destiny, and man is nothing more than a 'human animal'. One forgets that he is, or at least ought to be, a *person*, a responsible member of the human community. Unfortunately the collectivity does not concern itself with the social behaviour of the individuals who constitute it, so long as they create no scandal and do not openly transgress the laws that have been laid down.

There has always been a tendency to regard the sexual life of each individual as a purely private affair. At school, more pains are taken to teach us the tributaries of the Mississippi than the most elementary rules of life in a community. We are told that work 'ennobles' us, but not that our sexual life has a social aspect and entails a certain responsibility. The procreation of a thoroughbred who wins prizes at the races is watched over with care, and its mate is chosen with the utmost circumspection. But neither parent, teacher, doctor nor priest will concern himself with the sexual life of man. Even if we do not believe that sex is a negligible quantity, we contrive to make it appear so and treat it as *taboo*. Our first steps at school, in 'society' and in our military service are carefully watched over, but no one thinks of watching and guiding us when we first embark on the perilous sea of love. There are special schools for social deportment, but the pronouncements made by a few distinguished psychiatrists on the necessity for *schools of love* (of a purely theoretical kind, needless to say) have always been received with smiling scepticism.

It was therefore a great advance when those who were investigating this subject attempted to bring our sexual life into relation with the forms of society in which we live to-day. Most of these attempts were inadequate, and it is interesting to note how quickly they were abandoned by those who had initiated them.[1]

THE QUANTITATIVE THEORY OF SEX

This theory, though definitely rejected in scientific circles, still lingers in many publications on the sexual problem. Influenced no doubt by the now obsolete theory of psycho-physical parallelism, these 'quantitative sexologists' took the view that an un-virile psycho-sexual attitude must necessarily be the expression of a deficiency in physical virility; and conversely, that any defect in the genital tract must inevitably be accompanied by a lowered sexual activity. But the facts are very far from obeying so simple and logical a rule. We are often presented with phenomena which completely belie this unilateral schematism. In speaking of Don Juan we shall have occasion to develop this point in greater detail.

The touchstone of any theory of sexual psycho-pathology is the interpretation of the paradox of *homosexuality*. According to the nineteenth-century sexual schema, only effeminate men and virile women would tend to become homosexual. But this is not the case; any specialist could quote cases of homosexuality where the subjects showed no physical abnormality whatsoever. The men were perfectly virile, not only in their external appearance, but in their primary and secondary sexual characters and in all their behaviour except the sexual. This is true of one famous homosexual writer of to-day, and also of one of the greater modern Spanish poets, who was killed at the beginning of the late civil war. *Timid* men are very often completely virile

---

[1] We are thinking especially of Dr. A. Allendy, author of *Capitalisme et Sexualité*. In a later publication, *Les Conceptions modernes de la Sexualité*, Crapouillot, Special issue, Sept. 1937, the same author no longer makes the slightest reference to the relations that can exist between the sexual life of individuals and the structure of society. See also the ephemeral review *Le Problème Sexuel* (1934).

physiologically, but nevertheless incapable of a normal and adequate behaviour towards women. How often, on the contrary, a 'lady's man', a Don Juan, will be found to be more or less effeminate and poorly endowed with physical virility. All this will inevitably appear paradoxical so long as the facts are observed in the light of the out-moded and ultra-simple 'mechanical' theories of the last century.

Who has not seen a handsome, highly-sexed man turn pale or blush at the smile of a woman, or even lose countenance and flee from her presence like a schoolboy? How can such a phenomenon be explained by the *quantity of instinct*? As a matter of fact there is no exact correla-tion between the sexual vigour of a man or woman and their psycho-sexual 'energy'. Only too often there is a marked disparity between the two things. One can even go further, and point to men who are absolutely virile in every aspect of life, but who fail in one point only— their attitude to women. We shall find in the annals of the history of literature a case which will lead us to the problem of 'undiluted virility' (*ungemischte Männlichkeit*) spoken of by Wilhelm Michel.

A TRAGEDY OF VIRILITY: HEINRICH VON KLEIST

The history of literature is full of such cases, as indeed is everyday life. We have chosen that of the great German writer, Heinrich von Kleist, the author of *Kätchen von Heilbronn* and *Michael Kohlhaas*, because it strikes us as particularly significant.

A young man may be thoroughly *male* and yet be incapable of love. He can be so completely virile that not the smallest, most trivial element of femininity enters into the make-up of his personality. And yet, to reach the opposite sexual pole, to bridge the gap between himself and that unknown *not-self* which is woman (his comrades of the same sex being simply other editions of his virile ego), to understand his sexual partner in all her particularity and complexity, the young man, and *mutatis mutandis* the adolescent, requires a certain *psychological* preparation, he must possess a certain affinity with the psychology of woman, he must have a minimum of sympathetic intuition. For what is love—true love that dares to call itself by its name and urges us towards the opposite sex —what is it but the discovery in the partner of what we are not our-selves? It means stepping out of one's own ego, relinquishing one's own scale of values, and saying *yes* to the feminine scale of values. There are men, however, often over-sexed, who can never commit themselves in this way, who cannot achieve this exodus from their own selves and complete surrender to the non-self that is woman. They would like to confess this love for a woman, but the words stick in their throat. Such was the case of Amiel, as can be clearly seen in his *Journal Intime*. Such also was the case of Søren Kierkegaard, whom the Existentialist philosophy has brought into fashion again. His *Diary of a Seducer* and his frequent allusions to his 'terrible secret' (on account of which he even consulted a famous doctor) show this very clearly. And such, finally, was the case of Heinrich von Kleist. 'The sonorous beat of his iambics, the wails and imprecations in his letters, were but the impotent stuttering, the incoherent cry of a dumb man, because it could never reveal the deadly secret that was hidden within.'[1]

Kleist's *Geschichte Meiner Seele* has unfortunately not been preserved. In it we should have possessed a human document at least equal in value to Amiel's *Journal*. All we have are his works, at least as eloquent in self-revelation as those of Kierkegaard, and the outward facts of his life and of his death. Two outstanding character traits are always coming to the fore in his biography, traits which he shares with all those who, like him, are cursed with 'undiluted virility'. He is always seeking company, soliciting friendship, begging for love. In this he resembles Amiel. Both are always looking for something that will compensate for their feelings of inferiority—cause and effect of their inability to commit (*s'engager*) themselves. A man of this kind may bring himself to live with a woman. But since he always acts in conformity with his 'main directing lines', even in the normal sexual act he will only seek for a fresh confirmation of his already established *style of life*. He still remains incapable of voluntary self-surrender, and can never form that two-fold unity which comes into being when lovers meet. The carnal act demands not only the union of bodies but the fusion of souls; and of that, a man like Kleist, the eternal adolescent, is completely incapable.

And since the man who cannot escape from himself is bound to try to escape from his surroundings, Kleist takes to travelling. His life is full of changes of place and social setting. According to the Freudian psycho-analysts anyone who is unable to stay quietly home and loves to wander abroad and change his abode from place to place, is unconsciously trying to find a 'sexual object'. But in our opinion, what characterises this state of mind is a desire to flee from oneself rather than find anything else. Kleist probably felt that he ought to take that leap into the unknown which would initiate him into the love for a woman; but he preferred to take the decisive leap into death. He had an

[1] Cf. The chapter devoted to Kleist in *Das Leiden am Ich* by Wilh. Michel.

insatiable thirst for life, but was always finding himself excluded from life, so rather than venture the conquest of the non-ego he chose the abyss of non-being.

EXPLANATION OF HOMOSEXUALITY

A few general reflexions will help us towards a better understanding of Kleist. According to William Stern, the celebrated German psychologist who died in exile, a boy of fifteen feels closer in every way to a boy of his own age than to a girl. Everything feminine must necessarily seem to him alien and incomprehensible (except in the case where he has been specially prepared in this respect by a wise and far-seeing education). Whereas with boys of his own age he is on familiar ground, if only in regard to the physical formation of his body, everything to do with girls—their emotional and imaginative life, the budding secrets of their physical development—remains a strange and unknown territory. This is why young boys show a kind of resentment on the subject, and call girls 'stupid' and 'no good'. Boys take a pride in despising girls, and girls take a pride in being as independent of boys as they possibly can be. But since Alfred Adler carried out his penetrating investigations, we know that the attitude of the homosexual is simply an expression of the *masculine protest*, which consists in the subject asserting himself to be unaltered and unalterable by anything that may come from the opposite sex. This protest against the mutual dependence which nature has so surely established between the sexes exists to much the same extent in men and women. The number of women who are discontented with their role is probably much the greater, but on the whole they respond more successfully to psychological treatment than do men.

In Marlowe's *Edward II* we find the central character giving expression to this purely Adlerian conception of homosexuality. The king is tragically placed between his favourite Gaveston and his wife, Queen Isabel. In Act II, Scene 2, she exclaims,

> 'And when I come he frowns, as who should say,
> "Go whither thou wilt, seeing I have Gaveston."' [1]

But what in mature man is abnormal need not necessarily be so in an adolescent. The same thing is true of young girls at the time of puberty, when they are full of apprehension as to what awaits them in

---

[1] Cf. Oliver Brachfeld, 'Christopher Marlowe als Vorläufer der Individualpsychologie', *Internat. Zeitschr. f. Ind.-Psych.*, 1928.

their sex life. It was no doubt in view of these facts that William Stern and other specialists could speak of there being a 'normal' homosexuality in adolescents of both sexes during this period of transition to sexual maturity. We may add that it would be extremely dangerous to give publicity to such remarks, for they might easily lead to regrettable misunderstanding. The publication of such works as the Kinsey Report, very interesting but involuntarily tendencious, can do untold harm; this was true of the famous *Psychopathia Sexualis* of Krafft-Ebing. It would be quite wrong to think that because there is nothing abnormal in *apparently* homosexual leanings in certain adolescents, *every* adolescent must necessarily pass through this phase. The very opposite could be said of young people in Latin and Mediterranean countries. In Germany, on the other hand, the *Geschlechtsfindung*, i.e. the discovery by the subject of his authentic and definitive sexual role, takes place less easily and meets with many difficulties. It is best on the whole to speak of the homosexuality of adolescents as only *apparent*. It is very far from representing the definitive sexual orientation of most of the young people in whom it appears, and is to be regarded as only a passing phase in their sexual evolution. As soon as the feeling of helplessness before the opposite sex has disappeared, the *masculine protest* will disappear with it, as well as the absurd (though from the adolescent's own point of view the logical) desire to make oneself independent of the opposite sex.

Such is the case in *The Two Noble Kinsmen*, another Elizabethan play, where the transference of the heroine's affective orientation from her own to the opposite sex is very vividly portrayed.

Emily, sister of King Theseus, has lost her best childhood friend and continues to revere her memory, bringing flowers to her tomb every day. She is so inexperienced that she believes herself to be incapable of loving anyone of the opposite sex. However, Castor and Pollux, two young noblemen who are cousins and close friends, both fall in love with Emily at sight, and even challenge each other to fight in duel, their former love for each other having suddenly turned to hatred. The vacillations and hesitations of the three young people are shown with great subtlety by the unknown author. Castor and Pollux 'hostile to virgins' (here there are the mythological allusions dear to Bachofen) fall in love with Emily *simultaneously*; for as long as they both love her, neither will be able to win her, and their homosexual leaning to each other will be able to resist the pressure of the normal evolution. The

211

analysis of Emily's state of mind goes still deeper. She declares that she can love no one, so as to remain faithful to her dead girl friend lying in her tomb. (Once again puberal fixation of a love relationship with a person of her own age.) The young girl, who is gradually becoming accustomed to the inevitable but still hateful idea of choosing a husband, appears on the stage with a portrait in each hand, one of Castor, the other of Pollux. A monologue of hesitation begins. Emily dimly feels the approach of normal love in her heart, but cannot bring her choice to bear on either of the rival cousins. Thus by suspending her choice she is delaying the normal solution which will consist at the end of the play in her definitely choosing the victorious rival. Her transition from homosexual love (the transitory character of which is symbolised by its object being already dead and buried) to an attitude of indecision, and thence to a more and more definite selection of the normal love object—all this is described with the utmost subtlety and delicacy.

The co-ordination of the sexes in human nature is an inexorable law, and cannot be defied with impunity. Protests against it are always due to a sense of weakness and inadequacy ; but once again, we must remind the reader that feelings of inferiority can be produced as much by a *plus* as by a *minus*, and in both cases the result will be the same.

The timid Amiel and the bold Don Juan both suffer from the same trouble—an insecure ego which cannot find its feminine counterpart. The necessity for finding this counterpart is imposed on all of us by the fact that in our species sexuality bifurcates into two complementary currents and thus forms the *couple*, which is the fundamental human unit. The Don Juan differs from the timid type only in that he over-compensates his initial weakness. He was timid himself at the start. He tries to compensate for his terrible feeling of incompleteness by the excess and variety of his conquests. The timid man, on the contrary, means to defend his ego by completely excluding woman and sexual intercourse from his life. Moreover, he will compensate for this lack in his life by a purely superficial social intercourse with a type of woman who lacks sexual attraction, such as the blue-stockings who surrounded Amiel. There is thus only a step from timidity to Don Juanism. The Don Juan *over-compensates* the very feeling of inferiority which tortures the timid man and makes him ridiculous. The timid man very often has in him the makings of a seducer in the grand manner. Both are incapable of surrendering themselves to one woman only, in complete equality, and that is at the root of their trouble. To speak in this connection of 'inferior' and 'superior' types of timidity, as does Marañón, an exponent of the quantitative theory of sex, is to miss the point. Every man has in him a Don Juan *in spe*, who may or may not reach maturity; it will depend upon how much courage is there and what opportunities life supplies in each particular case. Both the timid man and the Don Juan are victims of a feeling of incompleteness; hence the emotional sterility which is the outstanding feature of all sexual perversions, whether sadism, masochism, onanism or necrophilism.[1]

TIMIDITY AND FEELINGS OF INFERIORITY

In one of his studies the late Professor MacDougall advanced the view that schizophrenia was at bottom an acute disturbance in the auto-estimative feelings. This was perhaps going too far, but there is certainly a close link between the feeling of inferiority and a syndrome closely allied to schizophrenia—timidity.[2]

Everyone knows the forced and unnatural smile of the shy person. It has the fixity of a mask and expresses no gaiety. There is something awkward and unauthentic about all the movements of the timid; they often remind us of marionettes moved by strings. Their behaviour seems to obey the same tendency as that which we find in dementia praecox and other variants of schizophrenia—namely the attempt on the

[1] It has been noted that all the Don Juans of literature are physically sterile. I have known several Don Juans in real life who were content to *enact* the preliminary ritual of the conquest. As soon as the woman yielded to them their eagerness fell to zero. I have shown elsewhere, 'Über die Furcht vor der Frau, in Sage, Märchen und Literatur', in *Intern. Zeitschr. f. Ind. Psych.*, 1928, how gynaecophobia, or the fear of woman, appears not only in all actual Don Juanism, but in the legend of Don Juan and other similar legends. 'To be a man'—that is more or less the consciously espoused motto of every Don Juan as of every pervert. In one of his short stories, Bruno Frank explains Frederick II's perversion by the same theme. It is the programme adopted by most Lesbians. Adler has shown how 'to be a man' can be regarded as the lowest common denominator of all attempts to compensate for a feeling of inferiority. Cf. *The Neurotic Temperament*, and more especially *El problema del homosexualismo y otros problemas sexuales*, with my introduction and commentary. Apolo Ed., Barcelona, 1936, and Cultura Ed., Santiago de Chile, 1937. The theory which regards perversions as merely variants of the one true perversion—the sense of impotence—was outlined for the first time in my contribution to the book *Selbsterziehung des Charakters*, Leipzig, 1930, which was compiled as a homage to Adler.

[2] Cf. Dr. F. A. Hampton's study on shyness in the *Journal of Neurology and Pathology*, 1928, VIII, p. 124. The author has based his comparison chiefly on external symptoms.

part of the patient to conceal his own ego, which he feels to be completely devoid of value. This mask, like their stereotyped movements, helps them at the same time to repel any attempt at a closer contact on the part of those around them.

A symptom that afflicts all timid subjects is what J. J. Rousseau, the most famous of that sad fraternity, described as the *esprit d'escalier*. The mental conflict they endure makes them incapable of doing the very thing they want to do; the more inferior they feel, the more they want to assert their own worth. When they are in the presence of a brilliant talker, the micromania which weighs on them will force them to hold their tongue. This reaction is not unlike the immobility of some animals when faced with danger, and of which the aim is 'not to be noticed'. But when this pressure on the auto-estimative level has been removed, when the subject finds himself alone, the tendency to assert himself will emerge once again. Then all the paralysed functions—intelligence, grace, wit, command of language—will come to life again, but 'in the staircase'! Timid persons of another type will compensate for their feeling of inferiority in exactly the opposite way; they become extremely loquacious, use a great quantity of words to say very little, and unload their stock of phrases as though they were firing a machine-gun. One often gets the impression that they rush into talk, urged by an unconscious fear that no one will listen to them. The loquacity which the experts of the last century numbered among the sexual traits of women, effeminate men, and homosexuals, is simply the direct outcome of the fear of not being taken seriously. And such a fear may well extend to the whole of the female sex, considering the centuries of contempt and under-estimation to which it has been subjected.

ADOLESCENT LEAGUES AT THE AGE OF PUBERTY

Here is another feature of adolescent behaviour which is found in adult males of 'undiluted' and unimpaired virility, as well as in those at the age of puberty.[1] A boy will often, in spite of the unconscious fear which accompanies it, feel a strong desire to approach the other sex, or rather a particular girl. He may even feel this (purely innocent)

[1] It should be noted in passing that the notion of psycho-sexual puberty is very different from that of purely physiological puberty. Thus, Oswald Schwarz of Vienna, well known in England, maintains that in many men puberty does not end till they have reached the age of 40, i.e. have built up a family and established their married life on a sure foundation, etc. And indeed, many old bachelors and Bohemians remain adolescent all their lives.

attraction for a younger or older sister. Whenever he is alone with her he will be friendly, affectionate, considerate, and obedient or even subservient. But as soon as another boy appears, a friend or a brother, his attitude will suddenly change; the masculine protest will appear, and he will turn against the girl, treating her with scorn and contempt and even physical roughness. How are we to explain this complete change of attitude? Can it be that there is a secret bond between the two boys, a kind of subconscious masculine solidarity? And since this tacit alliance takes place immediately, almost with any boy just because he *is* a boy, against the subject's own sisters, must it not be founded on something that is stronger than family ties? The fact is that very often there exists between two boys at the age of puberty a bond, similar to those which psychologists in pre-Hitler Germany denounced under the name of *Frauenfeindliche Jünglingen-(Männer-) Bünde*, Leagues of men and boys hostile to women. There is no need for them to form a club or a secret society, such as often happened in Germany. No, such alliances can have a purely *ad hoc* character and last only a few minutes; their existence is none the less certain. And the only explanation of such phenomena lies in the feelings of inferiority experienced when boys are brought face to face with the other sex, with that slight element of mystery, for which, as children, they have been insufficiently prepared.

This will explain what we have referred to elsewhere as the tragedy of 'excessive masculinity'. In most cases we are dealing with boys who meet few girls of their own age, or who have little occasion to mix with them and take them out. Not that these boys lack virility. On the contrary, it is often their very excess of virility which prevents them from approaching women. From their childhood up their souls have been starved of womanly contacts, they know nothing of the sweetness of surrender, their scale of values is inexorably and unilaterally masculine. The 100 per cent male (if he exists anatomically, which is doubtful) would be incapable of entering into a real relation with a woman. He may possess and enjoy a woman physically, he may even dominate and humiliate her, but for lack of mutual 'co-penetration' she will be serving him only as a means of masturbation. It might be possible to re-educate such men and teach them, late in the day, to become aware of and respond to womanly charm. This could be done, yet the victims we have been describing feel themselves condemned by God or by some mysterious law of nature to carry all their life the heavy burden of their timidity (wrongly so called), while they become increasingly fixed in their inability to understand the opposite sex. Theirs is not a case of 'superior' or 'inferior' timidity, as an out-moded treatment of sex problems would maintain. They are men who come near to the ideal of 100 per cent masculinity, but who lack the sensitiveness of feeling which would make it possible for them to approach members of the opposite sex not only physically but mentally and morally. Thus their masculinity will never be fulfilled, for it is only through woman that the youth becomes a complete man. And it is herein that lies the tragedy of the matter. For of what use is a virility that cannot find realisation in the one way that constitutes its *raison d'être?*

It must not be thought, as Dr. Marañón seems to do, that all timidity is of a sexual nature. That is taking too simple a view. Timidity is a general phenomenon; it appears as a result of feelings of inferiority and gradually extends over every domain of the subject's life. The urgent need to re-educate himself may induce the subject to *simulate courage* in certain departments of his life. This may succeed up to a point and enable him to throw a large number of his inferiority feelings overboard, as it were. But one weakness will remain in spite of everything —timidity towards women. It is the most invincible inferiority complex of them all.[1]

We all have to overcome our aversion to certain things, such as going into a shop to make a purchase, making a complaint or asking a favour; such minor efforts are a daily experience from childhood onwards. They are all manifestations of a feeling of inferiority, and are characterised by an attitude of indecision. But the need to overcome our feeling of inadequacy and helplessness before the opposite sex does not impose itself with the same urgency as do the minor difficulties of life. This explains why there are so many people of both sexes who are burdened with feelings of sexual inferiority. Sexually they are adolescents, even if in other domains of life they are already suffering from hardening of the arteries and calcification of the opinions. As we have seen, some writers consider that puberty may last till the age of forty;

[1] In his historical study *Philippe II*, 1927, M. Jean Cassou gives a vivid description of the adolescence of the unhappy Don Carlos, son of Philip II of Spain. 'In spite of the violence of his language and manners he was not known to have had any amorous adventure. . . . None of the princesses who were proposed to him attracted him, except the Archduchess Anne. It was for her sake, he said, that he would remain virgin. . . . And yet all night he would frequent the brothels, a false beard stuck on his face, in the company of other bad boys. By day he would take pleasure in humiliating and scandalising the women he met in the street. He would seize them by the waist and say "Kiss me, you whores!" . . . And yet no one knew at court whether or not he had ever had intercourse with a woman.'

others speak of puberty in the plural, as though there were different kinds of puberty in the course of our life. The truth is that it is not puberty that extends so far into our life, but simply this phenomenon which is far more common than is suspected—man's feeling of inferiority before woman. It is useless to try to overcome this feeling by means of physical love and a rough animal possession. So long as man does not achieve that mental fusion with his partner in love which will extend to the least details of their life in common, his feelings of inadequacy will render his masculinity an obsession to himself and a constant source of unhappiness.

It is obvious that what we have said about timidity in man also applies, within limits, to woman, for she too must learn in every detail the reciprocal process of adaptation to her partner. For a girl the opposite sex is also a *terra incognita*, though the role she will have to play in the field of sex is easier owing to its passivity. It is not she who takes the initiative in bridging the gap, and she need do no more than surrender passively to the young man. But this does not relieve her of the responsibility of preparing herself for an understanding of her partner which will transcend the purely physical aspect of sex.

Generally speaking, there is a marked difference between the timid man and the over-masculine man, for the latter has perhaps never suffered defeat at the hands of a woman. The only thing that prevents him from becoming 'normal' is his inability to enter into really intimate relation with her. The timid, on the other hand, are generally persons who have suffered disappointment. Naturally it is difficult to draw a hard and fast line between the two types of men who fail in their sex life. Both are the victims of powerful feelings of inferiority, but what distinguishes the 'undiluted males' is that they feel inferior through their lack of initiation into a realm of life which has remained closed to them. They pay very dearly for the ignorance of woman as such, in all her aspects, and therefore, *primus inter pares*, the sexual. The complex of the timid, on the contrary, is due to a real feeling of inferiority before women in spite of their possessing the mental preparation for a more intimate contact.

Who could speak the language of women better than a man like Amiel? He possesses many of the traits which are rightly called peculiarly feminine—vanity, instability, etc. And yet in spite of this nothing could have removed the fear which he had experienced as a child in the presence of one or more women. His case is particularly significant in this respect. He grew up surrounded almost exclusively by aunts and female cousins who were older, therefore bigger and stronger than himself. The feeling of being the smallest and weakest, and of being handed over to a number of large and strong women can easily create in the male child the 'absurd and mistaken opinion' (as Adler called it) that all women are stronger than oneself and are not to be trusted, or that it is dangerous to be dependent upon women. The unconscious 'directing line' which will henceforth determine such a man's behaviour may be expressed in the words 'Do your best to escape from woman's influence'. The timid man's conscious mind will tell him, 'You are really a fool, because most women are anything but evil and dangerous vamps'. But his unconscious mind, and hence his imagination, will always be haunted by the *femme fatale*, who is the product of bourgeois sexual morality, and represents the modern version of the medieval witch. We know how much stronger than the conscious mind is the affective side of man's personality, his unconscious, or rather the 'directing lines' of his personality. Is it surprising then if in such conditions the sexually timid man meets only with defeat when he tries to overcome his shyness by what seems to him an act of *superhuman* courage? Everything about the adventure will strike him as repulsive, uninteresting, even painful, for before entering upon the experience he is already convinced of his failure.

THE CASE OF ANDRÉ GIDE

The case of this ardent votary of homosexuality can be explained in much the same way as that of Amiel. Gide also suffered from the mental domination of a mother with too strong a character; as a child he too was often in the company of young girls who were bigger and stronger than himself. Is it not natural, then, that his heart should have conceived a deadly, though unconscious, hatred for those whom his reason was to recognise—too late!—as not at all dangerous? What can be done if the reasoning process is confined to the sphere of conscious thought? In the dark regions of the unconscious the directing lines established in childhood will inevitably continue their work. Gide believes that he can judge women 'objectively', just as he regards himself as 'condemned' to his anomaly, which, however, he persists in regarding as something perfectly *normal*. He is not the first to exclaim, 'Why condemn a being whose innate and irresistible inclination drives him to satisfy his instincts in a way that is different from that used by most of his fellow-creatures?' In another well-known case of the literature of sex, the same question had been asked by the Baroness Charlotte de Vaÿ and in still more poignant terms.

Why condemn a man for acting as a woman when he is born half woman? asked Zola in connection with a case of homosexuality which 'Dr. Laupts' had submitted to him. In his novel *Si le grain ne meurt*, Gide puts on record the fact that at a very early age he was guilty of violently aggressive behaviour towards the 'strong' women around him. This incident shows very eloquently how precocious in him was the attitude of struggle and protest, first against one particular woman, then against several 'strong' women by whom he felt oppressed, and finally, though no doubt below the level of conscious thought, against all women, against women in general.

It is interesting to follow the struggle which Gide's mother—the all too strong person in his family constellation—waged against the 'bad women' who might exercise an attraction on her son. And we need hardly add that these measures only helped to reinforce the boy's neurotic tendencies resulting from an unsuitable education. When he was twenty and had already achieved a certain degree of literary success, she would not allow him to go out at night unless accompanied by a friend who was to protect him from succumbing to the 'bad women' of the streets. I have not the space here to analyse Gide's autobiography in detail, and can only refer the reader to his *Journals* (now translated into English) and to my article 'André Gides Werdegang' in a summer issue of the *Zeitschr. f. Ind. Psychologie*, Leipzig, 1930. But I cannot refrain from recalling an amusing little adventure which he relates as having been undertaken by himself and his friend, Laurens, in view of 'renormalisation'. Gide's young friend successfully carried out his 'exploit' with a good-looking Moroccan girl. The next day it was to be Gide's turn, but before anything could happen his mother arrived post haste from Paris, having sensed from afar the danger that threatened her power as the only woman who really possessed her son's affection.

THE 'BARON' DE VAŸ

No less interesting, if it is viewed from the angle of inferiority feelings, is the case of the Baronne de Vaÿ. Her father, who had ardently desired a male heir to carry on the line, was deeply disappointed at the arrival of 'only a girl'. Unable to accept this humiliation he tried to sugar the pill by creating the illusion that he really had been blessed with a son and not a daughter. Instead of Sarolta (Charlotte) he called her

Sandor (Alexander), taught her to ride and hunt, to smoke a pipe and dress as a man. How could this unfortunate young woman escape the conviction that only what was masculine was worth while? How could she have been dissuaded from believing in the absolute inferiority that attached to being 'only' a woman? Was it not the logical outcome of such an upbringing that when she discovered the truth she attempted to bridge the gap that separates the two sexes, continued to dress as a man and refused to enter the serried ranks of depreciated womanhood? A return to femininity was unthinkable; her father had prepared the ground too well. Moreover, few people were in the secret, and the 'Baron' de Vaÿ was able to marry a woman, whose father, however, later brought the matter before the law courts.

It is extremely difficult to uproot an inveterate false valuation of the respective sexes, and to prevail upon those in whom it is ingrained to 'sink back' into the sexual condition they despise. We know a similar case where it was the mother who would not accept the fact of having given birth to a daughter, instead of the little Messiah who is the secret hope of every mother. The girl was brought up as her son, and many tears were shed by the child before the resulting disorders were eventually cured.

RAINER-MARIA RILKE

As a converse case, but still manifesting a protest against the normal sexual role, we may cite that of the poet Rilke. In this case the mother had always wished for a daughter, and therefore brought up her son as a girl, a step which brought in its wake the most unspeakable suffering for the poet, who was perhaps one of the greatest of our time.

For the selfishness of parents knows no limits; especially when, instead of accepting the rulings of fate, they try to impose upon their children the sex of their own choice. Nowadays, when the 'principle of virility' penetrates nearly every aspect of life connected with women, most couples only want sons; the birth of a daughter is regarded, if not as a catastrophe, at any rate as a disappointment. Cases such as those of Rilke's mother are therefore rare, and at first sight seem incomprehensible. One can understand a woman who has suffered all her life from the inferior status inflicted on her by society, wanting to spare her offspring the same fate and therefore indulging in the illusion that her girl can be brought up as a boy. The converse seems almost absurd. And yet, are there not parents of both sexes to whom the idea that their own children might surpass them in some way is intolerable? A selfish mother will realise that a son might have advantages in life which she had lacked, so she lets his hair grow long and dresses him as a girl. We know little of the psychology of Rilke's mother, but what indications we have point to interesting conclusions.

During his childhood Rilke was called by the French name *René*, which happens to be indistinguishable in sound from the female version *Renée*. It was not till later that he changed the name René-Maria to the German Rainer-Maria. This was when he had to leave his girlish little room for the rough atmosphere of a military cadet school. No wonder, then, that this sensitive poet should have interested himself in the fate of other unfortunates who are tormented with doubt as to their true sexual role. His name stands on the list of those who subscribed to the sexological review published by Dr. Magnus Hirschfeld, which espouses the cause of homosexuals who have fallen under the rigour of the law.

DOUBTS CONCERNING ONE'S SEXUAL ROLE

Here, then, is the root of so much feeling of sex inferiority. Unfortunately, the view that homosexuality and mental hermaphrodism are accompanied by certain bodily features is still being widely disseminated. The literature in question is not only degraded but, what is worse, often claims to be scientific. We cannot even exempt Dr. Hirschfeld from this charge; his views have been much attacked and are only pseudo-scientific. Among the so-called *stigmata of homosexuality* which he claims to have determined in the subjects who came to consult him, he notes, amongst other things, too great a distance between the big toe and the second toe, white hands, and other signs which nowadays we regard as completely devoid of sexual significance. Dictionaries of the symptoms of doubtful sex, such as Hirschfeld and his followers have compiled, can do an enormous amount of harm to young people of both sexes. What adolescent boy has not some feminine trait—such as a white, hairless arm, hips apparently too wide, a high-pitched voice, or a hesitating gait? Similarly a growing girl can easily have a slight excess of hair on the face, too deep a voice, too firm a walk. In such cases if the subject chances to look into a 'dictionary' (of which the general use should be severely banned in spite of its scientific appearance) he or she will inevitably experience feelings of sexual inferiority. At first there will be only curiosity and doubt. Then gradually the idea will emerge of freeing oneself from the special tasks peculiar to one's own sex, and adopting those of the other which, rightly or wrongly, are judged to be easier.

And there are many other minor factors in daily life which can induce doubt in our children as to the sexual role which nature has assigned to them. Girls are often dressed as boys, and *vice versa*: a boy's hair will be allowed to grow long, a girl's is cut short, names may be too masculine in the case of girls, too feminine in the case of boys: a boy may play with his sister's dolls while she interests herself in the more manly toys that have been given to him; and finally, a child of one sex may very easily be brought up in the style more generally used for the other. All these circumstances may form a starting point for what will later become a powerful inferiority complex.

But, it will be objected, have not many men worn garments as children which are now only worn by girls; have they not (if they are French) worn their hair in long curls and even had it done up in ribbons and chignons like their sisters? And yet, they have not become perverts, they have felt no doubt as to their sexual role, they have registered no masculine protest. This, however, does not invalidate our main contention. It would be stupid to claim that such details in a child's education are the cause of later sexual perversions, but they may become incorporated in already existing neurotic tendencies, colouring them in a special way and transforming them into neuroses and sexual perversions. For, contrary to the Freudian view that perversion is simply the 'opposite of neurosis', we hold that it is the most typical expression of neurosis. At the root of a perversion we shall infallibly discover an inferiority feeling of a general nature, devoid as yet of any sexual character. As a rule feelings of sex inferiority are a derivative from inferiority feelings of a more or less specific kind. Although still an ardent admirer of Freud, Adler disagreed with him sufficiently in 1907 to state (*Studie über die Minderwertigkeit von Organen*) that there was no organic minus value that did not automatically go hand in hand with a certain inferiority of the sexual organs. We could translate this statement into the purely psycho-sexual sphere, and say that there is no general feeling of inferiority which is not bound to have a repercussion of some kind in the subject's sexual behaviour.[1]

[1] In order not to overburden the text we have omitted a chapter on the feelings of incompleteness in woman, which appears in the Spanish editions of this book. In it we give a close analysis of the character of Hermione, heroine of the novel *Women in Love* by D. H. Lawrence.

CHAPTER XXIII

PSYCHO-GENESIS OF ART AND FEELINGS OF INFERIORITY

THE ARTIST AND THE WORK OF ART

IN dealing with the artist and the works he produces, the task of the psychologist is not such an easy one (relatively easy) as in the case of the neurotic or the delinquent. In the last analysis, art must be regarded as a socially useful activity, however asocial or even anti-social may be those who practise it. Crime and neurosis contain nothing of value to the community, whereas the artist creates something which becomes independent of him and acquires a value of its own—*the work of art*. This finished product is in general the only criterion we have for distinguishing the genuine artist from his imitation, the sterile charlatan. Both men may indulge in the same extravagant behaviour, wear the same loose bow-ties and lead the same Bohemian life; both may suffer from the same feelings of inferiority, even the same neurotic symptoms. The work of art, on the contrary, is something that is separate from its creator and his subjective character and has an existence in its own right. Psychology can tell us nothing of its 'objective vision'; it can at best only explain the process by which it came into being, its psycho-genesis. Aesthetics begin where psychology ends and, for lack of knowledge, must keep silent. For the neurosis which produces immortal works for the delectation and edification of humanity is of a different order from that which afflicts the unproductive and mediocre.

Obviously, from the point of view of psychology—a science which describes and interprets but does not evaluate—it would be impossible to authorise a given artist of established worth to keep or even cultivate his neurosis on the ground that he is a super-social personality, a creator who has to pay for his creation by his nervous complaints. The aim of psychology *qua* science of mental hygiene is to preserve as many individuals as possible from any kind of nervous disease. It cannot make exceptions in favour of super-social persons and allow them to escape from its net; it cannot take into account the works of art which such persons might or might not create. The fact that every neurotic is a kind of catalyst which tends to produce other cases of neurosis by mental contagion only confirms what we have just said. The objective appraisal of a work of art is an extra-psychological act, and must be completely detached from any personal evaluation of its author. The real interest of a work of art, the 'objective vision' of which it is the depositary, only begins where psychological analysis must end, and resign its job into other hands. The same is true of the achievements of science, or politics, or philosophy. A truth is equally true whether it springs from the brain of a lunatic or from that of a genius: the objective value that has been created breaks away from its creator and starts on a life of its own.

A concrete example taken from the history of music will help to make this clear. Beethoven, when he wrote the *Pastoral Symphony*, seemed to be trying to reproduce certain sounds in nature, the singing of birds, the murmur of the brook, etc. These features were very severely censured by contemporary criticism. We know now that the composer, who had been deaf for some years, did not want to copy or imitate nature, but was seeking a certain kind of 'security', in the Adlerian sense of the term. Being deaf, he re-created in his music the sounds he was condemned never to hear again, and he was able to do this, thanks to the marvellous phenomenon of mental compensation. Nevertheless, however imperious may have been Beethoven's need to find such compensatory security, we to-day listen with delight to this symphony, not because we look to it for any sort of security, but because of the pleasure it gives us as a work of art. What do the psychological factors which caused Beethoven to create it matter to us?

THE PSYCHO-GENESIS OF GENIUS

This brings us to the knotty problem of the psychology of the artist himself or, in other words, to that of the psycho-genesis of genius.[1] We shall not touch upon the sociological side of the subject which it was the fashion to deal with at great length some years ago, especially after the publication of the book by Lange-Eichbaum which so rapidly acquired popularity.[2] Adlerian psychology has thrown upon the

[1] Cf. my article in Catalan, 'Un nou teòric del geni: Alfred Adler' in *La Revista*, Barcelona, 1930.

[2] Cf. Lange-Eichbaum in the English translation, *The Problem of Genius*, Kegan Paul, 1931.

problem a light which was felt by some people to be a desecration of art, but which nevertheless represents a well-supported point of view, and one which has proved of great value to subsequent research.

We spoke just now of Beethoven. Among other notable figures in the musical world who suffered from auditory troubles the most frequently mentioned are Smetana, Humperdinck, Robert Franz and the musical critic Matheson. The thesis that there is a relation between a deficient sense of hearing and musical talent has been questioned on the ground that the *proportion of musicians who have become deaf is negligible.*

Elsa Bienenfeld[1] makes this objection, but the attempt has been made to use this purely statistical observation as a weapon against the Adlerian ideas.

The argument does not seem to us a refutation of the thesis that musical talent can be the result of over-compensation. We knew a boy of fifteen who showed no interest in music until his hearing was seriously impaired by an attack of otitis. After this he became intensely interested in everything audible, went regularly to the opera, attended concerts and a few months after the 'accident' organised a small chamber orchestra. He never became deaf, and his musical ear was perfect. I am convinced, however, that but for the illness which concentrated his attention upon his hearing he would never have found his way into the enchanted realm of music. The theory of musical talent as over-compensation does not claim that a *congenital* organic inferiority is indispensable for the development of such talent. Nor need we assume, as Elsa Bienenfeld seems to think we do, that 'an auditory inferiority in the musician's ancestors would lead to such results'. In the case mentioned it was an illness of the ear that concentrated the subject's attention on music. In other cases it is sufficient for the child to grow up in a musical atmosphere and become initiated into its pleasures at an early age. Families like those of Bach or the elder Strauss, which produced several generations of fine musicians, needed no auditory troubles for their members to be drawn to music. What matters is not the defect or inferiority, but the degree of interest in and attention to auditory material. Very often, but not always, this interest and attention awaken only as the result of an organic lesion.

A glance at cases suffering from deficiency in the visual sense will lead us to the same conclusion. Thus the examination carried out by Adler in an Art Academy showed that more than 70 per cent of the

[1] Elsa Bienenfeld, Ph.D., in 'Ertaubte Tondichter', in *Wiener medizinische Wochenschrift*, 1939, No. 39.

students suffered from a more or less serious deficiency or inferiority of eyesight. It has recently been considered possible to establish the fact that Albrecht Dürer squinted. We know that Adolf Menzel was extremely short-sighted, and could work only by bringing the canvas, etching plate or paper to within a few centimetres of his eyes. El Greco, like Manet, seems to have suffered from severe astigmatism. Mateyko was also myopic. Lenbach had only one eye. An old Italian painter, Guercino di Centa, was called so because he squinted, and Vasari is witness that Piero della Francesca ended by becoming completely blind, which leads one to suppose that from childhood he had suffered from some visual anomaly. Recent statistics compiled in various art schools give 40 to 60 as the percentage of budding artists who suffer from some kind of eye trouble.

Naturally, we cannot expect to find a large number of painters who have gone blind. No one would claim that an organic inferiority alone will lead to artistic achievement. But in many cases it may be the starting-point of such development. Very often an acute attack of conjunctivitis will suffice to direct a child's attention to visual objects. My friend, Ch. R., nearly went blind at the age of one. He never knew this, but later at the age of sixteen he developed a remarkable talent for painting. He was particularly expert in costumes, for after a brief survey of the subject he was able to remember the costumes of all the different historical periods down to the least detail. He was promised a brilliant career, but at the age of twenty-one he abandoned all his artistic activities. His eyesight had been singularly sharpened by the illness of his babyhood, but he lacked the other qualities of character, etc., that would have made of him a true artist. For it has never been claimed that *every* organic inferiority will *necessarily* lead to over-compensation, nor that over-compensation (obviously at work in the case of Ch. R.) will be sufficient to produce artistic achievement.

We see the same thing happening in the sphere of the other organs. Among actors—and not the least gifted—there are those who suffer from some defect of speech or diction. Among orators there is a large percentage of stammerers who can overcome their defect only under the stress of emotion—the very thing which makes them so eloquent in public. It is said of Camille Desmoulins that, although he stammered in private life, in public his speech 'flowed like liquid gold'. Moses himself, according to the Bible, was slow of tongue, while his brother Aaron possessed the gift of speech. Everyone knows that too much volubility in an orator is more tiring to an audience and less effective _

226

than a slow and apparently difficult delivery. Only the author who can overcome his inhibitions and (however much he may have prepared his speech beforehand) can give the effect of making the effort to think and find the right word at the time of speaking, will really be able to cast a spell over his audience.

To take an example from another sphere, where the inferiority in question was purely psychological and not in any way organic, we have it on record that at the age of four Linnaeus, the famous naturalist of the seventeenth century, used to be taken for a walk in the meadows every Sunday by his father. The father would name all the flowers they saw, but the child was inattentive and never remembered the names. One day the father lost patience and threatened to whip him if he did not pay more attention. This threat (equivalent to a psychological 'inferiority') apparently sharpened the small boy's attention to plants and their names. The *punctum minoris resistentiae*, which at the age of four was the naming of plants, was thus overcome under the threat of punishment, and resulted through over-compensation in Linnaeus' marvellous achievements as a botanist.

Unamuno, the great Spanish thinker and writer, relates as his earliest recollection a conversation between his father and a bearded stranger in a language he could not understand. After the stranger had left, the child learned that he was a Frenchman. It may well be that this early experience of a sense of inferiority at being unable to follow a conversation aroused the young Miguel's interest in languages. The fact remains that he became a philologist, was Professor of Greek at the University of Salamanca and read modern Greek, German and Danish with ease, as well as all the Romance languages. We know, since Adler's researches, that the interest of small children centres most easily around a defect, a weak point, an inferiority; and the experiences of Linnaeus and Unamuno, the psychological significance of which is pointed out here for the first time, certainly help to show that there is a very close connection between a child's earliest recollections and the future unfolding of its talent.

Since man is, according to most psychologists, first and foremost a visual being, an 'optic man' (*Augenmensch*, as Gundolf used to say), it is only natural that anomalies of the eyesight should have tended to develop an interest in visible things different in kind from that entertained by the painter or sculptor. A man who cannot see well will be better able than one endowed with normal vision, to recreate forms and configurations, if not with his hands then with his imagination. It may therefore be affirmed that the writer, and especially the novelist, must possess, in addition to the indispensable gift of language, a very strong *visual imagination*, which is the gift we often find in those who have gone blind.[1] The case of the modern Hungarian author, G. Szanto, has aroused great interest in his own country. Before the 1914–18 war, he was a painter; wounded in battle, he lost his eyesight, and when completely blind he became a writer of books in which the visual and even visionary element plays a great part. Greek and German mythology are full of examples that show in striking fashion that the ancients were dimly aware of the paradoxical relation between a physical defect and its compensation. Tiresias the singer, Homer the singer, and Ossian the rhapsodist are all represented as blind. The goddesses of fate, the Greek Moira and the Nordic Norns, spin the thread of human destiny without seeing it, and Justice, who really *ought* to see clearly, is represented as blindfold. In folklore, seers are always described as blind, as though the loss of physical vision were the necessary precondition to the mysterious power of piercing through the world of appearances into the realm of essences, hidden from ordinary mortals. The god Hephaistos, like his Nordic equivalent Weland, is lame; consequently, as a lame man cannot do much outside the house, he is represented as a horse-smith and jeweller. We read in the Iliad descriptions of the pictures he carves on Achilles' shield; they represent the battles in which, as a cripple, he cannot take part, but which he recreates by way of compensation with his artist's imagination. He is also a great braggart—the *enfant terrible* of Olympus.

Organic inferiority can therefore be the starting-point of a process of compensation which enables the individual to get the better of it

[1] Among writers known to have been myopic mention is generally made of Gustav Freytag. He would never wear spectacles and thus forced himself to develop what he called 'a swift intuition of many things that were not sufficiently clear to me'. The author of *Mon Frère et Moi* tells how his brother, Alphonse Daudet, went through life 'like a blind man possessed of a faculty for minute observation, of microscopic exactitude'. It was the blind Milton who wrote 'Hail, holy light . . .' and it is a curious thing that Schiller (the name means 'squinter'), who suffered all his life from inflamed eyes, should have described so vividly in *William Tell* the Swiss scenery he had never seen. His hero in this play is the man who *aims* better than anyone else, and one of the characters, Melchtal, is *blinded* by order of Gessler. Finally, there is the case of Marcel Proust, concerning whom I think I am the first to have observed that his *written* sentences grew progressively longer as his attacks of asthma became worse and his *spoken* sentences were forced to be shorter.

and sometimes to find *over-compensation*. This does not mean, needless to say, that every *minus-value* leads to achievements of a useful order. On the contrary, this is the exception rather than the rule. But the *possibility* of such compensation is always there; whether it is realised or not will depend on the autonomous, and we might almost call it the sovereign response of the individual. The compensation can be *real* or *fictitious*, by which we mean *useful* or *useless* to society. Generally speaking, however, we may say that over-compensation is subject to a certain number of very varied conditions. It is dependent upon the degree of feeling towards the community in which the subject lives, upon the social, economic and cultural barriers he will meet with; finally we must remember that there are polyvalent compensations (*compensaciones polifacéticas; mehrfache Kompensationen*), which mutually strengthen or weaken each other. In many cases the pronounced weakness or the purely physical resistance of the organ affected is an insurmountable obstacle.

It would be a mistake to regard this approach to the subject as one that reduces genius to a level of a nervous malady. Michelangelo created the Sistine Chapel not *because* he was a neurotic, but *in spite* of it. The same is true of Leonardo da Vinci. The question whether or not he was a neurotic is of no interest to the history of art, and it is doubtful if from any point of view the question can be formulated in these terms. It is not to the neurotic, but to the creative artist in him that we are indebted for the *Mona Lisa* and the *Last Supper*. As Wexberg has said, 'If there is a deep-lying relation between neurosis and artistic creation it can only be of a negative nature; it may well be that artistic creation is released as the result of a dialectical process resting on a division of the ego and acting as a kind of auto-cure of the individual.'

It was no doubt because artists constitute such a peculiar case that Adler did no more than indicate their place in his scheme of compensation. All he could assign to them was a dotted line extending from the socially useless to the superior type that is useful to society. In the era of bourgeois liberalism, however, it is clear that the utility of the artist was never considered comparable to that of the bank director or the brewer. Hence Adler's difficulty in facing the paradox that to the artist as such the notion of social utility is not strictly applicable. The Adlerian psychology dealt with the *isolated* artist of a period which is now obsolete, and it took no account of the changes in the function of art which were introduced with the development of mechanical reproduction. An artist, a scientist, or a writer who devotes himself entirely to his work, and who allows his creative work to 'devour' him, will very easily exaggerate the importance of what Adler calls the vital problem of work and will not even attempt to solve the twin problems of social and sexual adaptation.[1] To take an example from the world of contemporary science Lysenko is probably more adapted to his 'community' than is his opponent, who could easily be made 'neurotic' by coming into conflict with the power of the State. But it is perhaps the opponent who will have best served the cause of science.

No doubt such men are 'neurotics'. Have we the right, then, to make a distinction between the vulgar or inferior neurotics and those that are superior or super-social? And even admitting the justice of such a classification, what are the criteria by which we can establish it, especially in the lifetime of the person in question? The work of art, the scientific discovery, the new philosophical system—these might be taken as objective criteria to distinguish between the neurotic man of true ability and the neurotic charlatan. But both artistic and scientific reputations are subject to changes of fortune and many a genius has died unacknowledged by his contemporaries. The problem, therefore, admits for the present of no solution.

To sum up, we may say that no organic deficiency automatically produces a compensation. A compensation is neither inevitable nor even probable; it is at the most *possible*. A minus-value in the substructure of a human being *may*, therefore, produce a superstructure which would not otherwise have existed, and a work of art often comes into being like the pearl in the oyster, through the presence of a

---

[1] It is significant that just as Julien Benda denied the right to matrimony of the modern 'clerc' Søren Kierkegaard regarded it as treason for a pioneer of the spirit to get married. But was this belief not a neurotic symptom on his part, since we know that he dreaded marriage, broke off his engagement at the last moment, and probably regarded himself as condemned to an unmarried life because of his onanistic proclivities? *Symptom oder Leistung?* asks the modern psychologist. To renounce the world and retire into a convent from fear of marriage—a fear due to feelings of inferiority—is only a symptom in the bad sense of the word. But to do so while still feeling the desires and impulses of a normal man or woman, to practise renunciation not as an unconscious sop to one's own weakness, but solely in the service of a higher cause—that is an achievement, a merit. It is therefore only with such reservations in mind that one can subscribe to the following statement of Benda's: 'I have discovered that one of the great betrayals of the modern "clerc" is marriage or more precisely the state of father of a family, with the immense social interest and the inevitable conservatism which result from this state. ... Descartes, Spinoza, Kant, to say nothing of Montaigne and Voltaire, were not fathers of families; and I think their philosophy gained by it.'

lesion. In man, however, it is not the lesion itself which produces the compensatory process, but his feeling of the lesion, i.e. his feeling of inferiority. And the man of genius is by no means the product of his organic minus-value nor even of the mental compensations it leads to. As we have already stated, for the compensations to result in artistic or scientific activity which is worthy of the name they must work in with all kinds of non-psychological factors, of a political, social or economic order. It is a sociological fact that the 'cult of genius',[1] which was characteristic of the bourgeois liberal stage of social evolution, is on the decline; what psychology does is, in all humility, to point out that the inspiration of genius is due neither to divine favour nor to the 'mysterious play of heredity'.

If, from the psychological point of view, we dissociate ourselves from the cult of genius there can, on the other hand, be no question of regarding the work of genius as 'nothing but' a compensation for a defect, or 'nothing but' a sublimation, or again, as merely the result of a transference in the Freudian all too mechanical sense, i.e. of a transformation of psychic energy. The painfully vivid sense of the ego's insecurity in a hostile world owing to a sensory deficiency (visual in the artist, aural in the musician), or the impulse to acquire by means of the imagination what life has denied us in fact[2]—these give us only the psycho-genesis of the creative artist, not that of the work of art itself. Thus although culture and civilisation have their compensatory function, it would be an inadmissible error to regard them as compensation pure and simple on a gigantic collective scale. Feelings of inferiority and insecurity may well have *released* the cultural process; they can never supply its complete interpretation.

[1] 'Men must be loved, not admired', such is the conclusion of the remarkable work *Genie-Religion* by Edgar Zilzel.

[2] Balzac, Paul Valéry, and André Maurois all claim that this happens in the case of the creative artist. Watteau, who painted the marvellous *Embarquement pour Cythère*, was among the great men 'excluded from love'. Michelangelo . . . but the list would be interminable.

CHAPTER XXIV

RESENTMENT AND CATATHYMY

RESENTMENT AND INDIVIDUAL AND COLLECTIVE FEELINGS OF INFERIORITY

THE term 'resentment'[1] is sometimes taken as being synonymous with feelings of inferiority. This identification or rather confusion of the two terms is in our opinion completely mistaken, for they are based on two different conceptions and do not denote the same mental state.

The story of the fox and the grapes is often used to classify the notion of resentment. A man wants something that he cannot get, and because of this he declares it to be worthless, bad and not deserving to be coveted. In our opinion, however, the fox seems to represent a very intelligent type of person and not at all one burdened with resentment. According to the psychologists,[2] resentment takes place in two stages. The first stage consists in adopting a negative attitude in judging any values whatsoever. Kretschmer has given an admirable definition of this stage when he said that 'a feeling of scrutiny in a state of continual inner revolt was sufficient to justify a diagnosis of resentment'. With this sentence the word resentment, which Nietzsche loved to use, passed into the official ranks of psychiatry. In the second phase, a transmutation of values takes place in a catathymic fashion (from the Greek κᾰτᾰ́=down and θῡμός=soul), the subject assigning moral value to things that are devoid of value. According to Gaston Roffenstein, this

---

[1] We have chosen the English word 'resentment' as the nearest equivalent to the French word *ressentiment*. The reader will find, however, that as used in this chapter it acquires a shade of meaning slightly different from its usual connotation. It indicates a permanent state rather than a momentary reaction (Translator).

[2] It is a curious fact that the literature of resentment is even poorer than that of the feeling of inferiority. I can recall only a German book, *Pädagogik des Ressentiments*, published by J. A. Barth in Leipzig, which, however, does not speak of the subject, and Dr. O. Forel's recent short study, *Le Ressentiment—Problème de Ré-éducation*. Printed by A. Carrara, Morges, Switzerland, 1948. It had previously appeared in German in the *Revue de Psychologie Suisse* of the same year.

second phase has two fairly distinct stages, the first of which consists in the general negation of all values, and in stripping them of anything which made them 'superior'. This stage does not necessarily entail any insistence on one's own value as something superior; that attitude is reserved for the second phase.

But on closer examination all this is by no means identical with the feeling of inferiority. It would seem rather that what we have to do is to seek for the roots of resentment in the feeling of inferiority. 'Resentment', says Roffenstein, 'has its origin in an unconfessed minus-value or inferiority which may be imaginary or real, personal or objective.' This author, who died prematurely, is very far from accepting the somewhat exaggerated ideas of the late Max Scheler[1] on the subject. To call resentment a feeling of inferiority is to confuse the effect with the cause. Resentment could certainly not appear without a previous minus-value or feeling of inferiority, but this does not mean that every feeling of inferiority will necessarily grow into resentment. The exploited classes may well feel 'inferior' as compared to their rich masters, but that does not necessarily mean that they are ignorant of any good qualities which the latter may possess. The best thing for such people to do in the circumstances is to accept the situation as unalterable, to conform to it without rebelling inwardly against the inferiority which it confers upon them. Moreover, in most cases what happens is this: as soon as the subject recognises and admits his own inferiority, the resentment, which consists in refusing to recognise anyone as one's superior, ceases to have any *raison d'être*. Far more likely to arouse a spirit of resentment against the existing state of things is the feeling of personal insecurity. There can be no doubt that in Germany between the wars the acute economic insecurity and ensuing misery were the chief factors in carrying the masses first towards the parties of the extreme left, and then to the National Socialism of the extreme right.

The fact remains, however, that resentment and feelings of inferiority alike are *catathymic* phenomena. The term catathymy was used for the first time by H.-W. Maier to denote 'false judgments produced catathymically or on a basis of affective over-estimation'. In general, the term is used in psychiatry to mean the deformation of mental contents under the influence of affectivity. Thus catathymy is a quality which inferiority feelings and resentment (which is derived from them) have in common. In both cases, sane judgment is distorted, blinded by affec-

[1] Max Scheler, *El resentimiento en la moral*, Madrid, s.d., and *Vom Umsturz der Werte*, vol. I, 1919.

tivity, and becomes negatively directed on to a definite person. But in the case of the feeling of inferiority, this animosity is directed against one or more of the functions of the ego; while in the case of resentment, the subject, as he does not recognise his own inferiority, adopts a negative attitude to other people, or other things; he attacks the non-ego and tries to despoil it of its value. In both cases, there is a delimitation of the affective visual field and of the mental horizon; only, in the case of the feelings of inferiority the delimitation is of the subject's own person, of his ego, and consequently of his possibilities, whereas in the case of resentment the devalorisation—owing to the subject's deep-lying and unadmitted (unconscious) belief in his own inferiority —extends over the whole realm of the non-ego. Resentment may very easily lead to ideas of personal superiority and even to *folie de grandeur*. The feeling of inferiority, on the other hand, if it finds no compensation, implies a completely different attitude—that of self-minimisation or *micromania*. It can therefore be stated that resentment is precisely one of the many forms of compensation for the feeling of inferiority.

RESENTMENT, A MENTAL POISON

Thus the feeling of inferiority stands in judgment over the subject's own ego, like all the feelings which Janet described in his time under the various names of 'feeling of shame of the body', 'feeling of incompleteness', etc., all of which have the ego as their object. The object of resentment, on the contrary, lies *outside the self*. After suggesting the word 'rancour' (*rancune*) as possibly more suitable for the subject under discussion, Max Scheler says very characteristically,

'In resentment we have primarily a definite emotional reaction towards others, a reaction which repeatedly rises to the surface. This implies that the more it recedes from the zone of expression and action, the more deeply it penetrates to the centre of the personality. The tendency of the emotion to be always coming to life again and to persist is something very different from purely intellectual memory and the processes connected with it.'

(We may note in passing that the feeling of inferiority is also something very different from a purely intellectual consciousness of one's own inferiority.) According to Scheler, resentment, in the first place, consists in 're-living the emotion itself'; it is a re-feeling (*re-sentir*). Secondly, the term implies that the emotion in question is of a negative character, i.e. that it expresses hostility. It is in fact rancour, spleen, the bad feeling that has been kept under, which fills the soul with darkness, quite independently of any action taken by the self. It finally takes shape when the emotions of hatred and hostility have begun to recur at regular intervals. It has as yet no definite hostile aim, but it feeds every tendency of this nature.

There can be no doubt that this 'spleen' comes from something further back still, something of which all theoreticians should take account, whether they are philosophers, like Nietzsche and Scheler, or psychiatrists, like Kretschmer, and this something further back is always the feeling of inferiority or one of its variants. Has not Scheler himself asserted that 'at its base resentment is confined to slaves and subordinates, i.e. to those who languish under the yoke of authority against which they would rebel in vain'? Eliasberg and others have found this same resentment in domestic servants, and everyone knows how difficult it is to overcome in their case.

Nevertheless, whenever the feeling of inferiority finds a palliative or a compensation, it ceases to turn into resentment. A violently repressed impulse, which serves as a starting-point for resentment, may eventually lead to the development of an embittered or envenomed personality. If an ill-used servant can give full vent to his feelings in the servants' hall, he will not succumb to this inner poisoning which characterises resentment. But if, on the contrary, he has to put a smiling face on his misfortune, silently swallow his spleen, and bury the emotions of hostility and repulsion, resentment, says Scheler, will inevitably follow.

Resentment, then, arises from a lack of equilibrium in the individual's auto-estimation. The problem, therefore, is not one for philosophers and sociologists, but falls precisely within the province of the specialist in feelings of inferiority. For who better than the Adlerian psychologists know the need for some immediate little compensation, however anodyne, whenever the auto-estimative level has been lowered? The domestic servant relieving his feelings in the servants' hall is only utilising a form of compensation well known to the child psychologist.

We have already spoken of children who, when they have been scolded or punished, feel an imperious need either to shut themselves up in an empty room where they can curse to their heart's content the person who has inflicted this humiliation upon them, or to find immediate solace by buying sweetmeats. With adolescents and adults it is masturbation or normal sexual pleasure which will serve as compensations after such humiliations or other failures. Indeed, sexual pleasure and drink are the two most frequent methods for the *discharge*, or, to use a word which French psychologists are vainly trying to popularise, for the abreaction of adult feelings of inferiority. The art of the teacher, the spiritual adviser or the psychiatrist, when dealing with such characters, must therefore consist in finding the least harmful abreactions which will act as compensations for their feelings of inferiority. This kind of preventive pedagogy is undoubtedly the best prophylactic treatment for the disease of resentment.

Resentment, then, in Scheler's view, is a compensation; but it is not only a 'useless' but also an 'interior' compensation. He speaks of it as being a very infectious 'mental poison'. And indeed one might compare it to the naja's poison, dangerous only to others, but harmless to the serpent itself, though carried inside its body. The feeling of inferiority, on the contrary, is the sort of poison which produces auto-intoxication of the subject's whole personality. It is not a weapon in the struggle for survival, nor a reaction towards a hostile environment, nor (except by contagion) a danger to those around it; it is more like the scorpion's tail, with this difference, that it not only *can* inject the poison into its own body, but that it inevitably and continuously *does* so.

We must remember above all that resentment, like the feeling of inferiority, is extremely contagious. How, then, does Max Scheler describe this communication of resentment by one mind to another? 'Sociologically speaking', he writes, 'we can deduce the following very important principle. The abundance of the mental dynamite will increase with the degree of separation between the politically effective group and those groups in the community that have a just claim to the esteem or valuation of the public.' Now it seems to us idle to approach the problem from this point of view so long as one does not go back to the deep-lying origins of all collective resentment. The first question that arises is: How does resentment spread from one person to another? But before answering this we must deal with the more fundamental question—how does the feeling of inferiority, the cause of resentment, spread from one individual to another?

'SHARED' FEELING OF INFERIORITY

It can be stated forthwith that when the feeling of inferiority is shared it is far less acute than when it is experienced by the isolated individual. What is the reason for this curious phenomenon? It is easy enough to understand if we remember that every individual possesses, anyhow in a latent state, a large dose of community spirit or sense of solidarity. Now we know from what Adler has taught us that the best remedy for the feeling of inferiority is the feeling of community. If, therefore, those who feel themselves to be inferior or oppressed join together and form a community-through-necessity (*Notgemeinschaft*), it is only natural that this unit of solidarity should in a measure mitigate their suffering.

The facts indeed confirm this hypothesis; and were not Adler's theories entirely grounded on fact? A child who is late for school will often hang about, waiting for the arrival of another late-comer, before facing the sidelong looks of his schoolfellows and the rebukes of his master. The presence of the other culprit will give him courage, for it will no longer be alone, but *together* with another that he will face reprimand or punishment. In such a case there will come into being a certain tiny *community in misfortune*, even if the comrade in question is the worst pupil in the school and the most looked-down upon by the others. It is interesting to note how often the formation of such communities-through-necessity will make even the haughtiest child realise that his despised companions have a certain 'value'. Such situations can therefore lead by ricochet to a feeling of community.

The same thing happens when the members of any community or group identify themselves with one of their number who has been victimised by his superiors. A workman is wrongfully dismissed, and immediately his comrades go on strike. This identification, as it has been called, is in the first instance a purely selfish reaction, based on the thought 'Supposing it were to happen to me?' Thus people wrap themselves up in their selfishness, blind to the common danger because the education they have received, in school and out of it, has always directed their minds in a direction that is diametrically opposed to solidarity. It is infinitely easier to organise a collectivity *against* someone or something than *for* them. This explains why it has often been possible to obtain political ends in a catagogic manner, which one could never have gained in an anagogic way. German National Socialism, we are told, boasted of having developed the racial community feeling (*Volksgemeinschaft*), but it did so less by exalting its own 'racial' values than by denigrating other races and other nations, e.g. the Jewish 'race', 'negroid' France, etc.

Thus what first provokes an *individual* feeling of inferiority is a danger that threatens the individual in his particular situation. The

237

subject, if he does not succumb to neurosis, is then obliged to seek some sort of contact with his fellow-creatures. And this contact will bring to light the community spirit which years of individualistic education have not entirely stifled. In many, this awakening of the community spirit is so strong that it will shine in its full splendour. In others, even if it has been successfully dug out from under the mass of egotistical *débris*, it will awaken only for a short time. Quickly disillusioned, it will disappear again. Now the question arises whether a common danger, threatening each individual unit of a collective body, is sufficient to produce in the community as such a *collective* sense of inferiority. In other words, is a contagious feeling of inferiority already a collective one?

THE COLLECTIVE FEELINGS OF INFERIORITY CLASSIFIED

It is not easy to give an answer to the question which we have asked. We shall avoid terminological arguments and simply state the existence of two large classes of collective inferiority feelings. The first is that which we have just described, i.e. the sum of the individual feelings of inferiority, and could therefore be expressed by suitable mathematical symbols. But there is another kind, which does not arise simply in isolated moments of danger, but corresponds to a more or less permanent state of things. It appears by reason of the fact that the people in question belong to the same race, caste or social stratum. Examples taken at random are national minorities, the vast fraternity of 'the poor', the Jewish race, coloured persons, etc. Nor must it be thought that superior groups cannot also experience feelings of inferiority. The *being different* (which Stendhal regarded as the cause of hatred) is what engenders these feelings. They are not necessarily produced by any objective inferiority in relation to other groups, but always by the mental superstructure of those who experienced them. Typical instances of this are the feelings of a white man who chances to find himself in a 'coloured' restaurant in New York as the only representative of his race in a crowd of Negroes, or the child of rich parents among a crowd of guttersnipes, so much freer from parental control than he is. In all these and analogous cases, the feeling of inferiority comes from the sense of difference due to the fact of belonging to a different collective group. But even in these cases, the feeling does not cease to be *individual*, i.e. it is experienced and 'lived through' by one person alone. And yet, at the root of the experience in question, there is not an individual but a collective feeling of inferiority.

A second type of inferiority feeling which we should mention in passing is the 'feeling of strangeness' (*Fremdheitsgefühl*) experienced by uneducated or even semi-educated persons in the presence of strangers, of people speaking a different language and still more in the presence of coloured folk. This feeling is at the root of Chauvinistic anti-semitism. It is as though the auto-estimative level were threatened by the mere physical presence of a different sort of individual. This feeling is very confused and eludes all attempts at rationalisation. It is even difficult to find a name for it. On the whole the most appropriate is the German word *Unheimlichkeitsgefühl* (feeling of the uncanny).

There is a third class which can be regarded simply as one variety of the class of shared feelings of inferiority. Thus in the case of a school class under too strict a teacher, the whole collectivity feels itself inferior in relation to one individual. But when the same class considers itself inferior to another class in the same school, whether in scholarship or sport, we already have a feeling of inferiority felt by one group in relation to another group. This phenomenon is of frequent occurrence between competing teams in the field of sport. It may happen that the group suffering from a feeling of inferiority (a collective one, though each member participates in it to a different extent) will be unable to overcome its misgivings as to its own worth, and will be easily defeated by the opposing team, which has greater confidence in itself. In other cases, this same feeling of inferiority is the driving force that makes the team pull itself together and do better than in previous encounters. The inferiority complex becomes the agent of victory and the enemy team is beaten. What has been called the 'clash of the generations' between fathers and sons is in general nothing but the outcome of a feeling of inferiority on the part of the younger generation in the face of the literary, military, artistic and intellectual honours won by their forebears. We have here on the collective plane what used to be called *Herbertism*[1] in Germany, i.e. the mediocrity of the sons whose fathers had achieved exceptional distinction in any domain. *Collective Herbertism*, like its individual form, is due to the violent feelings of inferiority of the kind we have been describing. It is a curious fact that in many European countries the men of the first World War—combatants and non-combatants alike—subsequently felt themselves to be inferior to the generation that had preceded them and to that which succeeded them. This is undoubtedly what Remarque, author of *All Quiet on the Western Front*, meant when he said that the victims of the

---

[1] The name was coined from *Herbert*, the name of Bismarck's son.

war were not only those who had fallen in battle but those who had come back. And yet, some fifteen years after the war, when these men had discovered that this self-imputed inferiority amounted to nothing, they began to club together, to express new ideas, to publish new reviews ... by no means inferior in value and interest to those that had gone before or have come since. The *shock* of having forgone the intellectual (and material) pleasures of civilised life for a long spell produced in them such feelings of inferiority that it took fifteen odd years of work to dispel them. It is also curious to note that those who set great store by the fact of belonging to one generation rather than another,[1] are often the prey to serious doubts and misgivings concerning their own worth.

RESENTMENT HAS ITS SOURCE IN FEELINGS OF INFERIORITY

Now all these feelings of inferiority are communicated with more or less intensity from one individual to another. Every phenomenon resembling an inferiority complex is, after all, a social phenomenon. One neurotic will produce others in his *entourage*, and every neurosis is in essence a family neurosis. Even when large numbers of a collectivity refuse to consider themselves inferior and are at pains not to inculcate the collective inferiority complex of their group in their children, they will not succeed. I am thinking, for example, of the highly cultured Jews who dissociate themselves from and despise their brethren whose lives are entirely devoted to commercial gain. In spite of this they will continue to feel the weight of a public opinion which regards all Jews as contemptible. The inferiority thus assigned to them may lead them, by way of compensation, to develop a superiority complex. The Jews, the Germans and the Japanese would never have considered themselves superior to all other races (and even if they deny this conviction they cannot shake it off) had it not been for the position of inferiority that has been assigned to them. The fact of Jews being debarred from certain professions, in spite of their individual merits, solely because of their race, arouses in them the classic resentment, the 'Jewish hatred' of which Nietzsche wrote. And it is in vain that this resentment takes on the (at times very useful) mask of humanitarianism, such as the founda-

[1] I am thinking of those who believe in the theory of the 'clash of the generations', which was invented by Ortega y Gasset, but, significantly enough, only met with any serious success in Germany, where its principal representative is Wilhelm Pinder.

tion of hospitals, social welfare centres, scholarships, etc., not only for other Jews but for Gentiles as well. All judgment of value apart, we are bound to say that at the back of all this we find the typically Jewish inferiority complex and the resentment deriving from it. According to Nietzsche, Christianity itself was the direct outcome of this resentment, 'Am Judenherz frass Judenhass', and it is not by chance that in the Middle Ages the symbol for the Jewish people was the scorpion.

Mention may be made at this point of Karl Maylan's book *Freuds tragischer Komplex*. In this somewhat trivial and ineffectual work an 'Aryan' psycho-analyst tries to explain the birth of psycho-analysis itself by the supposed existence of a specific 'Jewish resentment'. In January 1931 I took part in a public debate with Maylan in the Steinicke Hall in Munich. By way of refutation I pointed out that in trying to destroy psycho-analysis with the help of psycho-analytical theories he was guilty of a *petitio principii* and that he was more of a materialist than Freud in explaining the latter's doctrine, which is after all a product of the *mind*, by the mere biological notion of *race*. The audience consisted chiefly of Nazis, and their applause revealed a certain resentment against Maylan, just as his ideas had shown resentment against Freud whom he wished to defy in the name of the 'aristocratic Aryan race'.[1]

According to Scheler (himself a Jew converted to Catholicism) the Sermon on the Mount is 'pure resentment' (which, we repeat, is not an ethical, but purely a psychological judgment). Saint Paul he also considers as a typical victim of violent resentment. For 'great pretensions, felt but repressed, great pride in conjunction with an inferior social position are extremely favourable circumstances for awakening the spirit of revenge' (Scheler). And what is revenge if not compensation due to what we have called the postulate of man's auto-estimative equilibrium, i.e. to a profound feeling of inferiority? And when Scheler states that 'envy, jealousy, and competition constitute the second starting-point for resentment', we would ask whether these emotions do not constitute resentment itself rather than its point of departure. For at the starting-point of all the phenomena we have been describing we shall always find the feeling of inferiority. And as for prudery, which Scheler describes as sexual resentment, what else is it but the feeling of sexual inferiority, which is always prior to the resentment it produces?

In order to see how slender is Scheler's whole theory of resentment and how little it is founded on psychological observation, it is sufficient to re-read what he has said on the subject of criminals. In his view, the

[1] Cf. *Neues Wiener Journal*, end of January 1931. *Psychoanalyse als Rassenfrage*.

criminal is never a man burdened with resentment, since 'he belongs to the active type of man. He does not suppress his hatred, his thirst for revenge, his envy, and his cupidity, but allows them to flow into crime.'

This seems to us a very superficial view and founded on a psychological mistake, the mistake of thinking that *activity* is equivalent to *normality*. True, we attribute a certain but very relative superiority to the active as opposed to the passive neurotic or criminal. But to jump from that to the assertion that non-repression frees the criminal from resentment is to go too far. Many criminals are completely free from cupidity, envy and revenge. The only defect from which they suffer is the fact of having become outlaws, at war with society. However great the activity deployed in the socially useless sphere, it is none the less a neurotic activity (criminal activity is only a variety of neurotic activity); nor is it necessarily devoid of resentment. At the back of such activity we shall never fail to discover a powerful feeling of inferiority. There are many cases where such feelings will spur the individual on to the most intense activity; and this activity shields him from the necessity of making himself useful in the social domain, to which he believes himself to be inferior. He will, nevertheless, be a compensated or overcompensated subject, qualitatively different from the man who possesses the same ability or agility from birth.

Generally speaking, and quite apart from the question of criminality, human achievements of a superior order attained through the process of compensation are qualitatively different from those that have been reached with the help of a superior congenital equipment. In the same way, what the Germans have called the *Leistungsmensch*, if considered not from the pragmatic but from the philosophical point of view, can never be regarded as equal to the *Seinsmensch*. And this is so, not only because we attribute congenital perfection to the ideal human being, but also for more pedestrian reasons. In the case of the *Leistungsmensch*, it has been found on close analysis that in spite of brilliant compensations, fully and heroically achieved, there always remains a certain psychic aftermath of the original feelings of inferiority. Not that the subjects will go on thinking about their deficiency or inferiority; indeed they may never have given the matter much thought even when they were striving to compensate for it. But a vague *physical consciousness*, as it were, of their inferiority as compared to the normal type will probably linger in them throughout life, following them like an unnoticed shadow, always ready to intrude itself once more upon their notice and cause them feelings all the more painful for having been forgotten so long. And this, incidentally, explains why persons afflicted even with purely *situative* organic inferiorities (i.e. those established by convention, such as red hair, left-handedness, ugliness, etc.) are so rarely free from feelings of resentment. It is no mere coincidence that painters and actors of genius have so often represented 'character studies' such as hunchbacks, dwarfs, misshapen or grotesque individuals or others afflicted with inferiorities of some kind or another.

The true affective 'fluid' that envelops and saturates the thought and activity of the subject with its peculiar 'logic of the heart' is not resentment; that is only a secondary consequence. In all cases of this kind it is —and we are not overstating our case on insufficient evidence—the feeling of inferiority.

In many cases the feeling of inferiority may lead to resentment, even (though Scheler denies this) when the subject has been able to abreact towards the cause of his humiliation. And the same thing may happen in favourable cases where the inferiority, real or imaginary, has found a compensation. In short, the compensation obtained does not in any way exempt the subject from the possibility of further resentment.

CHAPTER XXV

FEELINGS OF RACIAL INFERIORITY

'BEING different engenders hatred': so said Stendhal, and we added as a rider, 'But above all it engenders feelings of inferiority'. And are there any greater differences than those of race? Or rather we should say of social groups reputed as such, for the word 'race' is applied to-day in a way that strictly scientific anthropology would not allow.

Let us, to begin with, recall the law of 'little differences', which is that the smaller the difference that separates two human groups the greater will be the hatred which one will conceive for the other. Socialists have no bitterer enemies than Communists, though both ostensibly share the same ideal, not to speak of the enmity existing between the orthodox Stalinist and the heterodox Trotskyists or Titoists. Arabs and Jews both belong to the Semitic race and have much in common as regards language, customs and manners, and yet we see them separated by the most implacable hatred. Here again we see, in the collective sphere, a phenomenon which we have already described in the life of the individual. The reader will remember the case of the young amateur pianist who had no feelings of inferiority towards a brilliant professional player, but was 'terribly envious' of one of his friends who played only 'a little better' than he did himself. In the same way half-castes generally suffer from much more intense feelings of inferiority than do coloured people, for the difference that separates them from the whites is so much less. In *Magie Noire*, Paul Morand tells the story of an American mulatto family that is almost assimilated. The fact that they could almost pass as white folk makes their tragedy the more acute.

How many millions there are still who suffer from inferiority feelings simply because of the prejudice directed against them on account of the colour of their skin—black, yellow, mongrel, or simply dark. A great artist like Marion Anderson can still be hissed off the concert platform on account of her race. Fortunately, the Negro problem is receiving more and more attention in the United States and a number of outstanding books have recently been published on the subject.

244

Anyone who has lived in the colonies could tell us of the many racial inferiority feelings that occur there. I remember reading a striking report by Willy Haas on the inferiority complex of the Indian half-castes, which appeared in a well-known Swiss daily paper in 1947. The same complexes can be observed in Spanish Americans who, owing to their small stature as well as their dark skin, feel themselves inferior to the *Gringos*, i.e. the Northern Americans.

The great success which the present work has met with in Spanish America shows, in itself, how much interest these questions arouse in that part of the world. We have received considerable evidence of this, even the fact that a number of pirated editions are in circulation there. The time is ripe for the formation of an 'International League for the Prevention of Racial Inferiority Complexes'.

Some fifteen years ago the Hungarian actor, Ferenc Kiss, was highly praised by the Continental press for having built up his interpretation of Othello around the inferiority complex. And yet the same subject had been enacted on the stage centuries earlier in a play which still retains much of its charm, *El valiente negro de Flandes* ('The Gallant Negro of Flanders'). It is by Andrés de Claramonte, a minor poet in the long line of writers for the classical Spanish theatre. We do not know the exact date of his birth, but he was the director of the theatre at Murcia, a little town that flourished in the golden age of Spain. The problem of the feelings of inferiority is grasped in most masterly fashion and, as the Spanish scholar, Mesonero Romanos, noted in his time, the character of the Negro is drawn with the utmost skill.

The hero of the piece is a Negro called Juan de Mérida. His chief antagonist says of him that 'only the colour of his skin prevents him from being a true caballero'.

> *Sólo el color le falta*
> *Para caballera.*

In a fine monologue, Juan de Mérida complains of the 'baseness' inflicted upon him by the colour of his skin.[1] He wants to prove at all

---

[1]   *A colera y rabia me provoco*
   cuando contemplo en la bajeza mía
   pensamientos que van a eterna fama
   a pesar del color que así me infama
   ¡qué ser negro en el mundo infamia sea!
   ¿por ventura los negros no son hombres?
   ¿tienen alma más vil, más torpe y fea
   y por ello les dan bajos renombres?

costs that he is as good as other men. So he decides to have done with the 'infamy of colour' and to show the world his 'worth', which in Spanish means his courage.[1] If he cannot change his colour he will at least change his fortune. The colour of his skin, which now degrades him, will later, once he has achieved his useful compensation, be an honour. His rival, Don Agustin, is a captain, white-skinned but evil, for he has shamefully deserted a young girl whom he had compromised. Juan is tortured by the thought of his colour,[2] he suffers from a

[1] Con la infamia del color acabo,
      Y al mundo mi valor signifíco
      Pues aunque negro soy, no soy esclavo.

      .   .   .   .   .

      Si no el color, mudar quiero ventura

      .   .   .   .   .

      Si espanto soy, si noche soy agora
      el color que hoy me afrenta ha de ilustrarme:
      que la virtud triunfante y vencedora
      es licor celestial, que no hace caso
      del oro o del cristal en cualquier vaso.

[2] ¿Tanta bajeza es ser negro?
     ¿Tanto tizna el desdichado
          Color de mi rostro?
          ¿Qué esto es ser negro? ¿Esto es ser
     deste color? Deste agravio
     me quejaré a la fortuna
     al tiempo, al cielo y a ¡cuántos
     ne hicieron negro! ¡Oh reniego
     del color! ¡Qué nos hagan caso
     de las almas!—Loco estoy.
     ¿Qué he de hacer, desesperado?
                    . . . ¡Ah, cielos!
     ¡Qué ser negro afrenta tanto!

The psychological analysis is carried to such lengths that the Negro seems to understand that a being tortured with inferiority feelings as he is, is not a normal man. His mentality is a 'double' one and he is not to be trusted,

      Más no te fies de mi
      Que soy hombre de dos caras.

The process by which he overcomes his inferiority feelings is described with masterly skill, in spite of a few details which to-day seem rather puerile. When, with the strength of his arm and in spite of the resistance of the other sergeants, he earns the symbol of his new rank he exclaims:

      Bien me está
      la alabarda, y me ha infundido
      alma y espíritu nuevo
      para aspirar a ser mas,
      con generosos trofeos.

'proud and fierce envy'. The author at this point lacks our modern vocabulary; to-day he would talk of a 'cruel inferiority feeling'. After being made a sergeant, Juan is repeatedly promoted. After the exploit with the German captain he is raised to the rank of captain himself. Then, entering a Flemish encampment alone, he captures the Duke of Orange and turns what seemed to be a losing battle into victory. To the question who could have been so valiant he answers: 'It was I, for only a Negro could venture so much, just because he was nothing at all.'

Our Negro is brave, altruistic, a defender of the just and an implacable enemy of the wicked. When he is presented to the King he is overcome with confusion and can only murmur, '*Soy un negro, un negro soy*'. Henceforth his auto-estimative equilibrium is restored and he apostrophises Fortune: 'I need ask no more of thee, for the King himself has honoured me. I ask no greater joy, for—O Fortune—my colour has won me more than I could ever have imagined.' He rises not only socially but morally, and thanks to his burning sense of inferiority and its compensation of the useful kind in the society that surrounds him, he achieves the rank of general and becomes the first nobleman of coloured blood. The idea of achieving eminence after starting from the lowest depths of humiliation was one that belonged essentially to the Baroque Age in Spain; it was what Léo Spitzer called the 'antithetic feeling of life'. It was inevitable that this 'antithetic feeling' should have appeared at the moment of Spain's tremendous rise to power in her *edad de oro*. In any case what interests us most in this play is not only the fine moral idea it contains,

> *el color lo da la tiara*
> *el valor lo dan las cielos*

(Worth and courage are given us by Heaven; the colour of our skin

The *golden complex* has come to full flowering. Only once do we find a purely verbal compensation. When the Negro, dressed in white as a German, takes prisoner a captain of this nation and exclaims in a joyful play of words:

> *Yo más blanco que la nieve*
> *tu más negro que la pez.*

His prowess, he asserts, would be of no value

> *No ha sido exceso:*
> *Efecto ha sido de la envidia fiera*
> *Que ha dado en perseguirme.*

comes to us from the earth), but the psychology it reveals of the feelings of racial inferiority, which must have been wonderfully interpreted by Andrés de Claramonte, the obscure author-actor of the little town of Murcia.

World literature abounds in descriptions of inferiority feelings due to the fact of belonging to an 'inferior' race. And indeed even a member of the supposedly superior white race may be hiding an analogous feeling of inferiority when he finds himself alone among members of a coloured race. Where the situation is not one that has become habitual he will be overcome by strange and painful feelings which, in the language of the German professor, Pongs, could be called catagogic, i.e. they echo our most primitive ancestral instincts, which are thus suddenly called to the surface.

The experience of a white man or a small group of white men in the midst of coloured men is the clue to all these phenomena of racial inferiority feelings. Once again, it is not the colour, but the *difference* that begets such feelings; the numerical difference, too, or, in other words, the fact of being in a minority. Our thesis could be formulated thus: the members of a minority group always suffer from a collective feeling of inferiority towards the members of a majority group. The existence of such feelings in the majority group must not be assumed as certain and depends on a reversal of roles. But this would lead us to a fresh problem—that of *minority* feelings of inferiority.[1] For it is a curious fact that in the period between the two world wars one no longer spoke of 'nationalities' but of 'national minorities'. We shall try to illustrate this question, which is still a burning one in Europe to-day, by analysing what has been called the Jewish Complex.

[1] I would like to draw attention to the excellent booklet edited under the chairmanship of Charles S. Myers, C.B.E., F.R.S., on *Attitudes to Minority Groups*. It is a report prepared by a committee of psychologists and sociologists published by Newman Wolsely, 1946, and is a model of conciseness and good sense.

CHAPTER XXVI

THE JEWISH COMPLEX

To approach one of the thorniest problems of world-politics in an unbiased spirit is an ungrateful if not a dangerous task, and in dealing with the Jewish problem from a purely psychological standpoint one runs the risk of displeasing everyone—both Christian and Jew. Nevertheless, without adding fuel to the fire of political dissension we shall attempt to sum up here the most interesting conclusions that we have been able to reach from a prolonged study of what may be called the 'Jewish Complex', i.e. the inferiority feeling of a minority group of heterogeneous character distributed in varying density throughout practically the whole of the civilised world.

Racial prejudice is still a live issue to-day. In America, especially in New York State, the colour bar is being violently attacked, while on the subject of Anglo-Saxon negrophobia Sir Alan Burns has written an excellent book which I have had occasion to deal with elsewhere.[1] On the specifically Jewish problem I refer the reader to the publication *Attitude to Minority Groups* mentioned in a footnote at the end of Chapter XXV.[2] There remains, however, a great deal to be said on the subject.

Humiliated and pursued, at one time given century-long legal protection by the ethnical and religious majority groups around them, at another forced to live as wanderers on the face of the earth, the Jews, rich and poor, great and small, for the most part highly educated but often sunk in a primitive ancestral tradition—the Jews, in spite of all their variety, present to us as in 'pure culture' (*Reinkultur*) all the symptoms that are the subject of this book. It would seem that even the Jews who have settled in the new state of Israel are not altogether exempt from the complex we have been examining, though in many cases they have found the way to make something positive of it by transforming it into the *Golden Complex*. In a new state, born of the war, with no traditions of government, and where the majority of the subjects have barely escaped the terrible persecutions in their country

[1] Sir Alan Burns. *Colour Prejudice with Particular Reference to the Relationship between Whites and Negroes.* Allen & Unwin, 1948. The book was reviewed by me in *Revista Internacional de Sociología*, Nos. 26 and 27, Madrid, 1949.

[2] Reviewed by me in *Revista Internacional (loc. cit.).*

of origin, the leaders cannot be expected to be completely emancipated from the mechanism of this complex, which has often, both on the individual and the collective plane, led them into the opposite excesses of the compensatory superiority complex.

'As dying, and behold, we live': these words of St. Paul apply to the Jews with peculiar poignancy. Is it to be wondered at if, sociologically speaking, this paradoxical situation has produced a powerful complex of insecurity and inferiority? It started thousands of years ago, and was bound to survive in atavistic form. Not without cause some of the most clear-sighted Jews themselves spoke of the 'typically Jewish five-thousand-year-old hyper-sensitiveness'.

Much has been said about the physiognomical characteristics of the Jews, but the study of gesture also throws very interesting light on this matter. In spite of the paucity of research on this fascinating subject, it may be said that there is a certain national style in gesture and gesticulation. One need only recall the Latin word *gesta* (*res gesta*) derived from the verb *gero, gerere,* and which in the Romance languages has become *geste* (gesture) meaning both gesture and *panache*. Gesture, posture, physical attitude—all these play an extremely important part in the life of the Latin or Celt-ibero-Latin races. Like language—that other 'national style' (as Karl Vossler called it)—these external manifestations express the very soul of a people, for gesture is prior to logic and the control of emotion. The distinction is generally made between gesture derived from the emotions (*Affektbewegung*) and purely impulsive gesture (*Triebbewegung*).[1] In so far as the individual fails to obtain what he wants, the originally impulsive gesture becomes transformed into the corresponding emotional or affective gesture. There is therefore a striking analogy between what some have called 'affective gesture' and what others, such as Schiller de Harka, quoted above, have named (in speaking of nervous gestures) 'substitute' or *Ersatz* gestures.

Now we have at the hand of two of the pupils of Professor Boas of Columbia University an extremely interesting and suggestive study on this subject.[2] Their results, though purely empirical, are too significant not to be mentioned here.

With the help of some 5000 ft. of film, numerous drawings and close visual observation, the authors established, after a period of two

[1] Cf. L. Flachskampf, 'Spanische Gebärdensprache', in *Romanische Forschungen,* T. LII, No. 2-3, 1938.

[2] Efron and Foley, 'Gestural Behaviour and Social Setting', in *Zeitschrift für Sozialforschung,* 1937, T. VI, I.

years' investigation, a comparison between the gestures of Jews and Italians, both recently immigrated and more or less 'assimilated' to American life. Italian gestures, they found, are 'all of a piece', whereas those of the as yet unassimilated Jews very clearly express 'feelings of inferiority'. In gesticulation, Italians move their arms around the axis of the shoulder, whereas Jews gesticulate with the head, the hands and the fingers in a manner that is 'functionally different'. Italians show 'a clearly marked synergy', rarely making use of the fingers. Jewish gestures are much more complicated and have a zig-zag character which, when fixed on paper, describes tracings resembling a complicated lace pattern. Their movements also have the oft-noted sinuous character. In Italian gestures, on the contrary, elliptical or spiral lines predominate, connected with their more straightforward character; the movements are more or less symmetrical and performed by both arms. This is not so with the Jew, for with him one arm continues the movement of the other and the radius of movement is more restricted, as he rarely detaches the upper arm from the body (position of fear, being on the defensive, eternally on the alert). This contrasts markedly with the wide, free movements of the Italians, which start from the shoulder, whereas the Jew's start from the wrist or the elbow. Italian gesture is naturally centrifugal, Jewish gesture centripetal. The rhythm of gesture is on the whole homogeneous in the Italian, but irregular, asynchronic and often abrupt in the Jew, 'producing an effect resembling the artificial movements of marionettes'. The Jew uses his interlocutor's body as a fixed centre, around which he traces arabesques in the air. One of our observers once saw a Jew seize his interlocutor by the arm and continue to gesticulate with his other arm. Thus the Jew uses gesture to interrupt his partner and to attract the latter's attention. The Italian does not do this; at most he will touch his partner's shoulder in a 'frank' and friendly manner. Nor do his compatriots, when they talk together in groups, all gesticulate simultaneously, as do Jews. The latter, moreover, generally converse in compact groups (as though huddling together in gregarious fashion against some possible danger). This last circumstance, according to our authors, made it extremely difficult to photograph their gestures unobserved. Finally, they found Italian gestures to be 'physiographic', 'pictorial' or symbolic,[1] i.e.

[1] These symbolic gestures (which are totally lacking in Jews) are, it is claimed, the same, even in the assimilated Italians of New York, as those that were noted by Ancient Roman observers and described in the *Dictionary of Gesture* compiled by Di Jorio y Pitre.

imitative of *action*, whereas Jewish gestures were 'ideographic' and imitative of *thought*.

This brief summary is amply sufficient to show how interesting an extension of such a method could be for the study of different ethnical groups. We should add that the authors we have quoted, one of whom, Efron, is probably a Jew himself, have confined themselves to purely objective description and that their commentary on the gestures observed is completely free of any *parti pris*. There may be some connection between the 'sinuous' gestures of the Jews and the sinuous character which their enemies ascribe to them. But before establishing or refuting such parallelism a much more detailed study of the subject would be required; only then could we acquire an adequate knowledge of what, in Adlerian parlance, might be called the 'dialect of the organs'.

The Jews studied in the article we have summarised were mostly of humble social origin, hailing as they did from the ghettoes of Russia and Poland, and we have dealt with the subject at some length because hostility to Jews is so often supported by a dislike of their habit of gesticulating.[1] This is on a par with the reproach of miserliness and rapacity, as though these were national vices. Those who make such generalisations forget that for every 'rapacious' Jew it would be easy to find a generous one, or one of the most spiritual and unworldly type. In his famous novel *Jew Süss*, Feuchtwanger gives a masterly description of a lofty Talmudic Jew, wholly occupied with the things of the spirit. But naturally enough, this is not the type that will attract the attention of non-Jews, and its opposite will mistakenly be taken as more representative. Again, many people have taken the Jews to task for their tendency to political Radicalism, forgetting the resentment that inevitably arises from a precarious and 'inferior' sociological position. It is also frequently forgotten that if many Jews fill the ranks of the Communist movement in Russia, Germany, Hungary, etc., there are also plenty to be found on the other side of the fence, not only among the big conservative capitalists and the rich bourgeoisie, but also among the 'White' counter-revolutionaries.

[1] In the Nazi film of *Jew Süss* the actor who represented the central character gesticulated very freely, whereas the 'good Germans' abstained from any unnecessary movement. Now we were able to ascertain that when this frankly antisemitic and tendencious film was shown to Spaniards, the only character they liked was the Jew, whom they found to be 'almost a Spaniard', whereas they were repelled by the rigidity of the Germans. They were delighted too by the Synagogue chants, so similar to their own *cante Jondo*, but which the Nazi producer had used as an anti-semitic theme.

Considering, then, that Jews vary among themselves to an even greater extent than does any other ethnic group (whether a majority or a minority), it is clearly mistaken and unjust to tar them all with the same brush, as is the custom of crude anti-semitism. The only common characteristic they may be said to possess is of a purely psychological order. Accustomed as they have been for centuries to a problematic and insecure existence, forced as they have been to 'live dangerously', it was only natural that they should have sought in money and other movable goods a protection for their constantly threatened security. This inevitably aroused the envy of the majority groups amongst which they lived, giving rise to a vicious circle, that led from initial insecurity to the more or less illusory security of money, and thence to further insecurity. Even in highly cultured Jews who identify themselves completely with the ideals of the nation in which they live, this atavistic core remains; at a deep psychological level the rootless, homeless wanderer, the 'marginal man' still survives. It would be idle to ask whether this is due to some nomadic factor inherent in the race, or whether, on the contrary, this very nomadism is not the result of external and historical causes. In such complex cases it is impossible to distinguish hereditary factors from those of environment, to say nothing of imponderable elements of a purely personal nature. What is not open to question is the fact that in the course of history the Jews have always shown a willingness to submit to the existing Powers and to serve them with their money and their indubitable economic talent. It is only when the resentment due to their inferiority complex becomes too acute that they become corrosive elements in the body politic. Equally undeniable is their tendency, since the French Revolution, to become assimilated, and vital statistics show that among the more educated there is a constant fall in the birth-rate. In England, France and Germany the Jews would have disappeared completely as a separate race if their numbers had not been reinforced by fresh immigrations. Even without Hitler, according to a well-documented study by a German Jew published shortly before the advent of Nazism, the Jews of Berlin would have disappeared as such, for their numbers were falling in a 'catastrophic' manner. The anti-Jewish laws of 1937 and 1939 in Hungary revealed the presence of many Jewish ancestors in supposedly Gentile pedigrees. Indeed the process of assimilation has been retarded only by periodic persecutions. Complete assimilation was achieved in Spain when Ferdinand and Isabella expelled all the Jews who refused to become converted to Catholicism. A large number accepted conversion and thus became merged with the Christian community. Only in the island of Majorca did this assimilation fail to take place owing to the resistance of the Christian population.

The Spanish example of complete assimilation without any possibility of discrimination four centuries later might quite well have been followed in other countries.

The inferiority complex frequently leads the Jew to *dissimilation*, but it more often works in the opposite direction. It is common knowledge that well-to-do Jews tend to assimilation, because their inferiority feelings have already been compensated for by their wealth. The poorer, proletarian Jews, on the contrary, whose inferiority complex is only heightened by their precarious economic and social position, find compensation in a closer adherence to Judaism. Theirs is a double resentment—against the non-Jewish majority around them, and against the rich and especially the assimilated members of their own race. Jewish jokes about themselves also seem to be a kind of compensation or, as the Freudians would say, an abreaction against their racial inferiority complex.

This curious inferiority complex, which even the assimilated Jew rarely sheds, is one of the most puzzling among what we might call the collective inferiority feelings. It can be found in a great many individuals and lasts throughout many generations. Owing to the 'law of small differences' the Jewish complex is infinitely more complicated than that of the American Negro or of the Indian half-caste. The more insignificant the difference separating Jew from non-Jew, the more acute will be the inferiority complex. Nor can it be doubted that this inferiority complex prepares the ground for *feelings of guilt*, a subject that has been brilliantly analysed by Maryse Choisy. Owing to a kind of collective accident-neurosis (if I may use the term) the Jews are themselves in part to blame for anti-semitism. *Nicht der Mörder, der Ermordete ist schuldig.* This is the title of a work by Franz Werfel (a Jewish author later converted to Catholicism) which once attracted considerable attention. By an unconscious *arrangement*, such as Adler speaks of in the case of neurotics, the Jews themselves very often provoke anti-semitism as though they dimly felt the need of this challenge in order to awaken their instinct of self-preservation. Here again—and we shall return to this point—we can observe among them on a collective plane phenomena which, on the individual plane, are well known to be neurotic symptoms. 'I feel myself to be inferior and an outcast; it must be because those around me hate me and reduce me to this state. . . .'

In the religious art of the fourteenth, fifteenth and sixteenth centuries, especially in France,[1] the heraldic symbol of the Jewish people seems to have been the scorpion, an animal that was considered particularly venomous. Even to this day the same symbol might serve for this tragic people, for does not legend tell us that the scorpion thrusts its poisonous tail into its own body? And this is what happens, symbolically speaking, in the case of the Jews—and their number is not small—who are themselves anti-semitic. The subject was studied by Berneri, an Italian exile assassinated in Barcelona in 1937 as suspected of Trotskyism, in a little book entitled *Le Juif antisémite*. It contains a bibliography on the subject and seems to have been inspired by Otto Rühle's interesting book, *Karl Marx*, in which the author traces the ideas of Marx to the collective inferiority complex of the working-classes, allied to the inferiority complex of Marx himself. Berneri, in developing this idea, mistakenly identifies the inferiority complex we are studying with the Freudian castration complex. What is more relevant to our theme is the information he supplies that even in such definitely anti-semitic circles as the *Action Française* there were Jews openly known as such.

I have had occasion to make a close personal study of anti-semitic Jews who had become converted to Christianity. Some were uneducated persons, some university professors of the highest intellectual qualities. In all alike I saw the same mechanism at work—the desire to break away from 'the side regarded as devoid of value' and to belong to the 'side recognised as alone possessing value'. The spiritual aspect of their conversions seemed to be a psychological superstructure, a mere function of the desire for compensation.

I do not wish for a moment to cast any doubt upon the sincerity of these conversions. There can be no question of conscious hypocrisy. All I wish to do is to draw attention to what seemed to me the psychogenesis of the conversion, of which the mechanism was clearly released by inferiority feelings. These cases, moreover, revealed certain pathological features, such as the obsession of not being the offspring of a Jewish father but of some unknown Aryan, and the similar phantasies which sometimes resulted in a distortion of the philosophic outlook, phantasies that are familiar to anyone dealing with neurotics in general.

[1] Cf. Marcel Brulard, *Le Scorpion, Symbole du Peuple Juif dans l'Art Religieux des XIV, XV et XVI Siècles*. Boccard, Paris, 1935.

Marx has already given us a description of the 'bad conscience' of the bourgeois. In the case of the Jew, this condition is intensified in a peculiar manner. The Hungarian novelist Bela Zsolt (who died in 1949) gives in *Kinos ügy* ('A Painful Affair') a striking portrait of this state of mind, and F. Körmendi in his short novel *Juniusi hetköznap* ('A Day in June') describes that of a Jew who has been forced to emigrate by the anti-Jewish laws of his country.

The curious and somewhat paradoxical phenomena which we have briefly reviewed above would be incomprehensible except in the light of the psychology of the inferiority feelings. It explains the proverbial Jewish solidarity and also the fact that this solidarity is less powerful than Gentiles think it; it explains the equally proverbial generosity of the well-to-do Liberal Jew who contributes to public charities 'without distinction of religion' and the more limited beneficence of the Orthodox that is confined to Jewish causes. All this is connected with the 'psycho-pathology of kindness' (to use the happy phrase invented by Dr. Hesnard), and points not only to Jewish racialism, but to Jewish fascism which is only a derivative or variant of the latter.[1]

Another interesting manifestation of modern Judaism is the existence of a 'Jewish faith without religion'. This has been made the subject of a searching study by R. Bienenfeld.[2] This remarkable work, now unobtainable, has been commented upon with great penetration by the French Catholic psycho-analyst Dr. R. Laforgue.[3] Both these writers are very much intrigued by the part which Jews have played in modern life since the eighteenth century and by their profound influence on

---

[1] A case in point is that of the distinguished Frankfort sociologist Prof. Gottfried Salomon-Delatour (now at Columbia University). During his exile in Paris in 1937 he actually supported a kind of 'Jewish fascism', although the idea was in clearest contrast to his upbringing and his general outlook, and was in the nature of a 'foreign body' in his system of thought. He wrote the leading article in the short-lived German-Jewish Review *Ordo*, printed in German and financed by a Jewish millionaire. His article in the first issue began with the significant sentence, 'Never in the course of history has a people been so often betrayed as the Jewish people, and that by its own *élite*'. I call these words significant because they do contain a certain sociological truth: as soon as a Jewish family reaches social eminence it tends to segregate itself from the rest of the Jewish community. On the other hand, to *interpret* this very comprehensible fact as a ' betrayal' reveals a somewhat unacademic vehemence on the part of a sociologist.

[2] R. Bienenfeld, *Die Religion der religionlosen Juden*, Saturn Verlag, Vienna, 1938.

[3] R. Laforgue, 'Freud et le Monothéisme', in the excellent review, *Psyche*, edited by Mme. Maryse Choisy, Nos. 27–8, Paris, 1949.

modern thought.[1] Their explanations are entirely Freudian. Bienenfeld is only concerned with the 'Jewish super-ego', and Laforgue takes as his starting-point the terror which a child experiences at the sight of its father's sexual organs. These explanations strike us as far-fetched and fanciful. What we know of the mechanisms of inferiority feelings as described in this book offers not only a simpler, but a much more plausible explanation of the facts.

The pamphlet issued by the 'Council of Christians and Jews', which we have already mentioned, shows very clearly that the phenomenon of anti-semitism obeys all the laws of the psychology of minority groups. Whether we are dealing with Judeophobia or Negrophobia the rules of the game are the same—formation of an individual and collective inferiority complex by the minority group, leading either to the positive result of over-compensation or the negative result of under-compensation.

There is, however, a certain danger in asserting an absolute identity of structure in all cases. The psychology of a Negro, of a Jew, of a marginal man or a marginal woman, though all strongly marked by inferiority feelings, will vary according to individual differences even where the behaviour patterns are the same. There is a regrettable lack of research on the subject of resentment[2] in connection with the inferiority complex. After all, resentment is experienced chiefly when the individual feels himself wronged by *persons to whom he denies any claim to superiority*. Now Jews nearly always consider themselves superior to others, with the result that their social inferiorisation weighs all the more heavily upon them. The same could not be said of a Negro living in the U.S.A. or of an Untouchable in India. With Japanese persons living among Whites, the situation is again completely different. The further the Jews of Central Europe moved towards complete equality of status, the more high the positions they occupied in the State, the army, the universities, the stronger became their unconscious resentment, in accordance with the 'law of small differences'. And as, by ricochet, resentment in the inferiorised person arouses an even stronger resentment in his superior, the situation becomes more highly charged as it grows in complexity. (Witness the relations of

[1] R. Laforgue, *L'Influence d'Israel sur la Pensée Moderne*. Ed. de la Ligue internationale contre l'Antisemitisme, 1937.
[2] One good study, though inadequate to the scope of the subject, is Dr. Oscar Forel's *Le Ressentiment*, ed. A. Carrara, Morges, Switzerland, 1948. It first appeared in the *Revue Suisse de la Psychologie*.

domestic servants and their employers as studied by Eliasberg from the psychological, and by Max Scheler from the ethical point of view.)

A point on which Jews and Gentiles are agreed is that since the eighteenth century and particularly since the end of the nineteenth, the Jews have played a part in the life of modern society that is far greater than their numbers would warrant. The same thing is true of the Protestant minority in Hungary and even, within that body, of the Lutheran minority, who are outnumbered by the Calvinists. Again, the Greek minority in Rumania incurs the hatred of the other nationals, by a mechanism which is, on all essential points, the same as that of anti-semitic hatred. All these are cases of minorities which achieve compensation by deploying a greater effort than do the majorities amongst whom they dwell, majorities who, more confident in their position, are content to rest on their laurels.

The members of these minorities are obviously not more gifted originally than those of the majority. But since they meet with more difficulties in making their way, their quest for 'significance' becomes more intense, and under the pressure of the very circumstances which afflict them with feelings of inferiority they actually *become more gifted*. This arouses the jealousy if not the hatred of the competing members of the majority; the hatred sometimes manifests itself in violent forms and thus provokes, among the minority group, a fresh inferiority complex, often mingled with a sense of superiority, for the latter phenomenon is always a corollary to the former. The vicious circle becomes a spiral and produces reciprocal inferiority complexes. We may recall in this connection the many anti-semitic demonstrations in the universities of Central and Eastern Europe during the period between the two wars. At that time the *Pester Lloyd*, which was directed by Jews, conducted a campaign to show that these demonstrations were due to jealousy. (To-day we would say feelings of inferiority.) The journal urged the anti-semitic students to emulate their Jewish companions by spending more efforts on their studies instead of giving way to violence and horseplay. The advice was well meant but showed little knowledge of the psychological reasons for anti-semitism.

I come of a family with Jewish origins; my father was a convert, my mother of the Jewish faith. I was brought up as a Catholic, but educated in a Lutheran *lycée* in a town—Budapest—which was seething with racial strife, especially after the Bolshevism of Bela Kun; all this in a country, Hungary, that was itself a pronounced minority. I then spent twenty years in Catalonia where the Catalonian minority was constantly at loggerheads with the centralising Castilians. I think, therefore, I can claim that my personal experience has sufficiently sharpened my sensitiveness to such problems. Between the Hungarians and the Hungarian Jews of the capital there was a marked psychological contrast. I have known Jewish parents who made untold sacrifices for the social advancement of their children. If they were tradesmen they were proud to have intellectual children able to enter the so-called liberal professions. There was nothing of this tendency among the Hungarian Gentiles. 'Follow in your father's footsteps' was their motto, and most of the fathers were unwilling to see their sons outstrip them. Thus the Jewish minority which, incidentally, was determined not to acknowledge itself as such, was urged *upwards* by an eager desire for social position.

Such an urge cannot be explained by purely sociological factors. Its causes are *psychological*, and once again we are faced with the question, Why this quest for superiority? The question is all the more justified that in Hungary the Jews really did excel in nearly every sphere of life. They became Ministers of State, generals, university professors, in spite of the fact that army and academic circles were the most rigidly closed to them by tradition. The answer to our question seems to lie in Goethe's lines which we have already quoted in Chapter XIV of this book, where the great sage traces the presence of a particular advantage (*besonderen Vorzug*) in a living creature to the presence of some lack (*Mangel*) in its previous make-up.

Detractors of the Jewish race reproach it not only with its harsh features[1] (in spite of the beauty of its women), but with the fact of being 'a degenerate race', the notion of degeneracy being a rather outmoded relic of the Darwinian theory. It would indeed be hardly surprising to find that a social group of people whose ancestors have been

[1] According to the geographer, Jean Brunhis of the Collège de France, the only genuine Jews are the Sephardim, hailing from North Africa and Spain. The Ashkenazim, predominant in Central Europe, are said to be a Tartar tribe converted to Judaism, and it is the latter who have given rise to the tradition of the 'ugly' Jew. This may have a psychological explanation, for the deteriorating effects of suffering can be reflected in the human face. Travellers in Spain have claimed that the traditional beauty of the inhabitants had vanished as a result of their sufferings in the Civil War of 1936.

The late Sylvain-Lévy of the Collège de France was wont to say that in order to know the defects of any nation it was enough to look at its Jewish representatives, where they seem to exist, as it were, in caricature. In Palestine, Jews of Teutonic origin are twitted with the 'square-head' psychology of the Germans.

forced to live in ghettoes, with no possibility for exercise, were of poor physique. And yet we know that wherever Jews have been allowed to develop in freedom from the racial inferiority complex, their children are no less beautiful and well formed than those of other races. We know from what Koestler has written that the younger generation in Palestine is not only taller and more robust than its forebears but also has fair hair and blue eyes, as though in obedience to the Nazi theories of the Nordic superman.

In my opinion there is nothing to prove the existence of any general or important organic inferiority in the Jews. Much has been made of their flat-footedness, which some wags attribute to the forty years' wandering in the desert. Others have tried to make out that the Jews were more *musical* than other races, that the idea of an invisible God, but whose voice can be heard, proves the Jews to be an auditive people in contrast to the Greeks, who were a visual people. The attempt has been made to show that such a preponderance of the auditive faculty could not but come, according to the Adlerian theory, from some initial organic inferiority. Such theories, however, still await proof, and one cannot but feel that those who advance them are guilty of a *petitio principii*.

We therefore claim that we are justified in stating that biological factors play no part in producing the inferiority complex as it occurs in the Jews. The complex exists, but it is not the fruit of biological heredity. It is due to the influence of environment; if there is any heredity at work it is of a purely psychological order.

CHAPTER XXVII

NATIONAL FEELINGS OF INFERIORITY,
OR THE ETHNO-PSYCHOLOGY OF COMPLEXES

OUR study would be incomplete if we did not attempt to make, however briefly, certain reflections on the comparative psychology of nations from the standpoint of the complex that concerns us in this book. Given the complete lack of comparative studies on the subject, we shall necessarily confine ourselves to a few short remarks. We hope in some later studies, which will be in natura vili, to treat the subject at greater length.

At the time when Lazarus and Steinthal were publishing their valuable work on Völkerpsychologie in Germany, nothing was known as yet about the feelings of inferiority. Nor shall we find any mention of them in the vast contribution made to the subject by Wilhelm Wundt, the father of modern German psychology. And yet it would be very useful to extend the results of auto-estimative psychology to the study of that mysterious entity—the soul of a people. If we were in a position to compare the responses given by subjects of different nationalities to the same inferiorising situation, we should be much better equipped for analysing what is called national character and even such notions as people, nation and race. Universal human resemblances and national or ethnical differences would then appear in a completely new light.

It is indeed a curious fact that we still have no serious work on the comparative psychology of the nations. At a time when throughout the world there is still (in spite of the ideological conflict) such a clash of nationalities, when on the political if not the scientific plane such assiduous efforts are made to define the German, the Hungarian, the Venezuelan mentality, etc., this well-nigh total absence of scholarly work on ethno-psychology is a very surprising phenomenon. And what of the phase that still awaits us—viz. the study of international attitudes, i.e. the actual inter-psychology of peoples and nations?[1]

[1] Certain efforts have, however, been made in this direction. In addition to the American studies on international attitudes we have H. R. Harper's What European and American Students think on International Problems, Columbia Univ., 1931,

One could undoubtedly base a complete characterology of peoples and nations on the feelings of inferiority and community feelings. For this purpose one would only need to draw the *profile of the inferiority feeling* of each in order to know which are the situations in face of which a given nation 'feels inferior'; then the *profiles of the community feeling*, trying to estimate or measure the amount or dosage of this feeling as well as communitory forms peculiar to the people or nation in question. We have ourselves already attempted this extension of the Adlerian psychology to the field of ethno-psychology, but our results have not yet been published. It would not give us a complete characterology of the nations, but would furnish an interesting approach to the subject. In the meantime we still lack sufficiently certain data in this domain.

This absence of scientific data makes it very difficult to examine the feelings of inferiority in different peoples. Nations see themselves and each other under the form of abstract schemas, rather devoid of meaning, and always based on hurried generalisations. We see ourselves and each other only under the form of caricatures—John Bull, Marianne, Uncle Sam, etc. In what follows we shall therefore confine ourselves to short statements which will not be of a strictly scientific nature.

Private conversations which we have held with Japanese and Chinese intellectuals showed that the feeling of inferiority was not unknown in Asia. In 1932 we heard such opinions as these: 'It was the nineteenth army in its gallant defence of Shanghai against the Japanese that rid the Chinese of their inferiority complex.' On the other hand, Mme. Kikou Yamata once said to us in a conversation on the Sino-Japanese war, 'It is the war that has finally freed the Japanese of their feeling of inferiority . . .'

and also B.M. Cherrington's *Methods of Education of International Attitudes*, New York, 1931. We ourselves have organised similar enquiries in Spain and our friends the teachers M. and Mme. Perichaud have carried out analogous researches in two schools in the Paris area.

We would like to draw attention to the valiant but still too little known *Revue de Psychologie des Peuples* which, thanks to the labours of its Director, M. Abel Miroglio, has been appearing at Le Hâvre since 1946. Among the monographs published, *The Americans*, London, 1948, by Geoffrey Gorer deserves special mention. The author, who is preparing a book on the Russians, applies both psycho-analysis and the present-day methods of American anthropology. R. Bastide and Mme. Maryse Choisy also endeavour to apply psycho-analysis to ethno-psychology.

THE NEGRO INFERIORITY COMPLEX

Of all coloured people, it is the Negro who suffers most intensely from a sense of inferiority. The 'Negro Complex' has often been commented upon, and Sir Alan Burns in his well-documented book, *Colour Prejudice* (Allen and Unwin, 1948), deals with it at some length in one of the later chapters. He writes:

'The educated Negro is, unfortunately but perhaps naturally, obsessed by the white attitude to his race, and by his own inferiority complex. It is generally true that the better educated a black man may be the greater is the prejudice he encounters, while his education and culture make him more sensitive to insults. That the Negro suffers from an inferiority complex is generally admitted' (p. 140).

If this is so, it must be due not only to the Negro's greater sensitiveness to insults as he becomes more educated, but also to the social fact that he will then meet with greater difficulties in obtaining 'significance' (in Lewis Way's sense). A complete pariah is always more resigned than a semi-emancipated member of an inferiorised race or minority. On the other hand, the more successful the quest of an inferiorised person for significance, the greater will be his desire for *fresh* significance. A Negro (or a Jew, or even a Catholic in a Protestant country, or vice versa) who aspires to social position will, in the first place, find himself isolated from his own kind, and this isolation will increase as he reaches the higher rungs of the social ladder. Indeed, the small interval that separates him from the top will be more harmful to him psychologically than the greater distance he had to face when he started. Once more we see the operation of what we have called the 'law of small differences'.

Dr. Harold Moody, quoted by Sir Alan Burns, speaks of 'the inferiority complex with which our race is afflicted, not only in our masses but our intelligentsia as well' (*The Negro in the Future*, 1934, p. 2). And Miss Margery Perham has pointed out in the *Spectator* of August 23, 1935, that wherever Negroes are in close touch with white civilisations the dominating factor in their lives is the sense of inferiority. Sir Alan Burns brings support to this view in the following passage of his book:

'The Negro reveals the existence of his inferiority complex by the undue importance he attaches to inter-racial sporting contests, by his depression when a black is beaten by a white, and by exuberance of rejoicing when the tables are turned. When Joe Louis was defeated by Max Schmeling in 1936 the gloom among the coloured inhabitants of British Honduras was worthy of a major national disaster. A few weeks later, when Louis defeated Jack Sharkey, the event was celebrated with great rejoicings by the Negroes of New York; these rejoicings led to an affray in which one Negro was killed and four wounded. See *The Times* of August 20, 1936' (p. 39, n. 1).

And Professor D. Westermann (whom Sir Alan quotes on p. 95) in *The African To-day* (1934) speaks of the

'feeling of inferiority in the black man from which the educated classes in particular suffer, and which they try to counteract. The way of doing it is often naïve: the wearing of European clothes, whether rags or the most up-to-date style; using European furniture and European forms of social intercourse; using bombastic phrases in speaking or writing a European language; all these contribute to a feeling of equality with the European and his achievements.'

There is nothing in these descriptions which would not apply with equal truth to the inferiority feelings existing in the members of other minorities, especially of the racial variety as, e.g., the Jews. Sir Alan Burns speaks (*loc. cit.*, p. 137) of the 'jealous vanity that prompts him (the Negro) to criticise and pull down his brother Negro who has ascended a few rungs higher than himself on the ladder of culture and progress'. The same mechanism may be found in all minorities and inferiorised races. In the same way, it will be claimed, the unconquered sense of inferiority will lead the successful Negro to 'betray' his own race, on the principle that the *arrivé* is the worst enemy of the new-comer.

We doubt whether these accusations are as well-founded as their authors seem to believe. Be that as it may, we are convinced that a better and more widespread understanding of the mechanisms of inferiority feelings would substantially improve the situation and bring about a cure of such racial feelings. A psychologically inspired pedagogy would undoubtedly obtain beneficial results throughout the world.

THE SPANISH INFERIORITY COMPLEX

In every Spaniard there lurks a feeling of inferiority. They know it themselves. 'Azorin' in his first novel, *La Voluntad*, describes the type of man without will-power, the *abulico*; the writings of Costa give a perfect diagnosis of this national complex; and finally Unamuno, when he called the Spaniards the 'nation of twenty million kings', had perceived very clearly the superiority complex that was only compensating for burning feelings of inferiority. Spanish hypersensitiveness is proverbial, and has been compared cleverly enough—though with the qualifications required for such a use of psychiatric terms in daily life—to the state of mind of the schizoid or even of the schizophrenic subject. A definite phase in Spanish literature was initiated in 1898 by the feeling of collective inferiority due to the defeat of the monarchy in the Philippines and in Cuba.[1]

But all this is too vague and general. There is a particular brand of inferiority feeling that can be taken as peculiarly Spanish—though it may be found in private individuals of other nationalities. Leo Matthias, in his excellent book of travels, tells the story of a Spaniard staying in London who, on failing to find the way back to his hotel, quietly spent the night sitting on the pavement. At dawn he saw the front door of his hotel a few yards away from his resting place. Commenting on this little story, Spaniards will often remark, 'Well, naturally! He was quite right. . . . It is so unpleasant to have to ask anyone in the street for information. Especially abroad and in a foreign language, etc'. No one is so lost, travelling abroad, as a Spaniard . . . I am quoting the sayings of psychologically minded Spaniards.

Collective inferiority feelings which take the form of a 'categorical veto' or a *dressat*, to use the terminology of Künkel, are also more frequent among Spaniards than other Western Europeans. Nowhere else does one meet with such sayings as, 'We (Spaniards) have not got technical minds', 'We are individualists and therefore incapable of organising ourselves', etc. It cannot be denied that when such categorical vetoes are established in the public opinion and consciousness of a whole nation they will finally bring about a state of mind which we have every right to designate as a feeling of collective incapacity, impotence or inferiority.

One of the most characteristic traits of the Spaniard is his *masculine protest*. The value of virility is over-estimated to a degree that would be incomprehensible in other nationalities. It has nothing to do with

---

[1] Before the recent Civil War, I saw in the little town of Granollers a war memorial bearing the inscription, 'To the Victims of Spanish Imperialism in Cuba, the Philippines and Morocco.'

romantic gallantry. One example will suffice to emphasise the Spanish way of understanding virility. When Franco sent the Blue Division to fight with the Germans on the Russian front, a Spanish Division found itself under heavy fire from the enemy. The situation was nerve-racking. Finally, one of the Spaniards, unable to bear the nervous tension any longer, suddenly got up and began to sing and dance, calling out, 'Whoever does not do the same as me is *not very virile*.' (This is the account given me by an eye-witness, but we may suppose that a much coarser term was used.) Immediately, nearly all the others imitated him. . . .

Spanish instability is proverbial. *Ojos que no ven, corazón que no siente* (If the eyes do not see, the heart does not feel). But it is chiefly in connection with auto-estimation that this weakness comes into play. The football team that wins triumphantly against a powerful opponent will lose badly a week later against a much weaker team. 'Spaniards cannot fight', a tennis-player who had long lived in Spain once said to me. 'As soon as things go against them they throw in the sponge.' The Spaniard alternates painfully between the widely divergent experiences of euphoria and depression. All these are problems which have never received close attention. No one speaks so ill of Spain as the Spaniards themselves; but woe betide any foreigners who would dare to echo their sentiments. 'And if he speaks ill of Spain, he is a Spaniard', sang Bartrine, an ironic poet of the end of the last century. Juan Guixé, one of the few who have dared to face the nation's psychological problem, even speaks of a Spanish Zoilism, Zoilos being the archetype of envy. But what he really should talk about is the inferiority complex.

José Ortega y Gasset, one of the most penetrating intellects of contemporary Spain, has outlined a theory of auto-estimation in a brilliant little essay on the topography of Spanish *Soberbia*. It is printed in the volume *Goethe desde dentro*, Madrid, 1933, and is of the greatest interest to us in this connection. In it he describes the feeling of self-diminution we experience when the merits of others are preferred to ours as a kind of wound to the soul which shakes the whole personality, and he relates this to what Adler has called the 'dialect of the organs'.

'The feeling of believing oneself superior to someone else', he writes, 'is accompanied by the act of raising the neck and head—or by a muscular imitation of this act—which tends to make us appear physically taller than the other person. The emotion expressed by this gesture has been, in our language, cleverly called *altaneria*.'

From this Ortega y Gasset deduces the existence within ourselves of a kind of inner workshop or office which is always making out a very complicated 'estimative balance sheet', in which 'every single person of our social entourage is entered, accompanied by the logarithm of his or her hierarchical relation to ourselves'. As soon as we become aware of another person this inner workshop immediately sets to work in order to size up his value and to decide whether he is worth more, as much as, or less than ourselves. 'There is in man a feeling of the level he stands at which determines his way of behaving, and the character of a society will depend on the way in which the individuals that constitute it value themselves. *From this point better than any other one could embark upon a characterology of peoples and races*' (the italics are mine).

None but a Spaniard could have hit upon such an idea. A Frenchman or an Englishman would be as incapable of it as, say, of Comenius' *Orbis pictus*. Men, continues Ortega, could estimate their true value by making use of an idea that was dear to Nietzsche. They could go by their feelings of and about themselves (spontaneous evaluation), or by the judgments of others (reflective evaluation). Now it has been noted that in the Spaniard arrogance is the dominant factor in self-appreciation, and arrogance prevents the 'estimating eye' from seeing the good qualities of others: it can perceive only its own. Ortega concludes his essay with the following table:

Self-evaluation			
	Reflex	Normal	
		Abnormal = Vanity	
	Spontaneous	Normal	Founded on superior values
		Abnormal = Arrogance	Founded on low values = Spanish *soberbia*

Arrogance, he concludes, is the ethnic vice, the national passion, the besetting sin of the Spaniards. Among the Basques it exists in its purity. This pronounced 'level-consciousness' is also present in the Russians, but with them it is not due to pride or arrogance as with the Spaniards, but 'to a peculiar cosmic and religious feeling which reveals the affinity of the Slav to the Asiatic world'.

It is to be hoped that M. Ortega y Gasset may be induced to develop the ideas outlined in the essay from which we have quoted. The arrogance which he gives as the clue to the Spanish character is in our own view merely an interesting variety of compensation for the inferiority complex.

With regard to the Mexican aspect of this question all we have been told is that the inferiority complex which dominates the minds of the Mexican workers derives '*qua* class phenomenon' from economic inequality.[1] Investigation into the problem is not carried beyond an apodeictic statement of the facts.

The only nation of which the analysis has been attempted on historiographic lines is the *German people*.

---

[1] In Mexico, as in all countries with marked strata of Indian populations, one often hears about the Indians' feelings of inferiority. Many quotations from the press could bear witness to this. But it is curious to note that one of the communications made to the Pan-American Congress at Lima in 1938 (which received little notice in Europe) mentioned the Mexican *Indio*'s 'superiority complex, which rendered him incapable of taking part in the political life of the country'. And it is an interesting point that the Mexicans themselves attribute this fact sometimes to a feeling of inferiority and sometimes to a feeling of superiority. This apparent contradiction is explained as soon as one knows that the latter is a consequence of the former, being nothing but a compensation for it.

CHAPTER XXVIII

THE GERMAN INFERIORITY COMPLEX

C AN one really talk of a national feeling of inferiority? Is there
something which is common to all the individuals speaking the
same tongue, even if they live separated by different frontiers?
We have already stated the reservations that must be made in extending to collectivities the result obtained from analysing the minds of
individuals. All the same, there does seem to be such a thing as a collective inferiority complex. In previous chapters we have seen its operation in the working classes, in coloured races, and in the Jews. It is
obvious that the inferiority complex derived from a state of economic
and social dependence will be different in kind from that based on
racial discrimination. And if we can find in so strong and numerous a
people as the Germans a more or less hidden complex we may be sure
that it in its turn will be of a different order and operate on a different
plane. Thus even if we admit the existence of a *national inferiority complex*, there can be no question of making a comparison between, say,
the Spanish variety (which we have already examined) and that which
exists in Germany.

Let us first see what has been written on the subject.

Some fifteen years ago a young Hungarian, bearing the ancient name
of Wesselényi, published his first historical study, which immediately
aroused great interest in his own country and in Rumania.[1] It will be
worth our while to examine at some length the ideas of this young
author as they are very pertinent to the theme of the present book.

Since the publication of his book, the Baron Wesselényi has repeatedly asserted that he had no quarrel with Germany, still less with
the Germans, and that he bore them no ill-will. His aim was neither to
exalt nor to derogate the Third Reich, but only to serve the cause of
historic truth. His studies, however, led him to the conclusion that Nazi
Germany was following a course that quite clearly ran counter to the
'historic forces' of progress. With great objectivity he carried out his

[1] Baron de Wesselényi, *A Harmadik Birodalom Keletkése* ('The Birth of the
Third Reich'), Budapest, 1936.

research not only with the help of historical data but also with those of modern psychology. Especially did he endeavour to apply the idea of the inferiority feeling to a historic collectivity—modern Germany. He does not question the important part which Germany has played in modern European history. This role was the automatic result of the country's geographical position and thus a 'geo-political' necessity. Since the First World War, Germany's importance in international politics had not diminished, and the advent of National Socialism was a phenomenon for which the historian could not supply an explanation without the collaboration of the psychologist. These were some of the considerations which led Wesselényi to write his book.

In his view, the fundamental cause of the German catastrophe was the existence in the German soul of violent inferiority feelings. It was a case of a fixed idea existing, first in the minds of individuals and, since the state or nation consists of individuals, these separate inferiority complexes becoming integrated into one vast *national* and specifically *German inferiority complex*. This complex can only be understood in the light of the history of modern Germany.

According to our author, the Nazi rulers were perfectly well aware of the existence of this complex among their compatriots. What were they to do about it? This weakness, this low morale, had to be converted into a feeling of virtue, into something 'fertile' (from the ultra-nationalistic German viewpoint, of course). They therefore set about applying methods of collective psycho-analysis on a nation-wide scale. The procedure was amateurish, and we may add that it could not have been anything else, considering that Nazi chiefs such as Göring, who had received Adlerian treatment, had failed to be cured of their individual complexes, and had formed erroneous ideas on the subject. Hitler, Göring and Goebbels—not to mention minor figures such as Röhm, with his violent feelings of inferiority towards women—i.e. the triumvirate of the National Socialist Party, were all three neurotics. Hitler's case requires no further comment. The world press has dealt with it at sufficient length and with sufficient sordid details. His walk and general deportment were alone sufficient to show that he was a man very unsure of himself and of his personal 'valence'. Indeed, psychology tells us that brutality is in general a hyper-compensation for some original weakness. As to Göring, I know the Adlerian psychiatrist to whom he went for treatment, and shall refrain from naming him, if only because he carried out his job so badly. It is obvious that the Nazi chief's personal vanity, his love of adornment, his innumerable decorations, titles and uniforms were all so many compensations for his violent feelings of inferiority. And the same may be said of Goebbels, undersized and lame (like Byron, he took care to hide his defect), who allowed his wife's children by a former marriage to pass as his own. Such were the men who tried to cure the inferiority complex of their compatriots, when they were incapable of overcoming their own.

This psychological crisis in Germany was not unique. Wesselényi claims that many right-wing reactionary political movements were due to the same complexes, especially those reactionary movements that shook various European countries after the First World War. Here the Hungarian author's ideas coincide with those of Count Keyserling,[1] who, it will be remembered, in his book on psycho-analysis in America, maintained that an excessive nationalism is the result, not of overflowing national vitality, but, on the contrary, of a feeling of national distress.

What, then, was the genesis of the German inferiority complex? Our author has no difficulty in supplying an answer.

It arose towards the end of the Thirty Years War, and came gradually into being between 1650 and 1750. It was initiated—as in the case of individuals—by genuine physical insufficiency. The German physique at this time was so poor that it was reflected in the general economic position, which sank into a state of decadence. This was followed by symptoms of mental and spiritual inferiority. Germany, which had been a 'producer of culture' before the Thirty Years War, subsequently became a 'receiver of culture', and it was this lack of culture which gave rise to the national inferiority complex in the German people. Later, when Germany was once again in a position to contribute to the intellectual life of Europe, she must have noticed with chagrin that she had to compete with nations that had become very powerful during her period of physical collapse.

As the years went by the feeling of inferiority became more or less unconscious, but it emerged once more in the refractory spirit shown to the liberal ideals of the French Revolution, thus making Germany guilty of a historical error and placing her at the opposite pole of the great 'dominants' of human history. A century passed, and during the forty-odd years which preceded the world war Germany had still not

[1] Keyserling defended this thesis very eloquently in a course of lectures at the École de Sagesse in Majorca in 1937. His ideas are a useful adjunct to those of the late Sanchez Rivero, whose theories we have examined in an earlier chapter.

achieved harmony with the other Western Powers. We should add that the Germany of 1914 was ruled by a man who was the victim of the most pronounced inferiority complex, as Emil Ludwig and other authors have clearly shown. Nor was this a pure coincidence, for in history there is an intimate connection between the most heterogeneous facts.

According to Wesselényi, the Germans in 1914 were suffering from a kind of 'bad conscience'. They felt deep down, without ever admitting it openly, that they were 'guilty' in not yielding to the ideas of modern democracy. But the ruling elements at the time could not afford to surrender to the forces of progress. Their power rested on the uncertainty and insufficiency of the individual German citizen, and it would have crumbled if they had surrendered to the spirit of the times.

Wesselényi is a firm believer in the logic of history. The world events brought about by Germany are, according to him, the direct outcome of a morbid state of mind throughout the country. Without this widespread pathological state, National Socialism would never have triumphed as it did. The task it set itself was to transform this inferiority complex of the Germans into something on a higher moral level. Wesselényi is so scrupulously objective as to allow that from the historico-philosophical point of view National Socialism had 'the right to exist'. From the moral point of view, however, it was undoubtedly a '*negative* factor', a 'minus', for it was clearly the outcome of pathological mental facts. Its downfall was therefore certain, for the 'dominants' of historical progress would crush it without pity. (We may point out here that our author's work was published exactly three years before the outbreak of World War II.)

It will not be without interest to find this interpretation of history confirmed by German writers, especially those who were known to support the cause of National Socialism.

We are thinking of Professor W. E. Mühlman. In 1933 he wrote in *Sociologus* (an excellent review which only survived Hitler's advent to power by a few months) an article on *Die Hitler-Bewegung* (The Hitler Movement). In it he represented Hitler as the man who had 'restored' the psychology of the German people and cured them of their bitter and paralysing feelings of inferiority. This author's words are instructive from every point of view, and we shall therefore reproduce them here at some length:

'The Marxist Social Democrats of the period following upon the

war were fascinated by the bourgeois ideal. . . . Their aim seemed to be
to procure for the worker the security and lack of responsibility of the
bourgeois way of life (p. 129). . . . But it is impossible to deprive a
whole section of society of its deeply rooted energies—its readiness for
self-sacrifice, its joy in responsibility—and at the same time to raise its
level of auto-estimation (p. 131).

'After the defeat of 1918 and the humiliation of Versailles, the middle
classes were subjected to the constant threat of annihilation, and the ensuing spiritual crisis became a catastrophe affecting the whole nation.
This did away with the theory that the proletariat had a specific destiny
to fulfil, and reduced the social problem to the much wider problem of
the nation as a whole. When a whole nation is in torment, the "class
struggle" loses its meaning. The traditional social categories in Germany were disintegrating so rapidly that new social forms had to be discovered. But at the same time the crisis offered an unhoped-for opportunity to weld the Germans into a spontaneous unity of national will.
The new form of collective auto-estimation was therefore simply that
of the German workers—a form which comprised all those who were
ready to put their shoulder to the wheel. This is the real meaning of
the speech which Hitler delivered on Labour Day, May 1st, 1933, to the
German people.

'It may be objected that the antagonisms between the different social
groups have not been abolished and that this stage has yet to be reached
in practice. This is no doubt very true. But we must not ignore the fact
that *the passionate will of National Socialism has created a terrific psychological impetus* (the italics are mine). From those belonging to the
poorest strata of society we hear the admission, "For years we were
crawling on the ground; now we count for something after all." This is
the triumph of subjective will over objective misery, of faith over
scepticism. . . . Not without reason does Hitler, the great strengthener
of the people, insist that the people must excel itself by its will-power.
Only those who have lived through the passiveness and lethargy of the
depression that followed upon 1918 will understand this to the full.
The foreigner will be amazed at the sight of an impoverished people
hoisting flags on the housetops and organising festivals of joy. But the
spectator well versed in social psychology will see how inevitable all
this was after the events of the past years. The nation is breathing again
and gathering its strength on a mighty scale.'

Let us first of all note the words quoted from the 'little man', the 'man in the street'—*For years we were crawling on the ground; now we count for something after all.* That is the keystone of the Nazi edifice, the clue to Hitler's success—that he restores the people's will-power. Artificially, and with remedies that were even more dangerous than the disease, and eventually with disastrous results, Hitler did succeed for a time in freeing the German people of its inferiority complex.

And now we can see the meaning of the famous German theory of race. The deification of the Aryan, a being existing in reality only in the imagination of Nazi theorists, the 'nordification of the spirit', which is only another form of anti-semitic hatred, now appear to us in their true colours, viz. as compensations for a terrific inferiority complex. No doubt Nazism would not have taken on such monstrous proportions had it not been for the economic and political world situation at the time, but that does not do away with the fact that its explanation is first and foremost a *psychological* one. It was born of an immense psychological distress throughout defeated Germany. A hundred-and-one symptoms confirm our diagnosis. Never had the occult sciences, Oriental philosophy, the mysticism of psycho-analysis, graphology and Buddhism flourished so vigorously as in post-war Germany. It was all a gigantic 'evasion', to use a literary term; a terrific compensation, to speak the language of psychology. Of no avail, however; for the German soul could be saved neither by its literature, which had never been so brilliant, nor by the myths of the various political parties. It needed a more powerful, and a more pernicious remedy—Nazism. History as well as psychiatry has given us many examples of the mental contagion leading to collective psychoses. But only the modern methods of communication—the wireless, the aeroplane, the press, etc.— could enable the complexes of one individual who was a failure to become linked with the inferiority feelings of a nation of sixty million souls. Once he had risen to power, Hitler continued to suffer from his own inferiority complex. His sense of insecurity only increased behind the façade of his superiority complex. Constantly feeling himself threatened, he had to arm, arm to the teeth; he never succeeded in stepping out of the vicious circle created by his pathological state. 'Vicious circle' is perhaps not the right word. It would be better to speak of a vicious straight line—the straight line pursued by madmen and by all who are in flagrant opposition to the aims of human society. The universe, so Einstein tells us, contains no straight lines. Space is curved, and every earthly line must partake of this curvature. An imaginary straight line would only touch our planet at one point and then go out of our universe altogether. This is what happens to madmen and to abnormal politicians who pursue one set of ideas to the exclusion of all others. Hitler was driven by his 'vicious straight line' to go out of the universe of human values; he was unable to check his headlong and calamitous course, and thus brought to its doom the nation he wanted to save.

What conclusions are we to draw from the facts reviewed in this chapter? Can we or can we not accept the collective feeling of inferiority as an explanation of a great historical process? Does this feeling in the case of the German people, for example, yield the *whole* explanation of an infinitely complex historical phenomenon? The answer is an emphatic *No!* We do not believe that Wesselényi's analysis contains the whole of the truth. Every historical event is, to use a Freudian term, over-determined; it has several causes, any one of which would be sufficient to explain its occurrence. This may seem a paradox but is not one in reality. Every theory is like a piece of coloured glass. The facts seen through it all appear of the same colour. This involves no doubt a certain amount of falsification, but since we have no glass which enables us to see reality in all its variety of colour and shape, we must perforce use first one pair of coloured spectacles, then another. The role of a theory is the same, and if we make the reservation that it is to be used only as a working hypothesis, we may without further ado accept the theory expounded by Wesselényi that the *collective feeling of inferiority* may be regarded as a principle of historical explanation.

This raises the feeling in question to a principle of the philosophy of history. And such, indeed, was Adler's own conception towards the end of his life. In his last book, *Der Sinn des Lebens* ('What Life Should Mean to You'), we read in the chapter devoted to the Inferiority Complex:

'Just as a baby expresses by its very movements the feeling of its own insufficiency, its constant desire to perfect itself and to solve the problems of life, so the march of human history must be interpreted as the history of the inferiority feeling and of the attempt to work free of it. Ever since it was set in motion, living matter has tended to pass from a *minus* situation to a *plus* situation.'

Thus the feeling of inferiority emerges beyond its historical significance as a truly *metaphysical principle*. This is the culminating point of Adler's theory. To quote him once again:

'Man would be condemned to succumb to the forces of nature if he had not been able to use them for his own ends. Who can seriously question the fact that the feeling of inferiority is really a blessing for man (so ill provided for by Nature); a blessing because it is constantly urging him towards a *plus* situation, towards security, towards superiority? And the great but inevitable rebellion against this feeling of inferiority inherent in man is the basis for all human development; it is awakened and enacted in the childhood of every individual. . . . All movement goes from imperfection to perfection.'

CHAPTER XXIX

FEELINGS OF INFERIORITY
IN THE ANIMAL KINGDOM[1]

PARALLELISM BETWEEN THE ANIMAL AND THE HUMAN REIGN

LOVERS of animals on reading this book may have wondered whether some parallel of the inferiority feelings we have described exists among animals. Zoologists claim that the border-line between the two realms is becoming ever fainter; even from a purely biological standpoint the distinction between mineral, vegetable, animal and human has ceased to be definite. There is a continuous transition and animal psychology has enriched psychology in general by applying its own methods to human beings (cf. Watson's *Behaviourism*. In America, many authors still practise the behaviourism of approach—Hull, L. Welch, Norman R. F. Maier, etc.). The study of animals from the point of view of our subject may therefore lead to interesting confrontations and conjectures.

INFERIORITY FEELINGS AMONG UNDOMESTICATED ANIMALS

It is only natural that the wild animals should feel more helpless and insecure than the domesticated, but as yet no special study has been made of their inferiority complexes. Undoubtedly they are subject to the universal phenomena of fear and anguish. Before animals stronger than themselves, before the forces of nature or before man, the hunter, they must instinctively become aware of their weakness and helplessness. The form of fear which we have called inferiority complex is therefore not unknown to them. No need to quote classic cases such as those of the aged or mortally wounded elephant who retires into

1 This chapter was written for the Spanish edition of this book. Although it had been praised by an important psychiatric review of Pernambuco, it was omitted from the other Spanish, French and Danish editions. Since, however, animal neuroses and even psychoses are being produced *in vitro* in the American laboratories for the benefit of research in human psychiatry, I decided that it would be of interest to restore the chapter in the present edition.

solitude to die. Among deer and other gregarious animals, moreover, it has been observed that when a powerful male usurps the authority of the former chief, what we call 'loss of prestige' produces in the defeated animal a powerful feeling of inferiority which obliges it to live apart from the group in a state of hostility with the whole world. This neurosis is not essentially different from the human variety and generally comes to the fore more quickly and violently than in man. The 'bad temper' of such self-segregated animals is well known to country folk. The French name for the wild boar is *sanglier* from the Latin *porcus singularis*; the Spanish name comes from the Arabic *jabali* which also means singular or solitary, and popular poetry frequently refers to solitary animals that have been excluded or self-excluded from the community.

Undoubtedly too the *young* of animals are aware, as are human children, of their smallness, their lack of skill in finding food, and their general weakness in the struggle for life. Such reactions have been observed among anthropoid apes in the Zoos. In fact, animal reactions to inferiorising situations are of exactly the same order as in man— compensation in its two modalities of over-compensation and under-compensation (*dé-compensation*).

A film made many years ago by a party of explorers in Africa represents a large family of wild monkeys in flight. While they were crossing a river a very young monkey, less skilful than the rest, was stranded on a small island in mid-stream. The others could not help him and the island was gradually being broken up by the current. The little monkey was in great peril and called desperately for help, uttering stifled and terrified little cries. Finally the little animal, drawing courage from its despair, gave three little leaps on to some intermediate islands and thus gained the river bank.

In this quite commonplace example of animal psychology the monkey had all the *objective* means for overcoming its difficulty, but the fact of having always been able to invoke the aid of others made it behave like a pampered child, whose psychology it exactly reproduced. Experiences of inferiority are therefore not the prerogative of the human species, as these few brief examples will have shown. Many more examples could be taken from the works of Darwin and Bölsche, but we must now turn our attention to animal societies. As in all groups where hierarchies exist, we shall meet here too with the curious fluctuation of auto-estimation.

THE INSTINCT OF SELF-PRESERVATION AND FEELINGS OF INFERIORITY

In the animal, the feeling of valence (German, *Geltung*) certainly does not achieve the degree of consciousness that it does in us; it is built upon the 'confused consciousness' of its own size and the dimension of its own body. Without such a sensation no living being could survive, for it would not even know how to hide when threatened with danger. In the same way, a motorist must have a more or less exact feeling of the size of his car, or he could not drive through narrow streets and round corners. This diffused consciousness cannot be explained by reflexes, as the animal psychologist Öser has rightly pointed out. The theory of reflexes does not explain how a boa-constrictor eats mice when it is small, rabbits when it is larger, and a whole pig when it is fully grown. It cannot be seriously maintained that purely reflex mechanisms change in accordance with bodily growth. On the contrary, we must admit in the animal the existence of a feeling or 'diffused consciousness' of its own proportions. We all carry about with us a mental image of our own appearance and it may well be that in animals too there exists a *body image* (cf. Head, Pick) or *Körperschema* (Schilder).

We know of the animal's instinct for making itself appear bigger than it is as a means of survival in the struggle for life, and it may be that some residue of its confused self-feeling enters into this process. Again, only the existence of a body image could explain the fact that when migratory animals assemble they do so in groups of the same size. In our fish shops, the herrings, sardines, etc., displayed for sale are generally of the same size, and in nature itself one can observe very curious symbioses between animals of different species but of the same size.

Now in general, larger animals attack smaller ones without fear. The process is perfectly simple and logical, though later we shall see that there are some exceptions. An animal's vital space, i.e. that in which it finds warmth, food and a place for its offspring, is of primary importance to it, and there are many fish of 'fixed abode' who remain faithfully in the same place in the aquarium, even if they have to defend it against rivals of larger stature. Conversely, many large fish, if transferred to a new abode, are unsure of themselves and show signs

---

[1] Cf. Paul Schilder, *Das Körperschema*, 1923, and *The Image and Appearance of the Human Body*, Psyche Monographs, 4, Kegan Paul, 1935.

of weakness, as though they were suffering from 'psychic' inhibitions. They will retreat and allow themselves to be pursued and overcome by smaller fish, who go valiantly to the defence of their fixed abode and acquired rights. The newcomer is nearly always inhibited and, as it were, discouraged, and needs a certain period of time to become accustomed to his new geo-physical surroundings. Then his feelings of insecurity and inadequacy will disappear, and the primitive 'complex' will be overcome.

These facts show clearly the fallacy of reducing everything in the animal kingdom to the operation of the famous instinct of self-preservation. If this instinct were as preponderant as it is claimed to be, then animals would *always* run the risk of occupying the place where they find food and shelter, even at the risk of being annihilated by more powerful rivals, and this actually does *not* invariably happen. The animal may become discouraged and no longer dare to approach such places of vital importance to it. It will become immobile and will allow itself to waste away or die rather than conquer its fear. Similar phenomena have been observed in domesticated animals living in couples when one of the partners dies; the survivor loses its courage to live. Other animals will allow themselves to die of hunger when they are transported to new surroundings. Thus the instinct to remain in one's own place in defiance of the world and of all other creatures is in many cases more powerful and efficacious than the supposedly more fundamental instinct of self-preservation. It would seem, then, in the light of what is known of the psyche, that we are dealing here with something that is no longer an instinct but belongs to the psychic sphere.

The above leads us to very important consequences on the subject of the more or less diffused feelings animals may have of their own selves, of their own insufficiency and inferiority. In animals as in men the fundamental psychology is one of *courage* or *discouragement,* and these are the feelings which an animal's sense of its own size will give it, according to the situation or the adversary it has to face.

The close connection an animal feels with its accustomed vital space will influence it favourably, giving it courage in the face of larger and stronger animals. It will struggle for its place in the hierarchy of its group, valiantly defending its supremacy, and for a time the situation will remain unchanged. But defeat may be absolute. Lizards, once they are defeated, prefer to die rather than resume the struggle for their place in the sun. Heimroth refers us to the case of some geese who were driven by a swan from their pond in a zoological park and who did not dare to go near the water even many days after their more powerful rival had disappeared.

If, as we believe, we have shown that the instinct for self-preservation is subordinate to the auto-estimative feeling, let us now examine the latter in relation to the *reproductive* instinct. A hen that patiently submits to being pecked by the others will react aggressively as soon as her eggs are hatched. It is then she who will peck at the others. Öser, an Adlerian, has tried to explain this phenomenon by stating that the mother-hen feels herself to form a unity with her young, and this unity is necessarily a bigger entity than she was before. Once the chicks have been taken away from her she reacts as though she had suffered a diminution, and to such an extent that she spontaneously returns to the lowest place in the hierarchy of hens.

With regard to males, we know that they engage in battle for precedence in the social hierarchy when they are in rut. Now if a stag or an elephant is defeated in such an encounter, it will retire from the group and become a danger to any weaker living creature it may meet on its lonely wanderings. We are in presence here of a *definite vital discouragement*, of a powerful inferiority complex, which obliges the animal to follow a directing line leading to the sphere of 'social uselessness', to use the Adlerian terminology. It would not be hard to find analogous phenomena in the sphere of human social life, especially if we think of the *resentment* felt by the aged who are unconsciously aware that in the existing organisation of society there is no vital space for them.

THE HIERARCHY OF THE POULTRY YARD

The investigations made by Schjelderup-Ebbe[1] on the rigid hierarchy obtaining among poultry are of great importance. This hierarchy manifests itself on a graduated scale determined by the process of 'pecking the heads of the other hens'. Thus there will be one hen who pecks the heads of all the other hens in the farmyard. A second hen will peck all the other hens except the first; a third will peck all the others except the first two, and so on, down to the last hen, who gets all the pecks without being able to give one in return.

We have observed a similar phenomenon at the Budapest *Lycée*, where the boys, arranged in eight classes according to age, tacitly admitted the right of the top-class pupils, even if they were physically weaker, to beat or bully all those of the lower grades. The boys of the

[1] Thorleif Schjelderup-Ebbe, *Zur Sozialpsychologie des Haushuhns*, 1922.

lowest class were knocked about by everyone, those of the top class by no one. Typically, the most cruel were those of the second year, i.e. those who had just been emancipated from the lowest position. Schjelderup-Ebbe has noted that the hens standing low in the hierarchy, i.e. those who have only a few others to attack, are those who peck their victims most viciously; thus the parallelism with the human species is complete. Even among humans, resentment and inferiority feelings are most intense among those who stand rather low in the social hierarchy. This also explains the phenomenon of the criminal who turns policeman, and the arrogance of the *nouveau riche*.

It has also been noticed that when a hen does rebel against one immediately above her in the hierarchy she will display far less energy than when she is pecking an inferior, owing, precisely, to an inhibition of a psychic order, viz. the feeling of inferiority. We have had occasion to note a similar phenomenon in the human sphere, where schoolboys of seventeen allowed themselves to be bullied and terrorised by a much weaker comrade for the sole reason that this boy was the son of a Count who was also a Minister of State. The same boys reacted with all their energy against more physically powerful companions who were of the same social level.

To return to domestic animals, we find that their inferiority complexes have a more complicated structure than is the case in humans. This is because, however complex our social hierarchies, our interrelations develop on the human scale only, whereas domesticated animals find themselves implicated in three completely different social groups. (1) The group of their own kind. (2) The human group of the household, the poultry yard, or human *milieu* in general. (3) The animals of other species. Needless to say, these three large groups can be subdivided further, for among dogs, for instance, there are large and small, friends and strangers.

In this connection, I had occasion to make some interesting observations in Barcelona on two black cats in a neighbouring house with a large garden. In the same house there were two light-coloured cats, and the servants, who had a superstitious aversion to black cats, concentrated all their kindness on the other two, who therefore were larger and fatter from being better fed. Now when the black cats were with human beings, they immediately fled at the approach of the white cats; on the other hand, if they thought they were not being observed by any humans, they would attack the white cats and pursue them relentlessly. The mere presence of human beings, however, those powerful allies of the white cats, was sufficient to put the black ones to flight. The behaviour of these cats was exactly analogous to that of children who have been neglected or abandoned by adults. They do not lack the courage to attack other children even stronger than themselves, but they run away as soon as an adult appears on the scene.

I should add that I was not able to ascertain whether the behaviour of the black cats was due to physical or physiological factors as well as to psychological causes.

DOGS AND HORSES

The neuroses of dogs due to violent feelings of inferiority enable us to draw valuable conclusions concerning human psychology.

A well-bred dog once killed all its master's chickens and was duly thrashed for the offence. From this day it became 'neurotic' and was terrified of any human being of the male sex. When discouragement reaches this point, there are only two alternatives; either to kill the animal or to place it in the hands of compassionate persons who will know how to restore its confidence. If the latter course is adopted the dog will have achieved more or less consciously the object of its neurosis. It will never be beaten, but will be pampered because of its great timidity. In many discouraged children we can see exactly the same behaviour—the production of small neuroses leading to analogous results.

A small bitch, belonging to friends of mine, living with three other dogs in the same house manifests her inter-animal and inter-human relations in a very curious fashion. As soon as a member of the family, who make a great fuss of her, comes into the garden, she immediately abandons her 'canine' occupations and devotes all her attention to the humans. But she will not disturb herself in the same way for other human beings (the servants or the gardener), for she expects no caresses from them. She alone of the four dogs in the house behaves in this way. Thus she has 'relational persons' (Künkel's *Beziehungspersonen*) among the members of the family; but as soon as she is not aware of the presence of one of these persons, she continues to be just a dog among other dogs. I could not say what part her feminine sex plays in this curious behaviour, which differs from that of her three brothers, but at any rate her conduct shows a close parallelism to analogous human behaviour in similar situations.

Timidity and fear in horses resulting from a feeling of insecurity or inferiority is another well-known phenomenon. Psychologists of the horse have described this phenomenon as the animal's attempt to break off its community with the rider, especially when the latter takes no account of the organic or functional minus-values of the horse. In this case, we have an analogy with the timid and frightened child who has been brought up with the stick.[1]

Gredler[2] refers us to another characteristic situation in a small animal community. An innkeeper of Klausen possessed a magnificent horse, the finest and therefore the most pampered of the neighbourhood. It consequently grew to be so haughty that when in the summer it was put in a barn it would kick out at the other village horses. One day these other horses, as though by common consent, surrounded the proud horse and kicked it to death. In this case, as in many others, we can follow closely the play of inferiority feeling: feeling of one's own importance, desire to make this felt by others, mechanisms which, as we have seen, may lead to murder as a result of the rebellion of the oppressed on whom weighs a strong feeling of inferiority.

Among the equine diseases regarded, in the absence of any organic cause, as nervous, veterinary science gives the Latin name of *depertination* or *manie périodique* (Fr.) to a persistent opposition or obstinacy on the part of the animal. It occurs when the animal refuses to perform certain habitual services for no visible reason of a physiological order.[3]

Such cases will always seem incomprehensible and mysterious to the veterinary surgeon who has not the psychological training to make him take account of inferiority feelings closely analogous to those obtaining in human psychology.

According to Stein, however, a horse's obstinacy, as described above, is always due to some existing physical insufficiency. He writes:

'According to Adler we can establish two separate classes of minus-values (*Minderwertigkeiten*): relative inferiority and absolute inferiority. In the case of a horse, for instance, we have relative inferiority, when the animal, although perfectly healthy from the organic point of view, shows signs of minute alteration in its skeletal posture, which altered

[1] Leopold Stein, 'Beitrag zur Psychologie des Pferdes', in *Zeitschr. f. Ind. Psych.*, VI, I.

[2] Quoted by Zell, in *Das Gemütsleben in der Tierwelt*, Dresden, 1921, p. 92.

[3] Schneidemühl, *Vergleichende Pathologie und Therapie der Menschen und der Haustiere*, Leipzig, 1898, p. 752 *et seq.*

posture can become a minus-value in view of the tasks assigned to the horse by its master (racing, riding, being harnessed, etc.). Such an inferiority may be assumed to exist even when the horse shows a variation which makes it appear peculiarly fitted for being ridden, driven, etc., which variation, however, could be functionally eliminated by a skilful rider.'

Stein draws a parallel between such cases and certain situations in child life, where the subject's defects could be eliminated by an intelligent pedagogue, failing which, they will only increase. Stein also compares the situation in animal psychology with phonasthenia (weakness of the voice), a neurotic condition which occurs in some professional singers.

With regard to absolute minus-value, i.e. organic deficiencies, these can also occur in the horse. 'To this may later be added the feeling of inferiority . . . expressed in a dumb and diffused suspicion that *I am not capable of* . . .' (*loc. cit.* p. 53). 'This feeling of inferiority can easily lead to a complete change in the directing psychic line and produce very obvious functional disturbance.' Zürn mentions the case of a horse which suffered temporary paralysis of one leg; after it was cured the animal continued to limp.[1] Zürn tries to explain this phenomenon as a 'simulation', but it was more probably an unconscious 'arrangement', made in order to prolong a situation calling for less effort. In the literature on the subject many such cases are cited concerning 'intelligent' or artful horses.

We may therefore agree that the psychology of the horse betrays that 'teleological and immanent logic' which Adler regarded as a fundamental characteristic of all living things, and of man in particular. The same curious 'logic' is at the bottom of inferiority feelings of men and animals living in social groups. The rules of the game are the same in both cases. In animals there is also that tendency to superiority which Adler regarded as the most fundamental in man. It is expressed in many ways, especially in the horse according to the testimony of Stephen de Máday,[2] who, before becoming an Adlerian psychologist, was a captain of the Hussars and wrote one of the best books on equine psychology. The fact that, like human neurotics, animals are often content with the purely fictitious *appearance* of superiority can be seen in the behaviour of many dogs, who will bark furiously at passers-by from behind an iron gate, but are silent as soon as the stranger comes in through the

1 Zürn, *Die intellektuellen Eigenschaften des Pferdes*, Stuttgart, 1899, p. 20.
2 Stephen de Máday, *Psychologie des Pferdes*, Berlin, 1912.

gate. Other dogs, who follow passers-by and bark at them from inside a fence, cease to do so when they realise that no notice is taken of them. Others, on the other hand, scorn to use such methods for attracting attention to themselves.

In conclusion we may say that in spite of enormous differences the fundamental laws governing the behaviour of living creatures— whether animals or men—are, *grosso mondo*, the same. Life always stretches between two poles—community and a social isolation, the former being the normal situation, the latter being a function of many and varied sensations of insecurity, insufficiency and inferiority. Apparent defects of character are the result, even in animals, of an in-adequate and faulty adaptation to the immediate environment, and there is scope for the application of a system of psycho-therapy to animals. A change of surroundings is often a good cure, just as it is for human beings. And all other neurotic symptoms, such as cowardice, melancholy, bad temper, can be made to disappear from animals too by an adequate psycho-therapeutic treatment based on the knowledge of feelings of inferiority in human beings.[1]

[1] Dr. Rudolfina Menzel and Dr. Rudolph Menzel, 'Über die Geltung. Individual psychologische Gesetzmässigkeit in der Tierwelt', in *Intern. Zeitschr. f. Ind. Psych.*, III.

SUMMARY AND CONCLUSION

W E have reached the end of our 'inventory' and must now gather the scattered threads together.

Our object was to examine in monographic form the history of one of the most popular of the ideas that emanated from the Vienna school of psychological analysis known as 'depth psychology'. The notion of the 'feeling of inferiority' is not so much an *idée-force*, in Alfred Fouillée's sense, as a *mot-force*, for it corresponds to no exact and unequivocal conception. The term has become unduly inflated, and we could not deal exhaustively with the ground that it has been made to cover. For example, the various aspects of the feelings of inferiority in woman have not been included, and we have ourselves attacked the subject in a recent publication.[1]

Here under separate headings is a brief survey of the points raised in the present volume.

1. The idea of feelings of inferiority was in the air at the beginning of this century. Writers were preoccupied at this period with the idea of *degeneracy* and the large number of degenerates (*Minderwertige*) in civilised countries. At the same time, academic psychology was concerning itself with the various kinds of mental and motor inhibitions as expounded by Ranschburg. The old atomic psychology was gradually being replaced by the psychology of action, or functional psychology, the name of 'complex' being sometimes used in connection with a psychic function. The *Gestalt* psychology, still in its infancy, was being introduced by Ehrenfels. The idea of the body-soul unity (*Leib-Seele-Einheit*) appeared in medicine; and experimental psychology was gradually emancipating itself from the yoke of physiology. Under the influence of Freudian psychology, still in its early stages, sexologists such as P. Näcke were coming to the conclusion that human sexuality could not be studied without taking into account the mental factor, as it was then called.

Two important landmarks were the publication in 1907 of Alfred Adler's study on *Organic Inferiorities*, which aimed simply at completing, on purely empirical lines, the study then in vogue of degeneracy

[1] *Los complejos de inferioridad de la mujer*, published in Barcelona in 1949.

287

in general; while in 1910 the second edition of Carl Pelmann's *Psych-ische Grenzzustande* gave more precision to the idea of 'mental minus-value' (*geistige Minderwertigkeit*) and stated that these so-called de-generates exercised a considerable influence on our civilisation. Pelmann thus prepared the ground not only for Adler but also for the patho-graphic tendency which was represented by Lange-Eichbaum. J. Marcinowsky, another sexologist, should also be remembered, as in 'Die erotischen Quellen der Minderwertigkeitsgefühle', in *Zeitschr. f. Sexualwissenschaft*, he spoke of the 'erotic sources' of the feelings of in-feriority. He used the term 'feelings of inferiority' more frequently than did the Freudian school. The latter adopted it later, but avoided it very pointedly after the breach with Adler.

These, then, are the main trends of thought in German psychology which prepared the ground for Adler's teaching and for the idea which has been examined in this book.

2. If in Germany psychic *Minderwertigkeit* was regarded as a mere superstructure on organic inferiority, in France the term *sentiment d'infériorité* was already to hand since the publication of Stendhal's *Le Rouge et le Noir*. The same notion, moreover, had been prefigured in the writings of Montaigne, Hobbes, Mandeville and Vauvenargues. Add to this Janet's description of the *feeling of incompleteness*, and we shall see that even outside German-speaking countries conditions were ripe for the reception of the Adlerian ideas.

3. It is in vain that attempts have been made to trace feelings of in-feriority to an erotic source (Marcinowsky), to the 'castration com-plex' (Freud), or to the 'mutilation complex' (Baudouin). The feeling of inferiority has, from the first, been the most 'neutral' of ideas, and the easiest to fit into any existing psychological, philosophical or religious system.

4. We have shown throughout this book that the term 'feeling of inferiority' can be applied to the most varied phenomena, from simple inhibition to a sense of guilt, from the categorical veto to a feeling of social inferiority, from the sense of incompleteness described by Janet and D. H. Lawrence, to certain states of paranoia and schizophrenia.

The question whether it is the inferiority feelings that engender the neurosis or, as Dr. Ramón Sarró claims, the other way round, is an idle one. No doubt a vicious circle is established and 'mutual induction' takes place. In any case we found that a study of such phenomena has enlarged our knowledge of self-feeling and especially of *auto-estimation*.

Particularly useful in this connection was the word *valence* (borrowed from chemistry), the equivalent of the German *Geltung* and of the word *self-importance* as used in popular English and American writings on the subject. Finally, we showed how, in the language of affects, these terms could be co-ordinated with the notions of fear and anguish.

Another (purely theoretical) distinction we were able to establish was that between the 'feeling of *being*' and the 'feeling of *having*'. This opens up a vista of self-feelings of a negative character, ranging from a sense of frustration (the German *Beeinträchtigungsgefühle*) to the Christian's sense of inferiority towards God; from a sense of incompleteness to the Golden Complex. The series includes the confused feeling of insecurity in animals, passing on to the helplessness of the newly born infant, thence to the auto-estimative oscillations of the adolescent, and finally extends to adult complexes, which take the form called *dressats* by Künkel and *categorical vetoes* by the present writer.

We then extended the scope of our enquiry to deal with various social groups, and with racial minorities in particular. In this way we hope to have drawn attention to certain deplorable gaps in contemporary social psychology. The Adlerian psychology, supplemented by the notion of the 'community feeling', does not supply us with a complete sociology as his early disciples believed; but it has called attention to certain genuine situations of social inferiority.

Finally, our analysis can claim to have thrown a certain amount of light on the plight of modern man, artificially divorced as he is from nature and the social community, exposed to the upheavals of war and enforced migration (displaced persons), and even in time of peace to the harmful effects of industrial standardisation. We have pointed out also to what an extent modern man is conditioned by political and commercial propaganda resulting in feelings of impotence and inferiority. The powerful growth of the modern state, moreover, has over-emphasised the social side of man and led to a neglect of his qualities as an individual and, together with the decay of religion, has tended to rob him of his sense of personal responsibility.

5. The study of feelings of inferiority has contributed considerably to an understanding of the child-mind. Without it, such phenomena as 'infantile regressions and regrets' would be quite incomprehensible.

6. The same notion, combined with that of *compensation*, also rendered more comprehensible the behaviour which society regards as abnormal; it has enabled us to make a detailed comparison between neurosis, psychosis and crime, it has helped us to a better understanding of sexual perversions and toxicomania and, on a different plane, it has

allowed us to investigate the psycho-genesis of exceptional talent and even of genius.

Above all, the study of feelings of inferiority has helped us to penetrate more deeply into that obscure part of man's life—the realm of sex. In contrast to Freudian psycho-analysis, we found that behind all the physiological set-up auto-estimation was the prime mover of behaviour. Instinct, the quantitative material, is indeed the *sine qua non* of sexual conduct, the fuel of the motor, as it were; but the personal factor, which is of psycho-social order, is what determines the direction in which the engine will move. In a word, the study of inferiority feelings has supplied psychiatry or biography, as the new discipline has been called, with a very useful stock of information. The idea cannot indeed be erected into a unique and exclusive principle of *explanation*, but a proper knowledge of its application is a *sine qua non* to the psychiatrist, the doctor, the teacher and the sociologist, in fact, to anyone concerned in one or another branch of the new Science of Man.

7. Our study, then, would seem to show that *no human being can live without a minimum of auto-estimation*, and that the healthiest way of obtaining this minimum is for the subject to become harmoniously integrated into the structure of a *community*. An excessive *plus* of this auto-estimation is as hampering in life as a *minus*. The so-called superiority complex is invariably the result of an intense inferiority complex due to a lack of integration in the community. These facts will naturally assign fresh tasks to pedagogy and psycho-therapy, as well as to the new social techniques that are being developed to-day.

And yet, in spite of the importance of the subject, no substantial advance has been made in the study of inferiority feelings since Adler's first discoveries. His followers have been content to go on applying his results. The feeling of inferiority which began by being a 'psychic reflex', then a 'psychological superstructure', has in ordinary parlance become a 'complex'. True, the term 'feeling' is somewhat vague, but orthodox psycho-analysts are not altogether wrong in regarding the so-called inferiority complex as different from *their* complexes.

The somewhat vague notion of inferiority feeling has, however, slightly gained in clarity by the conception of the *masculine protest*. Freud accepted this notion himself, though with slightly ironic reservations, and the name was later changed by Marie Bonaparte into 'complex of virility'. Other protests which we have suggested have not, however, found favour with the specialists. The same can be said of Künkel's idea of a *dressat*, which is nothing but a deeply rooted feeling of *inferiority*, and of our conception of '*categorical vetoes*'[1] which differs only slightly from the preceding notion.

The distinction between 'feelings' and 'complex' of inferiority is not absolute. Adler himself never succeeded in defining it clearly. In the United States, moreover, there is a tendency to replace both by the word *attitude*. The same tendency appears in the new scientific treatment of public opinion and in the expression *public attitude*. The reader will remember in this connection our mention of Adler's collaboration with L. Ackerson in the article 'Inferiority Attitudes and their Correlations among Children'.

8. The way has been opened to a *new psychological theory* based on *auto-estimation*. We shall, therefore, conclude this chapter with a definition of the notion which has been the object of our study.

Thus we may state that the *feeling of inferiority is an auto-estimative disturbance*. It is a *diminution of the ego and its activities, characterised by an affective state of the negative order*, of which the subject is not always conscious, although his conduct is profoundly influenced by it.

Now, this diminution of the ego may take various forms. Sometimes it is a vague and diffused *sensation*, sometimes a more precisely delimited and more or less conscious *feeling*. It always has an estimative character connected primarily with the emotions but sometimes encroaching upon the intellectual sphere of estimative judgments.

The feeling of inferiority can exist in man without necessarily determining a clearly defined emotional *attitude*; in that case it remains in a subjacent state. But in most cases it determines an emotional *estimation*. I am thinking of Störring's *emotionelle Wertschätzung*. It then becomes a regulator of conduct. The feeling of inferiority does not, as some people think, arise from some previous comparison, but it may be prolonged and aggravated by such a comparison. It is probably prior to every other sensation or feeling. It 'falsifies' the ego and impairs the latter's 'authenticity'. It also causes a decline in sociability, though in its turn it will be prolonged and aggravated by social factors, on the pattern of the 'vicious spiral'. It is a malady of *being*, not of *having*. On the one hand it limits the radius of activity and inhibits the subject's will; but on the other hand it may, through the paradoxical operation of compensation and over-compensation, drive the subject to pseudo-activity, i.e. to the nervous agitation which masquerades as action. Thus the feeling of inferiority produces in the first place *discouragement*, and in the second, by ricochet, it may lead to fresh *encouragement*.

[1] Oliver Brachfeld, 'Les vétos catégoriques', in *Culture Humaine*, Paris, 1948.

9. We have not attempted in the course of these pages to clarify the relation between the feelings of inferiority and such phenomena as *shame* and *envy*, which belong to a traditional morality, nor to *inhibition* and *depression*, notions which are current in psycho-pathology. We have also left aside the *feeling of guilt*, so dear to the Freudian psycho-analysts, for they would have extended the scope of this work too far. The reader will also have noticed that we have spoken of 'feelings of inferiority' where classical psychology would have used the terms 'fear' or 'anguish'. The reason is that the new notion could not be added to already existing systems of interpretation because it opens up a new and *sui generis* perspective. 'Feelings of inferiority' is a global idea, a *Sammelbegriff*, which includes the most diverse notions, such as feelings of incompleteness, insecurity, etc., as well as those of guilt, shame, envy and fear. The exact implication of the new term is still too fluid for us to indulge in terminological niceties. The procedure we adopted, therefore, seemed to us preferable on purely heuristic grounds.

10. The analysis of inferiority feelings or complexes in the *individual* —whether child, adult, neurotic, sexual pervert, toxicomaniac or delinquent—can be regarded as having reached its final form. The time has come to systematise the results obtained and to introduce such alterations as will be needed to keep pace with the changing social and economic conditions which are daily creating new moralities of in-feriorisation.

But as far as the analysis of auto-estimative feelings on the *social* plane is concerned, most of the work has yet to be done. The psycho-logical analysis of social groups or collectivities exists as yet only in outline, and with the most insufficient data (witness the work of Henri de Man). This, no doubt, will be the task of a new Science of Man, which will include not only the physical and psychical aspects of the subject, as is done in the new psycho-somatic medicine,[1] but will also embody the viewpoint of the social sciences. If the present book has helped in some measure to prepare the way for this New Science by summing up the work that has been done up to date on the study of the feelings of inferiority, by delimiting their scope and application and thus clearing the ground for later research, then the somewhat thankless toil which its writing has involved will not have been entirely in vain.

[1] Not so new as some of its American votaries seem to think, for its foundations were laid by two Adlerians in the early twenties—Oswald Schwarz, well known in England, and the Catholic Adlerian, Rudolf Allers. In *Psychogenese und Psycho-therapie Körperlicher Symptome*, to which both these writers contribute, we find the whole of psycho-somatic medicine in embryo.

INDEX

293

INDEX

INDEX